Governance of Picture Archiving and Communications Systems:
Data Security and Quality Management of Filmless Radiology

Carrison K.S. Tong
Pamela Youde Nethersole Eastern Hospital, Hong Kong

Eric T.T. Wong
The Hong Kong Polytechnic Institute, Hong Kong

T0325199

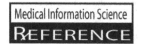
Medical Information Science
REFERENCE

MEDICAL INFORMATION SCIENCE REFERENCE

Hershey · New York

Director of Editorial Content:	Kristin Klinger
Director of Production:	Jennifer Neidig
Managing Editor:	Jamie Snavely
Assistant Managing Editor:	Carole Coulson
Typesetter:	Amanda Appicello
Cover Design:	Lisa Tosheff
Printed at:	Yurchak Printing Inc.

Published in the United States of America by
Information Science Reference (an imprint of IGI Global)
701 E. Chocolate Avenue, Suite 200
Hershey PA 17033
Tel: 717-533-8845
Fax: 717-533-8661
E-mail: cust@igi-global.com
Web site: http://www.igi-global.com/reference

and in the United Kingdom by
Information Science Reference (an imprint of IGI Global)
3 Henrietta Street
Covent Garden
London WC2E 8LU
Tel: 44 20 7240 0856
Fax: 44 20 7379 0609
Web site: http://www.eurospanbookstore.com

Library of Congress Cataloging-in-Publication Data

Tong, Carrison K. S., 1962-

Governance of picture archiving and communications systems : data security and quality management of filmless radiology / by Carrison K.S. Tong and Eric T.T. Wong.

p. ; cm.

Includes bibliographical references and index.

Summary: "This book examines information security management for the facilitation of picture archiving and communication systems"--Provided by publisher.

ISBN 978-1-59904-672-3 (hardcover)

1. Picture archiving and communication systems in medicine--Security measures. 2. Picture archiving and communication systems in medicine--Quality control. I. Wong, Eric T. T. (Eric Tsun Tat) II. Title.

[DNLM: 1. Radiographic Image Interpretation, Computer-Assisted--methods. 2. Computer Security--standards. 3. Image Processing, Computer-Assisted--methods. 4. Radiographic Image Interpretation, Computer-Assisted--instrumentation. WN 26.5 T665g 2009]

R857.P52T66 2009

362.17'70684--dc22

2008037010

British Cataloguing in Publication Data
A Cataloguing in Publication record for this book is available from the British Library.

All work contributed to this title is original material. The views expressed in this title are those of the authors, but not necessarily of the publisher.

Table of Contents

Section III:
PACS Total Quality Management

Preface

Picture archiving and communications system (PACS) is a filmless and computerized method of communicating and storing medical images. Quite a number of professionals including clinicians, medical physicists, radiographers, nurses, computer engineers, and manufacturers are involved in this emerging technology. Most of the professionals found PACS not only a new technology; it also leads the next digital imaging revolution. "Governance of Picture Archiving and Communications Systems: Data Security and Quality Management of Filmless Radiology" is a book intended for radiologists, networks technologists, information technologists and managers, hospital administrators, support and training consultants, quality managers, project managers, healthcare providers and suppliers. Anticipated growth in the take-up of picture archiving and communication systems (PACSs) by healthcare providers throughout North America, Europe, and Asia brings with it promise of a widening need for professionals to manage smooth transitions during, and uninterrupted services after, PACS implementations. Effective change management is vital in the installation of such systems; and the process needs to be planned before the new hardware and software are introduced. The purpose of this book is to explain the key techniques for effective governance of a PACS in filmless radiology operation.

This book is organized in four sections. Section I provides an introduction of PACS and Information Security Management. Chapter I describes the historical development of PACS and its infrastructure. Chapter II depicts the major components of ISO27000 Information Security Management System. Chapter III explains the High Availability Technologies used for the design of a PACS. Chapter IV provides a practical guide on the Implementation of ISO 27000 ISMS.

In Section II, the implementation of filmless hospital is described. Chapter V shows the planning for a filmless hospital. Chapter VI explains different designs of a filmless hospital. Chapter VII discusses the implementation procedure of a filmless hospital. Chapter VII presents the Quality Control, Quality Assurance, and Business Continuity Plan in PACS.

Section III describes the enhancement of key PACS quality dimensions through a Total Quality Management (TQM) approach. This approach comprises an application of Six Sigma, Reliability and Human Factor Engineering tools. This section subdivides into seven chapters that highlight the need to address key PACS quality dimensions individually and collectively. The quality dimensions addressed are: hardware, software, system, and human factors.

Over the last 20 years healthcare leaders seeking to improve quality and enhance patient services have an array of tools to help them in this task. These tools can be broadly grouped into two categories: (1) quality improvement tools—including Continuous Quality Improvement, Six Sigma, and Toyota Production System, and (2) hazard analysis tools—including Healthcare Failure Mode and Effect Analysis, Hazard Analysis and Critical Control Point, Hazard and Operability Studies, Proactive Risk Analysis. Each tool has common origin in the application of the scientific method to process analysis pioneered by Shewhart and Deming; each has unique attributes and advantages. However, a review of current PACS practices and previous research indicates the phenomenon of a fragmented approach in addressing PACS quality issues, thus offering limited discussion of more comprehensive views of PACS quality and practical guidance to its successful implementation and operation. Based on the experience of competing for a Quality Management Award in Hong Kong in 2005 and the subsequent PACS operations research, the authors have developed a cost-effective TQM approach for the enhancement of PACS quality. In this HSSH quality model, analytic and graphical tools are used to deal with each of the four PACS quality dimensions. In Chapter IX, practical PACS problems and feasible methods for the enhancement of the PACS quality dimensions are discussed.

Prior to a treatment of the key quality dimensions, it is essential to define the customer requirements of a PACS. The PACS customers include patients, hospital administrators, nursing staff, physicians, radiologists, quality and maintenance engineers, and so forth. Chapter X describes the process of capturing customers' requirements through a widely used Six Sigma tool: Quality Function Deployment (QFD). Essentially, the Voice of the Customer (VOC) is a market research technique that produces a detailed set of customer wants and needs, organized into a hierarchical structure, and then prioritized in terms of relative importance and satisfaction with current alternatives. Voice of the Customer studies typically consist of both qualitative and quantitative research steps. They are generally conducted at the start of a new product, process, or service design initiative in order to better understand the customer's wants and needs, as the key input for QFD, and the setting of detailed design specifications.

There are many ways to gather the relevant information, for example through focus groups, individual interviews, contextual inquiry, ethnographic techniques, and so forth. But all involve a series of structured in-depth interviews, which focus on the customers' experiences with current products or alternatives within the category under consideration. Needs statements are then extracted, organized into a more usable hierarchy, and then prioritized by the customers. It is emphasized that the PACS development team be highly involved in this process. They must take the lead in defining the topic, designing the sample (i.e. the types of customers to include), generating the questions for the discussion guide, either conducting or observing and analyzing the interviews, and extracting and processing the needs statements.

Although the concept of VOC may seem straightforward, it is actually quite complex. Surveys, focus groups, and interview processes are not easy to set up in a manner that gathers unbiased data. People often give the answer that they believe the interviewer desires to hear, as opposed to their actual opinion. This leads to biased results that often do not correlate well with the customer's actual transactions.

Customers have real needs, and healthcare organizations offer real solutions. VOC research is driven by this common interest and a sincere desire to share and listen. Customer driven organizations are the result of technology used to forward the idea that "the common good" can be explored best through democratic systems. Tools such as "Critical to Quality" trees and "Kano" models can help the PACS development team to uncover the specific requirements, and determine their relative importance to the customer.

Besides customer satisfaction, today healthcare demands a high PACS reliability. At the same time, it places ever-increasing demands on medical imaging services that push the limits of their performance and their functional life, and it does so with the expectation of lower per-unit production costs. To meet these demands, PACS design now requires a streamlined and concurrent engineering process that will produce a modern system at the lowest possible cost in the least amount of time. Not long ago, PACS primarily focused on image storage, retrieval, and viewing within radiology departments. Today, it is evolving into a mission-critical component of a broad enterprise system, including billing, management, and an electronic patient record.

Design for PACS reliability provides a systematic approach to the design process that is sharply focused on reliability and firmly based on the mechanisms of hardware and software failures. It imparts an understanding of how, why, and when to use the wide variety of reliability engineering tools available and offers fundamental insight into the total life cycle. Applicable from the concept generation phase of the system development cycle through system obsolescence, design for PACS hardware and software reliability, when integrated with Failure Modes and Effects Analysis (FMEA), Internet flow control and Human Factor Engineering (HFE), would form a coherent design process that helps ensure that the end product will meet PACS administrators' reliability objectives. Readers will learn to meet that goal and move beyond solidifying a basic offering to the healthcare industry to creating a quality PACS service.

The selection of probability distributions suitable for modelling PACS hardware or software failure characteristics is typically challenging. Such data often exhibit substantially larger variances than expected under a standard count assumption, that of the Poisson distribution. The over-dispersion may derive from multiple sources, including heterogeneity of PACS components, differing life histories for components collected within a single collection in space and time, and autocorrelation.

Chapter XI shows a novel reliability modelling technique for PACS hardware and software using a widely used spreadsheet. The process of fitting probability distributions to PACS failure data is usually computationally intensive, and it is not feasible to perform this task using manual methods. The authors found that among the failure distributions commonly used in the aviation and manufacturing industries, the Weibull model is used mostly—owing to its ability to represent various failure behaviour. As shown, the mathematically demanding process of verifying the distributional assumption has been simplified to a large extent through the method of matching of moments. This distribution is therefore recommended for PACS reliability predictions. Based on the reliability models constructed for the key PACS components, one can then improve the system reliability through the provision of equipment and/or software redundancy and practical arrangements such as the parallel and cross-linked connections are shown. While most PACS hardware failures are attributed to physical deterioration, software faults are mainly due to design problems. This is mainly due to the fact that most software developers would not spend too much time on non-productive tests and they do not want to see competitors launching a similar product earlier. In this chapter a case study on the detection of critical software errors during the acceptance test is given. The purpose is to illustrate a practical way of evaluating software reliability during PACS development and improvement.

The challenge facing PACS administrators is to design in quality and reliability early in the planning and development cycle. In this regard, FMEA is recommended for analyzing potential PACS reliability problems early in the development cycle where it is easier to take actions to overcome these issues, thereby enhancing reliability through design. FMEA is used mainly to identify potential failure modes, determine their effect on the operation of the system concerned, and identify actions to mitigate the failures. A crucial step is anticipating what might go wrong with a system or its components. While anticipating every failure mode is not possible, the PACS development team should formulate as extensive a list of potential failure modes as possible. The early and consistent use of FMEAs in the PACS design process allows the PACS team to design out failures and produce reliable, safe, and customer-oriented services. FMEAs also capture reliability data for use in future system improvement. The PACS-FMEA procedure is explained and illustrated through a case study in Chapter XII.

As shown in Section I, the implementation of DICOM into PACS requires the use of standard protocols such as Transmission Control Protocol/Internet protocol (TCP/IP). The IP architecture is based on a connectionless end-to-end packet service using the IP protocol. The advantages of its connectionless design, flexibility and robustness, have been amply demonstrated in the literature. However, these advantages are not without cost: careful design is required to provide good service under heavy load in an integrated system. Indeed, lack of attention to the dynamics of packet forwarding can result in severe service degradation or "Internet meltdown". This phenomenon was first observed during the early growth phase of the Internet of the mid 1980s, and is technically called "congestion collapse". In Chapter XIII, the simulation results of a proposed fluid flow model, realized by using inside tcl/tk script executed from Scilab (a free and open software), show that with a certain anticipated level of Internet traffic flow, one can find a practical TCP congestion control method by combining TCP with Active Queue Management (AQM) algorithms. It was found that the algorithms work reasonably well in complex environments involving multiple senders, multi-level routers, and multiple TCP flows.

Corporate culture can help drive healthcare results, but it takes a cultural analysis to differentiate which aspects of the culture can lead to superior performance. In Chapter XIV a cultural comparison adapted from Geert Hofstede's cultural Dimensions was carried out and the implications for the local PACS community were given. With access to people working for the same organization in over 40 countries of the world, Hofstede collected cultural data and analyzed his findings. He scored each country using a scale of roughly 0 to 100 for each dimension. The higher the score, the more that dimension is exhibited in society. Based on this cultural comparison, suggestions on improving the organizational structure and the communication process have been made. For a PACS regional network to be competitive and successful in a dynamic environment characterized by constantly changing customer demands and technological innovations, it must be capable of rapid adjustment in order to reduce the time and cost needed to deliver to the patient quality healthcare service. The factors critical to the success of a PACS regional network are also noted.

While Statistical Process Control (SPC) is extensively used in the healthcare industry, especially in patient monitoring, it is rarely applied in the PACS environment. Some of the anticipated benefits characteristic to PACS through the use of SPC includes:

- Decreased image retake and diagnostic expenditure associated with better process control.

- Reduced operating costs by optimizing the maintenance and replacement of PACS equipment components.
- Increased productivity by identification and elimination of variation and out-of-control conditions in the imaging and retrieval processes.

Statistical process control (SPC) involves the use of mathematics, graphics, and statistical techniques such as control charts to analyze the PACS process and its output, so as to take appropriate actions to achieve and maintain a state of statistical control. The objective of SPC differs significantly from the traditional QC/QA process. In the traditional process, the QC/QA tests are used to generate a datum point and this datum point is compared to a standard. If the point is out of specification, then action is taken on the product and action may be taken on the process. To move from the traditional QC/QA process to SPC, a process control plan should be developed, implemented and followed. Implementing SPC in the PACS environment is not a complex process. However, if the maximum effect is to be achieved and sustained, PACS-SPC must be implemented in a systematic manner with the active involvement of all employees from the frontline staff to the executive management.

The present study demonstrates for the first time that use of this monitoring tool can be extended to the PACS. The way in which one could construct, choose and interpret control charts associated with PACS condition monitoring is provided in Chapter XV. To illustrate the benefits of implementing the proposed TQM approach in PACS, a successful case based on the HSSH model is given in Chapter XVI. Besides shows the winning details of a project aiming at the 2005 Hong Kong Quality Management Award, the real purpose is to show how the Quality Management Award criteria could be used as a guide to focus improvement methodology on the whole department. A brief description of the judging criteria is given, followed by an outline of the Grand Award holder's submission and the Project Leader's explanation of project-related issues during the Judging Panel interview.

A review of the application of the suggested approaches to deal with PACS security and quality management aspects would indicate potential issues for future research and these are given in Chapter XVII. For instance, the HSSH model is particularly useful in examining Human Factors issues in microsystems in healthcare, such as the emergency room or the operating theatre PACS—mismatches at the interface between the components in these PACS microsystems may lead to medical errors. The authors are of the view that the HSSH quality model may have some unexploited potential in PACS overall enhancement. A chart showing the sequence of each section and the corresponding chapters is shown below.

Flow chart showing the sequence of different Sections

Section I   Introduction of PACS and Information Security Management

Chapter 1   Introduction of PACS

Chapter 2   ISO27000 Information Security Management System

Chapter 3   High Availability Technologies for PACS

Chapter 4   Implementation of ISMS

Section II   Implementation of Filmless Hospital

Chapter 5   Planning for a filmless hospital

Chapter 6   Design of a filmless hospital

Chapter 7   Implementation of a filmless hospital

Chapter 8   Quality Control, Quality Assurance, Business Continuity Plan

Section III PACS Total Quality Management

Chapter 9   PACS Quality Dimensions

Chapter 10   Customer Oriented PACS

Chapter 11   Design for PACS Reliability

Chapter 12   PACS Failure Modes and Effects

Chapter 13   PACS Network Flow Control

Chapter 14   Human factors and Culture

Chapter 15   PACS Monitoring

Section IV Future PACS Directions and Planning of Future Hospitals

Chapter 16   Quality Management Benefits

Chapter 17   Epilogue

Section I
Introduction of PACS and Information Security Management

Chapter I
Introduction

INTRODUCTION OF PACS

Picture archiving and communications system (PACS) is a filmless and computerized method of communicating and storing medical image data such as computed radiographic, digital radiographic, computed tomographic, ultrasound, fluoroscopic, magnetic resonance and other special X-ray images. A PACS consists of image and data acquisition, storage, display stations integrated with various digital networks.

A PACS handling images from various medical imaging modalities is called a full PACS. Small-scale systems that handle images from a single modality (usually connected to a single acquisition device) are sometimes called mini-PACS. A hospital-wide PACS is a PACS which entirely replaces conventional x-ray film by displaying digital images on a network of workstations throughout the hospital. This kind of hospital is called a "Filmless Hospital" (Strickland, 2000). In healthcare environment, the practicing of radiology without X-ray film is called "Filmless Radiology".

PACS replaces hard-copy based means of managing medical images, such as film archives. It expands on the possibilities of such conventional systems by providing capabilities of off-site viewing and reporting (tele-education, tele-diagnosis).

Typically a PACS network consists of a central server which stores a database containing the images. This server is connected to one or more clients via a local area network (LAN) or a wide area network (WAN) which provides and/or utilizes the images. Client workstations can use local peripherals for scanning image films into the system, printing image films from the system and interactive display of digital images. PACS workstations offer means of manipulating the images (crop, rotate, zoom, brightness, contrast and others).

Modern radiology equipment feeds images directly into PACS in digital form. For backwards compatibility, most hospital imaging departments and radiology practices employ a film digitizer.

The medical images are stored in an independent format. The most common format for image storage is DICOM (Digital Imaging and Communications in Medicine) (NEMA, 2008).

There are many benefits of introducing PACS technology into the conventional paper and film-based operation in hospital. Using PACS, it is possible to manipulate a digital image for value-added diagnosis, treatment or surgery. The efficiency of radiographers and radiologists is improved. Errors of radiographers are considerably reduced during data input. Film waiting time for clinicians is minimized and there are no film losses. A PACS can be as simple as a film digitizer connected to a display workstation with a small image database, or as complex as a total hospital image management system. No matter what the scale of a PACS is, like other information systems such as banking, security is always one of the major problems that have to be addressed.

Information security (Calder, 2006) is a large research topic. It consists not only of the disclosure of patient information but it also covers accuracy, accessibility, misuse, mishandling and management of data. In banking and finance industries, billions of dollars have been spent on daily security issues on their information systems which handle our properties and money. Comparing to the healthcare industry, less than one percentage of the annual hospital budget was spent on the security of clinical information systems on which saving of our lives depends.

Before 1999, there was no standard for information security. In 1999, British Standards Institution (BSI) published their BS 7799 standard for Information Security Management System (ISMS) was then adopted by International Organization for Standardization as ISO 17799 which is a code of practice for ISMS. In 2000, BSI published the requirements of BS 7799 ISMS as part II of BS 7799 standard. In 2005, both standards were re-arranged as ISO 27000 series of ISMS standards

The purpose of this book is to provide some information on security issues and handling of security in PACS. It emphasizes the design of a secure PACS and the implementation of ISO 27000 standard on PACS.

HISTORY OF PACS

The principles of PACS (Huang, 1999) were first discussed at meetings of radiologists in 1982. Various people are credited with the coinage of the term PACS. Cardiovascular radiologist Dr Andre Duerinckx reported in 1983 that he had first used the term in 1981. Dr Samuel Dwyer, though, credits Dr Judith M. Prewitt for introducing the term.

In UK, Dr Harold Glass, a medical physicist working in London in the early 1990s secured UK Government funding and managed the project over many years which transformed Hammersmith Hospital in London as the first filmless hospital in the United Kingdom. Dr Glass passed away a few months after the project went live but is credited with being one of the pioneers of PACS.

One of the earliest research projects related to PACS in the United States was a teleradiology project sponsored by the US. Army in 1983. A follow-up project was the Installation Site for Digital Imaging Network and Picture Archiving and Communication System (DIN/PACS) funded by the US. Army and administered by the MITRE Corporation in 1985. Two university sites were selected for the implementation, the University of Washington in Seattle, and Georgetown University/George Washington University Consortium in Washington, D.C., with participation of Philips Medical Systems and AT&T. The U.S. National Cancer Institute funded UCLA, one of its first PACS-related research projects in 1985 under the title of Multiple Viewing Stations for Diagnostic Radiology.

Baltimore Veterans Administration Medical Center

The Baltimore VA Medical Center (Siegel, Kolodner, 2001), operating with approximately 200 beds, has been totally digital except in mammography since its opening in 1994. All examinations are 100% archived in PACS with bidirectional HIS/RIS (Hospital Information System/ Radiology Information System) interface. Currently the system serves three other institutions in the region: the VA Medical Center Fort Howard Hospital (259 beds), the Perry Point Hospital (677 beds), and the Baltimore Rehabilitation and Extended Care Facility. Surveys of clinicians have consistently indicated a preference for the filmless system over conventional films. An economic analysis also indicates that filmless operations costs are offset by reduced equipment depreciation and maintenance costs. The general statistics are as follows: radiology department volumes increased by 58%, lost examinations decreased from 8% to 1%, productivity increased by 71%, repeated examination decreased by 60%, and image reading time decreased by 15%. These results suggest that the medical centre and the networked hospitals as a whole have increased healthcare efficiency and reduced operational cost as a result of PACS implementation.

Hammersmith Hospital

When the Hammersmith Hospital (Strickland, 2000) in London, England decided to build a new radiology department, a committee was set up and chaired by the Hospital Director of Finance and Information. A top-down approach was adopted for the hospital-wide PACS project. The hypothesis of the project was that there would be cost savings arising from PACS and at the same time PACS would contribute to increased efficiency in the hospital. Hammersmith Hospital includes the Royal Postgraduate Medical School and the Institute of Obstetrics and Gynaecology. It has 500 beds and serves 100,000 people. The justification of the project was based on direct cost/saving and indirect cost/saving components. In direct cost/saving, the following components were considered: archive material and film use, labour, maintenance, operation and supplies, space and capital equipment, and buildings. Indirect cost/saving comprised of junior medical staff time, reductions in unnecessary investigations, saving of the time of radiologists, technologists, and clinicians, redesignation and change of the use of a number of acute beds, and reduction in the length of stay. Currently the system consists of a 10-terabyte long-term archive, and a 256-giga-byte short-term storage servicing 168 workstations. Since the start of system operation in 1993, the PACS has improved hospital-wide efficiency, the number of filing clerks has been reduced from 8 to 1, 3.3 radiologists have been eliminated, physicist/information technology personnel has increased to 1.5, and no films are stored on site. PACS has a number of advantages over conventional films. These include time savings, space savings, economies in consumables and personnel, reduced patient irradiation, efficiency of data management, accessibility of images, teaching benefits and system reliability.

Samsung Medical Center

Samsung Medical Center, an 1100-bed general teaching hospital, started a four phases PACS implementation plan since 1994. The medical centre had over 4000 outpatient clinic visits per day and performed about 340,000 examinations per year. The departments of orthopaedic surgery, neurosurgery, neurology, emergency room and surgical intensive care unit were selected for the first phase of PACS implementation. The PACS in Samsung serves the following functions: primary and clinical diagnosis, conference, slide making, generation of teaching materials, and printing hard copies for referring physicians. A total of 218 PACS terminals are currently installed throughout all departments, operating rooms and wards, boasting the largest scale worldwide. All examinations and diagnosis are performed digitally except mammography.

Hong Kong Hospital Authority (HA)

In Hong Kong, there are 44 government funded public hospitals under the administration of Hong Kong Hospital Authority. Since 1999, all the territory's hospitals under the HA network have used a proprietary Clinical Management System (CMS) with Electronic Patient Records (ePR) that tracks a patient's medical history by allowing all hospitals and clinics to access a patient's entire medical history. In 2005, a PACS module was added to integrate radiological images with the existing ePR system backbone as part of any patient's ePR. The radiological information and images have also been centrally available to doctors across all the HA's hospitals. In the long term, private medical practitioners would be given access to the system as well. This is part of HA's strategy to foster a closer co-operation between the public and private health sectors in Hong Kong. In the future, HA intends to implement filmless radiology in all of its hospitals.

National Health Service (NHS) in UK

PACS has been available in the UK since the early 90s, so some installations in trusts in England including Norfolk and Norwich University Hospital, Princess Royal Hospital, Telford, St George's Hospital, London, pre-date the work of NHS Connecting for Health's National Programme for IT. Since 2008, NHS PACS has lived in NHS Trusts across England including the following areas:

*   Barnsley Hospital NHS Foundation Trust
*   Essex Rivers Healthcare NHS Trust
*   Hull and East Yorkshire Hospitals NHS Trust
*   Mid-Yorkshire Hospitals NHS Trust
*   Nottingham University Hospitals NHS Trust
*   United Lincolnshire NHS Trust
*   Ashford and St Peters NHS Trust
*   Royal Free Hampstead NHS Trust

The initiative has the added benefit of saving money, with trusts where the programme is being used reporting an average saving of £250,000 in its first year.

INTRODUCTION OF ISO 27000

The international standard on information security management is ISO 27000 (British Standards Institution, 2005) and the origin of this standard goes back to the days of the UK Department of Trade and Industry's (DTI) Commercial Computer Security Centre (CCSC). Founded in May 1987, the CCSC had two major tasks. The first was to help vendors of IT security products by establishing a set of internationally recognized security evaluation criteria and an associated evaluation and certification scheme. This ultimately gave rise to the ITSEC and the establishment of the UK ITSEC Scheme. The second task was to help users by producing a code of good security practice and resulted in a "Users' Code of Practice" that was published in 1989. This was further developed by the National Computing Centre (NCC), and then later a consortium of users, primarily drawn from British Industry, ensured that the Code was both meaningful and practical from a user's point of view. The final result was first published as a British Standard's guidance document PD 0003, then a code of practice for information security management, and then after having followed a period of further public consultation recast as British Standard BS 7799:1995. A second part BS 7799-2:1998 was added in February 1998. Following an extensive revision and public consultation period, which began in November 1997, the first revision of the standard, BS 7799:1999, was published in April 1999. Part 1 of the standard was proposed as an ISO standard via the "Fast Track" mechanism in October 1999, and published with minor amendments as ISO/IEC 17799:2000 on 1st December 2000. BS 7799-2:2002 was officially launched on 5th September 2002. In 2005, BS 7799-2 finally entered the ISO Fast Track mechanism and emerged on 14th October 2005 as ISO/IEC 27001:2005 after significant re-ordering of controls and general restructuring.

Tseung Kwan O Hospital

Tseung Kwan O Hospital is a newly built general acute hospital in 1999 with 458 in-patient beds and 140 day beds. The hospital has several clinical departments including medicine, surgery, paediatrics & adolescent medicine, eye, Ear, nose & throat, accident & emergency and radiology. A PACS was built in its radiology department in 1999. The PACS was connected with the CR, CT, US, Fluoroscopy, DSA, and MRI system in the hospital or clustered hospital. The hospital has become filmless since a major upgrade of the PACS in 2003.

A BS 7799 ISMS was introduced to TKOH PACS in 2003. When it was introduced, a PACS security forum was also established with members from radiologists, radiographers, medical physicist, technicians, clinicians and Information Technology Department (ITD). After a BS 7799 audit was conducted at the beginning of 2004 and it was upgraded to ISO 27000 in 2006, TKOH PACS was the world's first system with an ISO 27000 certified ISMS established.

ELEMENTS OF PACS

PACS is a electronic system which could manage the communication, display, and archiving of diagnostic image information

DICOM Standard

DICOM (Digital Imaging and Communications in Medicine) (NEMA, 2008) (Huang, 2004) is the industry standard for transferral of radiological images and other medical information between computers. Patterned after the Open System Interconnection of the International Standards Organization, DICOM enables digital communication between diagnostic and therapeutic equipment and systems from various manufacturers.

Such connectivity is important to cost-effectiveness in healthcare. DICOM users can provide radiology services within facilities and across geographic regions, gain maximum benefit from existing resources, and keep costs down through compatibility of new equipment and systems. For example, workstations, CT scanners, MR imagers, film digitizers, shared archives, laser printers, and host computers and mainframes made by multiple vendors and located at one site or many sites can "talk to one another" by means of DICOM across an "open-system" network. As a result, medical images can be captured and communicated more quickly, physicians can make diagnoses sooner, and treatment decisions can be made sooner.

The DICOM 3.0 standard evolved from versions 1.0 (1985) and 2.0 (1988) of a standard developed by the American College of Radiology (ACR) and National Electrical Manufacturers Association (NEMA).

ACR-NEMA, formally known as the American College of Radiology and the National Electrical Manufacturers Association, created a committee to draft a set of standards to serve as the common ground for various medical imaging equipment vendors in developing instruments that can communicate and participate in sharing medical image information, in particular in the PACS environment. The committee, which focused chiefly on issues concerning information exchange, interconnectivity, and communications between medical systems, began work in 1982. The first version, which emerged in 1985, specifies standards in point-to-point message transmission, data formatting, and presentation, and includes a preliminary set of communication commands and data format dictionary. The second version, ACR-NEMA2.0, published in 1988, was an enhancement to the first release. It included hardware definitions and software protocols, as well as a standard data dictionary. Networking issues were not addressed adequately in either version. For this reason, a new version aiming to include network protocols was released in 1992. Because of the magnitude of the changes and additions, it was given a new name: Digital Imaging and Communications in Medicine (DICOM 3.0). The latest version was released in 1996, consisting of 13 published parts. Each DICOM document is identified by title and standard number in the form: PS 3.X-YYYY where "X" is the part number and "YYYY" is the year of publication. Thus, PS 3.1-1996 means DICOM 3.0 preliminary specification document part 1 (Introduction), released in 1996, and PS is an internal ACR-NEMA code. Although the complexity and involvement of the standards were increased by manifold, DICOM remains compatible with the earlier ACR-NEMA versions. The two most distinguishing new features in DICOM are adaptation of the object oriented data model for message exchange and utilization of existing standard network communication protocols.

Although the standard committee is influential in the medical imaging community, in the beginning, medical imaging equipment manufacturers were slow to respond and comply with the ACR-NEMA standards. As the specification of DICOM 3.0 becomes widely accepted, the manufacturers have taken a very cooperative manner and have begun to develop new versions of software and equipment totally based on this standard. Modalities that do not conform to the DICOM standard either follow the ACRNEMA standard or have their own format. To accommodate the former, a conversion from ACR-NEMA to DICOM should be developed. And for the latter, a translator is needed to convert the manufacturer's specifications to either the ACR-NEMA or DICOM standard. A set of software modules, collectively called the encoder library, is needed for these purposes. A well-developed encoder library should have the following characteristics:

1. Generic for multimodalities and various vendors's imaging equipment.
2. Portability to various hardware platforms.
3. Software architecture based on the top-down and modular principles.
4. Standard programming language, such as C.

The ACR-NEMA standard consists of image format and point-to-point communication standard. Since point-to-point communication has been completely replaced by DICOM network protocols, we will not consider it further. Instead, we focus on its data format, as many existing PACS systems and components are still using ACR-NEMA format standard. Let us use an encoder to explain how images are converted from a manufacturer's modality to ACR-NEMA format standard. According to the ACR-NEMA 2.0 data dictionary, each image should contain two parts: a command group and a data set. The data set can be further divided into information groups: identifying, patient, acquisition, relationship, image presentation, overlay, and image pixel data. The data in these groups, when transmitted across equipment, constitutes a message. When an image is generated from an imaging modality by a manufacturer, it consists of an image header that describes the nature of the image, and the image pixel values. Since the image header has no standard, its content is pretty much up to the manufacturer. For this reason, not every piece of header information from a modality will have a corresponding group-element category specified in the ACR-NEMA format. On the other hand, not every element defined in the ACR-NEMA dictionary will cover data types included in the image headers of various equipment vendors. Therefore, a minimum set of groups and a minimum set of elements within those groups as the core data structure should first be defined. In other words, all images, regardless of modality and manufacturer, should bear this minimum set once it has been formatted. Additional groups and elements are then defined based on the header information provided by the specific modality and the manufacturer. Additional information can be defined in two shadow groups: display shadow group and a raw header shadow group. The display shadow group stores the information that is vital to support workstation display and provide fast access. The raw header group retains the entire header information to permit the retrieval of data item not formatted, should it become necessary. Additional groups and elements, such as acquisition information (group 0018), relationship information (group 0020), image presentation (group 0028), and overlay (group 6000-60 IE; even numbers only) will be applied depending on the type of in formation provided by the manufacturers. Dependent on the modality, the numbers of groups and elements to be formatted differ considerably. To provide a systematic way for an encoder program to extract and map data from the image header to the ACR-NEMA format, a configuration file which describes the included groups and elements, is needed for each modality. The encoder of a modality reads in a specific configuration file and calls various module' in its program to convert image data to the ACR-NEMA format. The last data group to be converted should be the pixel data group (7fe0), which is attached to the end of the message. In addition, for each modality, these encoders are grouped in a library with all the necessary modules for encoding. This library resides in the acquisition gateway computer to perform the data conversion once the image data has been received from the imaging modality. The general algorithm of converting raw image data into ACR-NEMA format is as follows. First, an image is acquired from a modality. If it is not in the ACR-NEMA format upon arrival at the acquisition gateway computer, it goes through the encoding process and is converted to the standard format. After that, the formatted image is sent to the PACS controller for archiving, and subsequently, is transmitted to display workstations.

The DICOM 3.0 standard provides several major enhancements of the earlier ACR-NEMA versions. Among these are:

1. DICOM 3.0 is applicable to a networked environment.
2. It specifies how devices claiming conformance to the standard react to commands and data being exchanged.
3. It provides guidelines on levels of conformance.
4. It structures as a multiple part document.
5. It uses information objects to describe entities (images, graphics, studies, reports, etc.).
6. It uses the entity-relationship model for uniquely identifying any information objects.

Two fundamental components of DICOM are the information object class and the service class. Information objects define the contents of a set of images and their relationship, and the service classes describe what to do with these objects. The service classes and information object classes are combined to form the fundamental units of DICOM, called service object pairs (SOPs). This section describes these fundamental concepts and provides some examples.

PACS DESIGN

PACS Design Concept

A picture archiving and communication system consists of image and data acquisition, storage, and display subsystems integrated by various digital networks. It can be as simple as a film digitizer connected to a display workstation with a small image data base, or as complex as a total hospital image management system. PACS developed in the late 1980s, were designed mainly on an ad hoc basis to serve small subsets of the total operations of many radiology departments. Each of these PACS modules functioned as an independent island, and was unable to communicate with other modules. Although this piecemeal approach demonstrated the PACS concept and worked adequately for each of the different radiology and clinical services, it did not address all the intricacies of connectivity and cooperation between modules. This weakness surfaced as more PACS modules were added to hospital networks. Maintenance, routing decisions, coordination of machines, fault tolerance, and the expandability of the system became sources of increasingly difficult problems. The inadequacy of the early design concept was due partially to a lack of understanding of the complexity of a large-scale PACS and to the unavailability at that time of certain PACS-related technologies.

PACS design should emphasize system connectivity. It should be a general multimedia data management system that is easily expandable, flexible, and versatile in its operation calls for both top-down management to integrate various hospital information systems and a bottom-up engineering approach to build a foundation (i.e., PACS infrastructure). From the management point of view, a hospital-wide PACS is attractive to administrators because it provides economic justification for implementing the system. Proponents of PACS are convinced that its ultimately favourable cost benefit ratio should not be evaluated as a resource of the radiology department alone but should extend to the entire hospital operation. This concept has gained momentum. Several hospitals around the world have implemented large-scale PACS and have provided solid evidence that PACS improves the efficiency of healthcare delivery and at the same time saves hospital operational costs. From the engineering point of view, the PACS infrastructure is the basic design concept to ensure that PACS includes features such as standardization, open architecture, expandability for future growth, connectivity, and reliability. This design philosophy can be constructed in a modular fashion with an infrastructure design described in the next section.

PACS Infrastructure Design

The PACS infrastructure design (Nesbitt, Schultz, Dasilva, 2005) provides the necessary framework for the integration of distributed and heterogeneous imaging devices and makes possible intelligent database management of all patient related information. Moreover, it offers an efficient means of viewing, analyzing, and documenting study results, and furnishes a method for effectively communicating study results to the referring physicians. The PACS infrastructure consists of a basic skeleton of hardware components (imaging device interfaces, storage devices, host computers, communication networks, and display systems) integrated by standardized, flexible software subsystems for communication, database management, storage management, job scheduling, interprocessor communication, error handling, and network monitoring. The infrastructure as a whole is versatile and can incorporate rules to reliably perform not only basic PACS management operations but also more complex research job and clinical service requests. The software modules of the infrastructure embody sufficient understanding and cooperation at a system level to permit the components to work together as a system rather than as individual networked computers.

The PACS infrastructure is physically composed of several classes of computer systems connected by various networks. These include radiological imaging devices, device interfaces, and the PACS controller with database and archive, and display workstations. Figure 1 shows the PACS basic components and data flow. This diagram will be expanded to present additional detail in later chapters.

Figure 1. Schematic diagram of a PACS

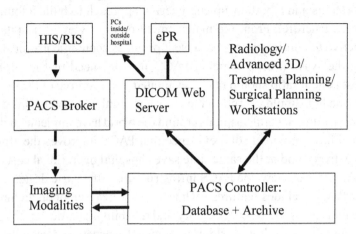

Where HIS is Hospital Information System,
    RIS is Radiology Information System,
    ePR is electronic Patient Record,
    DICOM Web Server is a Web server for distribution of medical images in Digital Imaging and
    Communication in Medicine (DICOM) format,
    ➤ is the flow of image data,
    ➤ is the flow of patient demographic data

IMAGING MODALITIES

Introduction

Interoperability of medical imaging modality, PACS and HIS is a crucial point for determining the effectiveness of the performance of a digital diagnostic radiology department. The common imaging modalities (Dreyer, and Kalra., 2005) used in radiology department include the following technologies.

Computed Radiography (CR)

Storage phosphor based luminescence imaging plates (IP) (Seibert, Filipow, and Andriole, 2000) (Huang, 2004), which consists of a photostimulable phosphorus layer made of $BaFX:Eu^{2+}$ (X = Cl, Br, I), europium activated barium fluorohalide compounds, for computed radiography are a new medium for filmless radiography. This technology is based on the principle that after the X-ray exposure, the photostimulable phosphor crystal is able to store a part of the absorbed X-ray energy in a quasistable state. Stimulation of the plate by a helium-neon laser beam having a wavelength of 633 nm leads to emission of luminescence radiation, the amount of which is a function of the absorbed X-ray energy. The luminescence radiation stimulated by the laser scanning is collected through a focusing lens and a light guide into a photomultiplier tube, which converts it into electrical signals and displays it on a monitor.

The special advantage of this technique is its higher sensitivity than classical film radiography and the potential for automated for automated image processing due to the digital readout of the IP's.

Digital Fluorography

Digital fluorography (DF) is another method that can produce a digital X-ray image without substantial changes in the radiographic procedure room. This technique requires an add-on unit in the conventional fluorographic system. Recall that fluorography is the procedure of displaying fluoroscopic images on a video monitor by means of an image intensifier coupling with a video camera. This technique is used to visualize motion inside body compartments (e.g., blood flow, heart beat), and the movement of a catheter during an intervention procedure, as well as to pinpoint a body region for making a film image for subsequent detailed diagnosis. Each exposure required in a fluorographic procedure is very minimal compared with a conventional X-ray procedure. Digital fluorography is considered to be an add-on system because a digital chain is added to an existing fluorographic unit. This method utilizes the established X-ray tube assembly, image intensifier, video scanning, and digital technologies. The output from a digital fluorographic system is a sequence of digital images displayed on a video monitor. Digital fluorography has an advantage over conventional fluorography in that it gives a larger dynamic range image and can remove uninteresting structures in the images by performing digital subtraction. When image processing is introduced to the digital fluorographic system, dependent on the application, other names are used: digital subtraction angiography (DSA), digital subtraction arteriography (DSA), digital video angiography (DVA), intravenous video arteriography (IVA), computerized fluoroscopy (CF), and digital video subtraction angiography (DVSA) are examples.

Computed Tomography (CT)

Computed Tomography (CT) (Herman, 1980) imaging is also known as "CAT scanning" (Computed Axial Tomography). Tomography is from the Greek word "tomos" meaning "slice" or "section" and graphia meaning "describing".

CT was invented in 1972 by British engineer Godfrey Hounsfield of EMI Laboratories, England and by South Africa born physicist Allan Cormack of Tufts

University, Massachusetts. Hounsfield and Cormack were later awarded the Nobel Peace Prize for their contributions to medicine and science.

The first clinical CT scanners were installed between 1974 and 1976. The original systems were dedicated to head imaging only, but "whole body" systems with larger patient openings became available in 1976. CT became widely available by about 1980. There are now about 6,000 CT scanners installed in the U.S. and about 30,000 installed worldwide.

The first CT scanner developed by Hounsfield in his lab at EMI took several hours to acquire the raw data for a single scan or "slice" and took days to reconstruct a single image from this raw data. The latest multi-slice CT systems can collect up to 4 slices of data in about 350 ms and reconstruct a 512 x 512 matrix image from millions of data points in less than a second. An entire chest (forty 8 mm slices) can be scanned in five to ten seconds using the most advanced multi-slice CT system.

During its 30 year history, CT has made great improvements in speed, patient comfort, and resolution. As CT scan times have gotten faster, more anatomy can be scanned in less time. Faster scanning helps to eliminate artefacts from patient motion such as breathing or peristalsis. CT exams are now quicker and more patient friendly than ever before. Tremendous research and development has been made to provide excellent image quality for diagnostic confidence at the lowest possible x-ray dose.

Magnetic Resonance Imaging (MRI)

Magnetic resonance imaging (MRI) (Huang, 2004) has become the primary technique throughout the body in the routine diagnosis of many disease processes, replacing and sometimes surpassing computed tomography (CT). MRI has particular advantages in that it is non-invasive, using non-ionizing radiation, and has a high soft tissue resolution and discrimination in any imaging plane. It may also provide both morphological and functional information. The resultant MR image is based on multiple tissue parameters any of which can modify tissue contrast. In its development, MRI has incorporated a multidisciplinary team of radiologists, technicians, clinicians and scientists who have made, and are continuing to make, combined efforts in further extending the clinical usefulness and effectiveness of this technique. The first successful nuclear magnetic resonance (NMR) experiment was made in 1946 independently by two scientists in the United States.

Felix Bloch, working at Stanford University, and Edward Purcell, from Harvard University, found that when certain nuclei were placed in a magnetic field they absorbed energy in the radiofrequency range of the electromagnetic spectrum, and re-emitted this energy when the nuclei transferred to their original state. The strength of the magnetic field and the radiofrequency matched each other as earlier demonstrated by Sir Joseph Larmor (Irish physicist 1857-1942) and is known as the Larmor relationship (i.e., the angular frequency of precession of the nuclear spins being proportional to the strength of the magnetic field). This phenomenon was termed NMR as follows:

- "Nuclear" as only the nuclei of certain atoms reacted in that way;
- "Magnetic" as a magnetic field was required;
- "Resonance" because of the direct frequency dependence of the magnetic and radiofrequency fields.

With this discovery NMR spectroscopy was born and soon became an important analytical method in the study of the composition of chemical compounds. For this discovery Bloch and Purcell were awarded the Nobel Prize for Physics in 1952.

Interestingly, Dr Isidor Rabi, an American physicist who was awarded the Nobel Prize for Physics in 1944 for his invention of the atomic and molecular beam magnetic resonance method of observing atomic spectra, came across the NMR experiment in the late 1930's but considered it to be an artefact of his apparatus and disregarded its importance. During the 50's and 60's NMR spectroscopy became a widely used technique for the non-destructive analysis of small samples. Many of its applications were at the microscopic level using small (a few centimeters) bore high field magnets.

In the late 60's and early 70's Raymond Damadian, an American medical doctor at the State University of New York in Brooklyn, demonstrated that a NMR tissue parameter (termed T1 relaxation time) of tumour samples, measured in vitro, was significantly higher than normal tissue. Although not confirmed by other workers, Damadian intended to use this and other NMR tissue parameters not for imaging but for tissue characterization (i.e., separating benign from malignant tissue). This has remained the Holy Grail of NMR yet to be achieved due mainly to the heterogeneity of tissue. Damadian is a controversial figure in NMR circles not least for his exuberant behaviour at conferences. Although criticism has been levelled at his scientific acumen it should not overshadow the fact that his description of relaxation time changes in cancer tissue was one of the main impetuses for the introduction of NMR into medicine.

On the 16th March 1973 a short paper was published in Nature entitled "Image formation by induced local interaction; examples employing magnetic resonance". The author was Paul Lauterbur, a Professor of Chemistry at the State University of New York at Stony Brook. One would not think that from reading the title that it represented the foundation for a revolution in imaging. Indeed the paper was nearly not published having been initially rejected by the editor as not of sufficiently wide significance for inclusion in Nature. In this seminal paper Lauterbur described a new imaging technique which he termed zeugmatography (from the Greek zeugmo meaning yoke or a joining together). This referred to the joining together of a weak gradient magnetic field with the stronger main magnetic field allowing the spatial localization of two test tubes of water. He used a back projection method to produce an image of the two test tubes. This imaging experiment moved from the single dimension of NMR spectroscopy to the second dimension of spatial orientation, forming the foundation of MRI.

MR also owes a debt to computed tomography (CT) as it was developed initially on the back of CT but quickly outpaced that technique. The impact that CT had in the medical community is not to be disregarded as it stimulated interest both of clinicians and manufacturers to the potential impact that this new technique. It had already demonstrated the advantage of tomographic sections through the head or body of a patient allowing diagnosis of disease processes in a non-invasive way. In the late 70's and early 80's a number of groups, including manufacturers, in the US and UK showed promising results of MRI in vivo. This was, and still is, a technological challenge to produce wide bore magnets of sufficient uniformity to image the human body. In the UK these included the group from the Hammersmith (Professor R Steiner & Professor G Bydder) collaborating with Picker Ltd. at Wembley (Dr Ian Young), two independent groups in Nottingham (Professor P Mansfield and Dr W Moore), and in Aberdeen (Professor J Mallard & Dr J Hutchinson). The first commercial MR scanner in Europe (from Picker Ltd.) was installed in 1983 the Department of Diagnostic Radiology at the University of Manchester Medical School (Professor I Isherwood & Professor B Pullen). Further applications of MRI are currently being assessed. The manipulation of gradients and enhanced software give not just exquisite anatomical detail but also provide functional information as in perfusion and diffusion studies of the brain in vivo.

Two and three dimensional MR angiography provide a roadmap of vessels in any part of the body, together with the ability to obtain functional velocity profiling of blood flow. This non-invasive technique is likely to replace conventional diagnostic x-ray angiography in the near future.

Nuclear Medicine (NM)

Although CT is sectional imaging, nuclear medicine scanning is projectional. Therefore, the principle of nuclear medicine is needed to explain what the concept of CT is. The formation of an image in nuclear medicine relies on the administering of a radiopharmaceutical agent that can be used to differentiate between a normal and an abnormal physiological process. A radiopharmaceutical agent consists of a tracer substance and a radionuclide for highlighting the tracer's position. The tracer typically consists of a molecule that resembles a constituent of the tissue of interest, a colloidal substance that is attacked by reticuloendothelial cells, for example, or a capillary blocking agent. A gamma camera is then used to obtain an image of the distribution of the radioactivity in an organ. The radionuclide is chosen on the basis of its specific activity, half life, energy spectrum, and ability to bond with the desired tracer molecule. Its activity is important because, in general, one would like to perform scans in the shortest possible time while nevertheless accumulating sufficient nuclear counting decay statistics. As always, the half life must be reasonably short to minimize the radiation dose to the patient. The energy spectrum of the isotope is important because if the energy emitted is too low, the radiation will be severely attenuated when it passes through the body; hence nuclear statistics will be poor or scan times will be unacceptable. If the energy is too high, there may not be enough photoelectric interaction, and absorption in the detector crystal will be low. Typical isotopes used in nuclear medicine have γ-ray emission energies of 100-400 keV.

Positron Emission Tomography (PET)

In PET (Myers, Cunningham, and Bailey, 1996), a positron instead of single photon is used as a radionuclide source. The positron emitted from a radionuclide is rapidly slowed down, and is annihilated by a combination yielding two 511 keV γ-rays oriented about 180° to each other. The PET system utilizes this unique property of positrons by employing a detector system that requires simultaneous detection of both photons from annihilation, and thus avoids the need for collimators. With a pair of detectors, placed on the two opposite sides of the patient, only events that are detected in coincidence are recorded. Simultaneous detection of two annihilation photons by the detector system thus signals the decay of a positron anywhere along a line connecting the two points of detection. Because of this multiple coincidence logic, PET systems have higher sensitivity than SPECT. The correction of attenuation is easier in PET than in SPECT because the probability that annihilated photons will reach both detectors simultaneously is a function of the thickness of the body between the two opposite detectors. The correction factor can be obtained by means of a preliminary scan of the body with an external-ray source, or a correction table based on a simple geometric shape resembling the attenuation medium to be used. Patient movements, oversimplified geometric shape, and non-uniform medium will cause errors in attenuation correction. Thallium drifted sodium iodide NaI(Tl), bismuth germanate (BGO), and cesiumfluoride (CsF) are being used as detector materials. Because of the high energy of the annihilation photon, detector efficiency plays a crucial role in selecting a scintillator for a PET system. Bismuth germanate is considered to be the most prominent candidate for PET detector material because of its high detection efficiency, which is due to its high physical density (7.13 g/cm³) and large atomic number (83), as well as its nonhygroscopicity (which makes for easy packing) and its lack of after glow. A typical whole body PET scanner consists of 512 BGO detectors placed in 16 circular array banks with 32 detectors in each bank. During scanning, the system is capable of wobbling to achieve higher resolution via finer sampling. The image spatial resolution for the stationary and wobbled modes are 5-6 and 4.5-5 mm, respectively. A recent PET engineering development is the whole body imaging technique which produces tomographic images of the entire body with equal spatial resolution in orthogonal image planes. Since the body longitudinal axis is, in general, longer than the other two axes, the patient bed is required to advance during the scanning process to permit the entire body length to be scanned. A complicated data acquisition system in synchrony with the bed motion is necessary to monitor the data collection process.

Ultrasound (US)

Ultrasound is sound with a frequency greater than the upper limit of human hearing, this limit being approximately 20 kilohertz (20,000 hertz). Medical sonography (ultrasonography) is a useful ultrasound based diagnostic medical imaging technique used to visualize muscles, tendons, and many internal organs, their size, structure and any pathological lesions. They are also used to visualize a fetus during pregnancy. Ultrasound scans are performed by medical healthcare professionals called sonographers. Obstetric sonography is commonly used during pregnancy.

HOSPITAL INFORMATION SYSTEM (HIS) AND RADIOLOGY INFORMATION SYSTEM (RIS)

Hospital Information System (HIS)

A hospital information system (HIS) (Huang, 2004) is a computerized management system for handling three categories of tasks in a healthcare environment:

1. Support of clinical and medical patient care activities in the hospital.
2. Administration of the hospital's daily business transactions (financial, personnel, payroll, bed census, etc.).
3. Evaluation of hospital performances and costs, and projection of the long-term forecast.

Radiology, pathology, pharmacy, clinical laboratories, and other clinical departments in a healthcare centre have their own specific operational requirements, which differ from those of general hospital operation. For this reason, special information systems may be needed in some health centres. Often, these subsystems are under the umbrella of the HIS, which maintains their operations. Others may have their own separate information systems, and some interface mechanisms are built to transfer data between these systems and the HIS. For example, the radiology information system (RIS) was originally a component of HIS. Later, an independent RIS was developed because of the limited support offered by HIS for the handling of special information required by the radiology operation. Large-scale hospital information systems mostly use mainframe computers. These can be purchased through a manufacturer with certain customization software, or home grown through the integration of many commercial products, progressively throughout years. A home grown system may contain many reliable legacy components, but with out-of-date technology. Therefore, in interfacing HIS to PACS, caution is necessary to circumvent the legacy problem.

Radiology Information System (RIS)

RIS (Smith, 2005) (Huang, 2004) is designed to support both the administrative and the clinical operation of a radiology department, to reduce administrative overhead, and to improve the quality of radiological examination delivery. Therefore, RIS manages general radiology patient demographics and billing information, procedure descriptions and scheduling, diagnostic reports, patient arrival scheduling, film location, film movement, and examination room scheduling. The RIS configuration is very similar to the HIS except it is on a smaller scale. RIS equipment consists of a computer system with peripheral devices such as alphanumeric terminals, printers, and bar code readers. In most cases, an independent RIS is autonomous, with limited access to HIS. However, some HISs offer embedded RIS subsystems with a higher degree of integration.

The RIS interfaces to PACS based on the HL7 standard through TCP/IP over Ethernet on a client/server model using a trigger mechanism. Events such as examination scheduling, patient arrivals, and examination begin and end times trigger the RIS to send previously selected information associated with the event (patient demographics, examination description, diagnostic report, etc.) to the PACS in real time.

Structured Query Language (SQL)

SQL, Structured Query Language, is a database query language that was adopted as an industry standard in 1986. A major revision to the SQL standard was completed in 1992, called SQL2.

Stored Procedure

Benefits of Stored Procedure include the followings:

- **Precompiled execution:** SQL Server compiles each stored procedure once and then reutilizes the execution plan. This results in tremendous performance boosts when stored procedures are called repeatedly.
- **Reduced client/server traffic:** In some situation, if network bandwidth is limited, stored procedures can reduce long SQL queries to a single line that is transmitted over the wire.
- **Efficient reuse of code and programming abstraction:** Since the stored procedures can be used by multiple users and client programs, the software development cycle can be shortened.
- **Enhanced security controls:** User's permission can be granted or limited to execute a stored procedure independently of underlying table permissions.

Health Level 7 (HL7)

Health Level 7 (HL7) (Smith, 2005) (Huang, 2004), established in March 1987, was organized by a user-vendor committee to develop a standard for electronic data exchange in healthcare environments, particularly for hospital applications. The common goal is to simplify the interface implementation between computer applications from multiple vendors. This standard emphasizes data format and protocol for exchanging certain key textual data among healthcare information systems, such as HIS, RIS, and PACS. HL7 addresses the highest level (level 7) of the Open System Interconnection (OSI) model of the International Standards Organization (ISO), but does not conform specifically to the defined elements of the OSI's seventh level. It conforms to the conceptual definitions of an application to application interface placed in the seventh layer of the OSI model. These definitions were developed to facilitate data communication in a healthcare setting by providing rules to convert abstract messages associated with real-world events into strings of characters comprised in an actual message.

PACS BROKER

The database to database transfer method allows two or more networked information systems to share a subset of data by storing them in a common local area. For example, the ADT data from HIS can be reformatted to HL7 standard (Huang,

2004) and broadcasted periodically to a certain local database in HIS. A TCP/IP communication protocol can, be set up between HIS and RIS to allow HIS to initiate the local database and broadcast the ADT data to RIS through either a pull or a push operation. This method is most often used to share information between HIS and RIS.

DISPLAY WORKSTATIONS

Diagnostic Workstation

A diagnostic workstation (Huang, 2004) is used by the radiologists for making primary diagnosis. The components in this type of workstation must be of the best quality possible. If the workstation is used for displaying projection radiographs, multiple 2K monitors are needed. On the other hand, if the workstation is used for CT and MR images, multiple 1 K monitors will be sufficient. A diagnostic workstation requires a digital Dictaphone to report the findings. The workstation provides software to append the report to the images. In addition to having the entire image processing functions, the diagnostic workstation requires a rapid (1-2 s) image retrieval.

Review Workstation

A review workstation is used by radiologists and referring physicians to review cases in the hospital wards. The dictation or the transcribed report should be available, with the corresponding images. A review workstation may not require 2K monitors, since images might have been read by the radiologist from the diagnostic workstation, and the referring physicians will not be looking for every minute detail. Diagnostic and review workstations can be combined as a single workstation sharing both diagnostic and review functions like an alternator.

Analysis Workstations

Analysis workstations differ from diagnostic and review workstations in that the former are used to extract useful parameters from images. Some parameters are easy to extract from a simple region of interest (ROI) operation, others (e.g., blood flow measurements from DSA, 3-D reconstruction from sequential CT images) are computation intensive and require an analysis workstation with a more powerful image processor and high performance software.

Web Server

The Internet was developed by the federal government originally for military applications. Through the years, its utilization has been greatly extended. The Internet can be loosely defined as a set of computers, connected together by various wiring methods, that transmit information among each other through TCP/IP network protocols using a public communication network. An intranet, on the other hand, is a private entity that transmits information through a secured network environment. The World Wide Web is a collection of Internet protocols that provide easy access to many large databases through Internet connections. The Web is based on the hypertext transfer protocol (HTTP), which supports the transmission of hypertext document on all computers accessible through the Internet. The two most popular languages for Web applications that allow for the display of formatted and multimedia documents to be independent of the computers used are HTML (hypertext markup language) and Java language (just another vague acronym) from Sun Microsystems. In Web terminology, there are the Web server and the clients (or sites, or browsers). A Web site can use trigger processes to access information on a Web server through HTTP. During the past several years, the application of Web technology has been extended to healthcare information. Some Web sites now support access to textual information from Electronic Medical Record (EMR) systems. These Web-based EMR systems (Dreyer, 2005) can be categorized according to their characteristics (e.g., completeness and detail of information model, coupling between the Web-based and legacy hospital information systems, machinable quality of data, customization). The use of the Web server as a means to access PACS image data is being considered and implemented by both academic centres and manufacturers. In the next section, we present the design of a Web-based image file server in the PACS environment as a means of accessing PACS images and data for both intra and inter hospital applications.

Consider the image file server, let us see what properties it needs to be qualified as a Web-based file server. First, the server has to support Web browsers connected to the Internet. Second, the server must interpret queries from the browser written in HTML or Java, and convert the queries to DICOM and HL7 standards. Third, the server must support the DICOM Query/Retrieve SOP to query and retrieve images and related data from the PACS controller. And finally, the server must provide a translator to convert DICOM images and HL7 text to HTTP.

The Web server is a nice concept utilizing existing Internet technology available in everyone's desktop computer to access PACS images and related data. There are, however, drawbacks to using the current Internet for image retrieval. First, the response time for image transmission from the Internet is too slow because of the constraints imposed by the WAN speed. As a result, it is feasible to use the Internet for such applications only if the number and the size of images retrieved are small. The proposed next generation Internet (NGI) may alleviate some of these constraints. On the other hand, Web technology is well-suited for intranet applications, especially if the intranet uses a well-designed high speed LAN (e.g., gigabit Ethernet or ATM). Another problem is that Web technology is not designed for high resolution gray-scale image display, especially when real time lookup table operation is required. In this case, the waiting time for such an operation is intolerably long.

ADVANCED WORKSTATION

Surgical Navigation Workstation

The basic principle behind computer assisted orthopaedic surgery is relatively simple. Digital images of the patient's anatomy are gathered prior intraoperatively and provide the surgeon with anatomical landmarks on which to base bone cuts and final placement of orthopaedic implants. In most systems the actual surgical instrumentation can also be incorporated into the digital model, allowing for precise positioning and movement that surgeons are not generally afforded in minimally invasive procedures. The benefits provided by Computer Assisted Surgery (CAS) are increased accuracy in needle biopsy, implant placement, reduced outliers in surgical outcome and the ability to employ less invasive surgical techniques.

In general, CAS systems can be broken down into three categories. Preoperative image based systems usually utilize computer tomography (CT) scans to provide a 3D digital image of the patient's anatomy prior to the surgical procedure. The digital model is then loaded into the OR's computer and visualization system, providing an anatomical map for the surgeon to follow throughout the procedure. Intraoperative image based systems generally rely on a composite of two dimensional images provided by fluoroscopic imaging equipment after the patient is actually positioned on the operating table. The final and newest category is image-free systems that require no pre-scanning of the patient, thereby eliminating the added cost and patient transport required for CT and fluoroscopic scanning. The image free systems provide real time anatomic information intraoperatively based on a constant collection of landmark locations being updated to the software supporting the digital model.

Radiosurgery

Of general interest is the use of new technology applied to the practice of medicine. Specific interests are relevant to the precise and accurate applications of radiation and other interventional therapies for cancer patients. One example is the use of stereotactic radiosurgery. This is an accurate (to within 0.5 mm) and highly focused use of radiation on normal and diseased tissue in the brain. Other interests include the following: the development of new techniques for accurate localization of tumours and normal tissue in the central nervous system and other areas of the body; improvement of techniques for patient immobilization and positioning; and application of computers and other technologies toward these ends.

An active research area is the assessment of tissue response to stereotactic radiosurgery in the brain. This involves the use of several medical imaging technologies such as magnetic resonance imaging, positron emission tomography, and computed tomography to measure the time course of radiation effects. Spatial correlation of radiation dose with the observed imaging changes and clinical response over time is exploited.

A second area of research is high precision stereotactic guidance of probes or radiation in order to affect changes in the brain. A typical approach is the use of an electrode to cauterize a small region of cells in the globus pallidus to help treat Parkinson's disease. In this invasive procedure, a wire electrode is threaded into the globus pallidus where a well-defined electric current is injected. Under investigation is whether a highly focused beam of radiation can be substituted for the electrode in order to provide a non-invasive approach to treating the disease. In another study, an oxygen electrode is stereotactically guided to measure the oxygen levels in selected brain tissues. This approach can be used to validate new, non-invasive imaging technologies that measure oxygen levels.

A third area of research is the use of infrared stereo-optic camera systems to monitor motion and direct the positioning of cancer patients before and during radiation treatments. Such devices can help to dynamically coordinate the targeting and shape of radiation beams while the patient breathes. They also can monitor the motion of radiation treatment machines relative to the patient.

TELERADIOLOGY

Teleradiology is a subset of telemedicine (Boland, Schlakman, Thrall, 2005) dealing with the transmission and display of images in addition to other patient related information between a remote site and an expert centre. The technology requirement for teleradiology is more stringent than that of general telemedicine, because the former involves images. Basically, telemedicine without teleradiology requires only very simple technology: a computer gathers all necessary patient information, examination results, and diagnostic reports, arranges them in proper order at the referring site, and transmits them through telecommunication technology to a second computer at the expert centre, where the information is displayed as soft copy on a monitor. In modern hospitals or clinics, the information gathering, and the arrangement of the information in proper order, can be handled by the hospital information system (HIS). In a private practice group or an individual physician's office, these two steps can be contracted out to a computer application vendor. Another requirement of telemedicine is to design communication protocols for sending this prearranged information to the expert centre. Special hardware and software components are needed for this task. Hardware and telecommunication choices vary according to required data throughput. The hardware component includes a pair of communication boards and or modems connecting the two computers, one at the referring site and the other at the expert centre through a telephone line. The type and cost of such hardware depends on which telecommunication service is selected. Depending on the transmission speed required, the line can be a regular telephone line, a DS-0 (digital service, 56 Kbit/s), an ISDN (Integrated Service Digital Network, from 56 Kbit/s to 1.544 Mbit/s), or a DS-1 or private line (T-l), with 1.544 Mbit/s. The costs for these lines are related to the transmission speed, and the distance between sites. For telemedicine applications without images, a regular telephone line, DS-0, or a single ISDN line would be sufficient.

Teleradiology and PACS

When the teleradiology service (Boland, Schlakman, Thrall, 2005) (Huang, 2004) requires patient's historical images as well as related information, teleradiology and PACS become very similar. Most current teleradiology still uses a digitizer as the primary method of converting a film image to digital format, although the trend is moving toward the DICOM standard. In PACS, direct digital image capture using DICOM is mostly used. In networking, teleradiology uses slower speed wide area networks (WAN) compared with the higher speed local area network (LAN) used in PACS. In teleradiology, image storage is mostly short-term, whereas in PACS it is long-term. Teleradiology relies heavily on image compression, whereas PACS may or may not. In clinical applications, a single image is not sufficient for diagnostic purposes. In general, a typical examination generates between 10 and 20 Mbyte.

REFERENCES

Boland, G., Schlakman, J. T., & Thrall, J. H. (2005). Teleradiology. In Dreyer K.J., Mehta A., Thrall J.H. (Eds.), *PACS: A Guide to the Digital Revolution,* (pp. 523-530). 2nd ed., Springer Verlag. ISBN: 0387260102; ISBN-13: 9780387260105

Calder, A. (2006). *Information Security Based on ISO 27001/ISO 17799: A Management Guide.* Van Haren Publishing. First Edition ISBN-10: 9077212701.

Dreyer, K. J. (2005). Web distribution. In Dreyer K.J., Mehta A., Thrall J.H.. (Eds.), *PACS: A Guide to the Digital Revolution,* (pp. 373-382). 2nd ed., Springer Verlag. ISBN: 0387260102; ISBN-13: 9780387260105

Dreyer, K. J., & Kalra, M. K. (2005). Digital imaging fundamentals. In Dreyer K.J., Mehta A., Thrall J.H. (Eds.), *PACS: A Guide to the Digital Revolution,* (pp. 183-228). 2nd ed., Springer Verlag. ISBN: 0387260102; ISBN-13: 9780387260105

Herman, G. T. (1980). *Image Reconstruction from Projections: The Fundamentals of Computerized Tomography.* Academic Pr. ISBN-10: 0123420504; ISBN-13: 978-0123420503

Huang, H. K. (2004). Digital Medical Image Fundamentals. In Huang, H. K. (Ed.), *PACS – Basic Principles and Applications,* (pp. 23-48). New York: John Wiley & Sons. ISBN: 0471251232; ISBN-13: 9780471251231

Huang, H. K. (2004). Digital Radiography. In Huang, H. K. (Ed.), *PACS – Basic Principles and Applications,* (pp. 49-78). New York: John Wiley & Sons. ISBN: 0471251232; ISBN-13: 9780471251231

Huang, H. K. (2004). Computed Tomography, Magnetic Resonance, Ultrasound, Nuclear Medicine, and Light Imaging. In Huang, H.K. (Ed.), *PACS – Basic Principles and Applications,* (pp. 79-118). New York: John Wiley & Sons. ISBN: 0471251232; ISBN-13: 9780471251231

Huang, H. K. (2004). Industrial Standards (HL7 and DICOM) and Work Flow Protocols (IHE). In Huang, H. K. (Ed.), *PACS – Basic Principles and Applications,* (pp. 171-194). New York: John Wiley & Sons. ISBN: 0471251232; ISBN-13: 9780471251231

Huang, H. K. (2004). Integration of HIS, RIS, PACS, and ePR. In Huang, H. K. (Ed.), *PACS – Basic Principles and Applications,* (pp. 307-330). New York: John Wiley & Sons. ISBN: 0471251232; ISBN-13: 9780471251231

Huang, H. K. (2004). PACS Data Management and Web-Based Image Distribution. In Huang, H. K. (Ed.), *PACS – Basic Principles and Applications,* (pp. 333-352). New York: John Wiley & Sons. ISBN: 0471251232; ISBN-13: 9780471251231

Huang, H. K. (2004). Telemedicine and Teleradiology. In Huang, H. K. (Ed.), *PACS – Basic Principles and Applications,* (pp. 353-380). New York: John Wiley & Sons. ISBN: 0471251232; ISBN-13: 9780471251231

Myers, R., Cunningham, V., & Bailey, D. L. (Eds.), (1996). *Terry Jones Quantification of Brain Function Using PET.* Academic Press. 1st edition. ISBN-10: 0123897602; ISBN-13: 978-0123897602

National Electrical Manufacturers Association (NEMA) (2008). *Digital Imaging and Communications in Medicine (DICOM).* PS 3.01~18-2008

Nesbitt, K. M., Schultz, T. F., & Dasilva, R. (2005). PACS architecture. In Dreyer K. J., Mehta A., Thrall J. H. (Eds.), *PACS: A Guide to the Digital Revolution,* (pp.249-268). 2nd ed., Springer Verlag. ISBN: 0387260102; ISBN-13: 9780387260105

Smith, G. (2005). Introduction to RIS and PACS. In Dreyer K. J., Mehta A., Thrall J. H. (Eds.), *PACS: A Guide to the Digital Revolution,* (pp. 9-26). 2nd ed., Springer Verlag. ISBN: 0387260102; ISBN-13: 9780387260105

Siegel, E. L., & Kolodner R. M. (2001). *Filmless Radiology.* Reprint ed., Springer Verlag.

Strickland, N. H. (2000, July). PACS (picture archiving and communication systems): Filmless radiology. *Archives of Disease in Childhood 2000, 83,* 82-86.

Chapter II
ISO 27000 Information Security Management System

INTRODUCTION

The protection of information for a healthcare organization, in any form, while in storage, processing, or transport, from being available to any organization or person that is neither authorized by its owner to have it nor for patient caring, is the objective of information security management in healthcare. There are many standards on information security management. The international standard for information security management is ISO 27000. The objective of this chapter is to provide an introduction of ISO 27000 and its application in PACS.

INTERNATIONAL STANDARDS ON INFORMATION SECURITY MANAGEMENT SYSTEM

The Develop of International Information Security Management Standards

The BS 7799 ISMS was not the first one to be proposed as an ISO standard. The original version, BS 7799:1995 was submitted in the summer of 1996 but was narrowly defeated. Those countries who voted in its favour were not dismayed, however. Australia and New Zealand for example recast it (by changing the UK legislative references to corresponding Australian and New Zealand references) and re-published it as AS/NZS 4444. The Netherlands embraced it wholesale and established a certification scheme, which went live early 1997. This international interest encouraged the British to develop the standard further.

Certification Schemes

Indeed, much to the British chagrin, the Dutch were the first to establish a certification Scheme. It included revolutionary ideas on entry and advanced level certification, and self as well as third party certification. The "advanced level" certification recognized that in real life it might be necessary to apply safeguards other than those listed in BS 7799. BDD/2 applauded this idea, and married it with its own ideas on third party certification to create the "c:cure" scheme.

BS 7799 Part 2

Because BS 7799:1995 was a code of practice, how could an assessor associate a pass or fail verdict? Indeed, if non-BS 7799 controls could be included, how would an assessor know which safeguards were to apply and which were not. The answer lay in the creation of BS 7799 Part 2 which spells out precisely what an organization and the assessor need to do in order to ensure successful certification.

Almost by accident, the creation of Part 2 led to the dramatic conclusion that the concept of an ISMS is perhaps of far greater and fundamental importance than the original Code of Practice. By the inclusion of a variety of feedback loops (as shown in the slide on the right), an ISMS allows managers to monitor and control their security systems thereby minimizing the residual business risk and ensuring that security continues to fulfil the corporate, customer and legal requirements.

Less than two years after its creation, the UK "c:cure" certification scheme found itself challenged by alternative schemes predicated on EA7/03, a document entitled "Guidelines for the Accreditation of Bodies operating Certification/Registration of Information Security Management Systems". This is a document agreed and recognized throughout Europe and the members of the European co-operation for Accreditation. It has formed the basis of various third party audits undertaken within the USA, mainland Europe, Africa and the UK and is recognized in other parts of the world. In view of the wider acceptance of EA7/03, as of 2nd October 2000, the DTI withdrew its support for c:cure and the effectively the c:cure scheme has been terminated, to be replaced by the internationally accepted norm.

The Creation of ISO/IEC 17799

Following the publication of BS 7799:1999 in April 1991, Part 1 of this new version of the standard was proposed as an ISO standard via the "Fast Track" mechanism in October 1999. The international ballot closed in August 2000, and received the required majority voting. In October 2000, eight minor changes to the BS text were approved and the standard was published as ISO/IEC 17799:2000 on 1st December 2000.

The Revision of Part 2

BS 7799 Part 2:2002 was published on 5th September at the BS 7799 Goes Global Conference in London. The new edition of BS 7799 Part 2 has been produced to harmonize it with other management system standards such as ISO 9001:2000 and ISO 14001:1996 to provide consistent and integrated implementation and operation of management systems. It also introduces a Plan-Do-Check-Act (PDCA) model as part of a management system approach to developing, implementing, and improving the effectiveness of an organization's information security management system.

The implementation of the PDCA model will also reflect the principles as set out in the OECD guidance (OECD Guidelines for the Security of Information Systems and Networks, 2002) governing the security of information systems and networks. In particular, this new edition gives a robust model for implementing the principles in those guidelines governing risk assessment, security design and implementation, security management and reassessment.

As a consequence of references to the OECD guidance being incorporated into BS 7799-2:2002, publication was delayed until 5 September 2002. This was to coincide with the publication of the OECD guidelines and also to ensure that the rules from UKAS regarding transition from BS 7799-2:1999 to BS 7799-2:2002 could be developed and put in place.

2005 Versions of the Standards and ISO/IEC 27001:2005

In 2005, BS 7799-2 finally entered the ISO Fast Track mechanism and emerged on 14th October 2005 as ISO/IEC 27001:2005 after significant re-ordering of controls and general restructuring. There is a lot of similarity between the two standards and apart from two differences the others are relatively insignificant. The first difference that is worthy of note is the adoption of ISO/IEC 17799:2005 as the basis of the SOA. The second is the introduction of a new requirement concerning ISMS metrics and the need to measure the effectiveness of the information security controls. ISO/IEC 17799:2000 has been substantially revised and a new version was published in mid-June 2005 as ISO/IEC 17799:2005. Subsequently ISO/IEC 17799:2005 was renumbered as ISO/IEC 27002:2005 in July 2007, bringing it into line with the other ISO/IEC 27000-series standards.

The ISO/IEC 27000-series standards have been reserved for a family of information security management standards which is known informally as "ISO 27000", similar to the very successful ISO 9000 family of quality assurance standards. The other family members of the standard either already published or working in progress are as following:

- ISO/IEC 27000—will provide an overview/introduction to the ISO27000 standards as a whole plus the specialist vocabulary used in ISO27000.
- ISO/IEC 27001:2005 is the specification of Information Security Management System requirements standard against which over 4,400 organizations have been certified compliant.
- ISO/IEC 27002:2005 (ISO/IEC 17799:2005, 2005) is the code of practice for information security management describing a comprehensive set of information security control objectives and a set of generally accepted good practice security controls.
- ISO/IEC 27003 will provide implementation guidance for ISO/IEC 27001.
- ISO/IEC 27004 will be an information security management measurement standard to help improve the effectiveness of your ISMS.
- ISO/IEC 27005:2008 is a new information security risk management standard released in June 2008.
- ISO/IEC 27006:2007 is a guide to the certification or registration process for accredited ISMS certification or registration bodies.
- ISO/IEC 27007 will be a guideline for auditing Information Security Management Systems.
- ISO/IEC TR 27008 will provide guidance on auditing information security controls.
- ISO/IEC 27010 will provide guidance on sector-to-sector interworking and communications for industry and government, supporting a series of sector-specific ISMS implementation guidelines starting with ISO/IEC 27011.
- ISO/IEC 27011 will be information security management guidelines for telecommunications and will be released soon.
- ISO/IEC 27031 will be an ICT-focused standard on business continuity.
- ISO/IEC 27032 will be guidelines for cyber-security.
- ISO/IEC 27033 will replace the multi-part ISO/IEC 18028 standard on IT network security.
- ISO/IEC 27034 will provide guidelines for application security.
- ISO/IEC 27799, (ISO 27799, 2006) although not strictly part of ISO27000, will provide health sector specific ISMS implementation guidance.

THE ESSENCE OF INFORMATION SECURITY

Confidentiality

Many forms of access control (Calder, 2006) are basically about protecting confidentiality. Encryption is another example of a control, which can provide for the confidentiality of information. Controls may be applied at every level of an information security management system, the physical level (e.g. locks on doors, filing cabinets, safes etc), and the logical level (e.g. individual data fields in a database, data in applications and in hardcopy form such as paper documents). In every case the threats and vulnerabilities should be identified, the associated risks assessed, and a system of controls selected, implemented and applied to protect against these risks.

Integrity

Integrity is ensuring that information is accurate and complete in storage and transport; that it is correctly processed and that it has not been modified in any unauthorized way. We also wish to establish the integrity of the networks and systems that we connect to, to ensure that they are who we intend them to be. Many data handling devices contain automatic integrity checking facilities to ensure that they, including disk drives and other media, and telecommunications systems, do not corrupt data. Integrity controls are essential in operating systems, software and application programs in order to prevent intentional or unintentional corruption of programs and data during processing. Integrity controls need to be included at the procedural level to reduce the risks of human error, theft or fraud, e.g. controls for input/output data validation, user training and other operational type controls.

Availability

Availability is ensuring that information is available to those who are authorized to have it, when and where they should have it. In practice the availability of information requires a system of controls: for example information backups, capacity planning, procedures and criteria for system acceptance, incident management procedures, management of removable computer media, information handling procedures, equipment maintenance and testing, procedures for monitoring system use, and business continuity procedures. Monitoring, reviewing and checking security, incidents, service levels, and system performance in a timely and on-going manner can be a preventative control to ensure availability.

Sensitive or Critical Information

ISO/IEC 27000 (ISO/IEC 27001, 2005) defines a number of controls, which are applicable to both sensitive and critical information. What is sensitive or critical information and how do we recognize it? For every organization the definition will be different. Some means should be found to assess the value or utility of information in the context of the individual organization in order to be able to label information as sensitive or critical when needed and the rest as non-sensitive or non-critical. In healthcare organization, the data availability means the chance to save lives while the data integrity means the quality of healthcare. The data confidentiality is the quality management of the healthcare organization. There is also a time element: a patient's radiological images or laboratory test reports will be very important to be available before the surgery, but have less importance after surgery. Sensitivity will also be reflected in the level of classification given to the data. Part of the risk assessment process involves the valuation of information assets in order to calculate the risks and the level of security required to protect these assets using an appropriate system of controls.

- **Contingency planning** is a generic/all-encompassing term meaning the preparation of secondary arrangements in case primary arrangements fail. It comprises a suite of techniques designed to identify and minimize risks. Contingency planning concepts apply to healthcare business, medical equipment, IT, political, personal and other situations.
- **Crisis planning** specifically concerns planning for the immediate aftermath of a disaster evacuating staff safely, putting out the fires, treating casualties and so forth. This is probably the most critical period of all since normal processes and controls have more or less completely failed at this point. Some individuals have reverted to primitive survival instincts, while others may be physically and/or mentally traumatized to the extent that they are incapable of normal behaviour. A good crisis plan provides sufficient structure and guidance to stabilize the situation and enable the actual recovery processes to commence.
- **Business continuity planning** usually means preparing to keep the healthcare business going in some form, or perhaps restarts it, despite a disaster. Typical business continuity plans would include advance agreements or contracts to take over alternative office space in case of a physical disaster such as a major office fire, and IT disaster recovery plans.
- **Medical information system disaster recovery planning** concerns making arrangements to recover critical medical IT services onto fall-back/standby systems and network equipment.

Ten Major Sections

ISO 27000, is a detailed security standard. It is organized into ten major sections, each covering a different topic or area:

1. Business Continuity Planning

The objectives of this section are: To counteract interruptions to business activities and to critical business processes from the effects of major failures or disasters.

In a filmless radiology project, the business continuity plan may involve the continuous of radiological service using traditional X-ray films and disaster recovery procedures. In the design of the BCP, the required people, equipment, site, and time should be estimated and prepared.

2. System Access Control

The objectives of this section are:

1. To control access to information
2. To prevent unauthorized access to information systems
3. To ensure the protection of networked services
4. To prevent unauthorized computer access
5. To detect unauthorized activities.
6. To ensure information security when using mobile computing and telenetworking facilities

The design of PACS, like other information systems, can be classified into centralized and distributed systems. The system access control for a centralized PACS is more efficient.

3. System Development and Maintenance

The objectives of this section are:

1. To ensure security is built into operational systems;
2. To prevent loss, modification or misuse of user data in application systems;
3. To protect the confidentiality, authenticity and integrity of information;
4. To ensure IT projects and support activities are conducted in a secure manner;
5. To maintain the security of application system software and data.

Most of PACS are in clinical and production environment in which system development often occurred. System maintenance involving both preventive maintenance and corrective maintenance are more common.

4. Physical and Environmental Security

The objectives of this section are:

1. To prevent unauthorised access, damage and interference to business premises and information;
2. To prevent loss, damage or compromise of assets and interruption to business activities;
3. To prevent compromise or theft of information and information processing facilities.

Like other equipment in a hospital environment, physical and environmental security is more conscious. In most of well developed medical centres, the physical and environmental security policies have been included in the comprehensive hospital management schemes.

5. Compliance

The objectives of this section are:

1. To avoid breaches of any criminal or civil law, statutory, regulatory or contractual obligations and of any security requirements
2. To ensure compliance of systems with organizational security policies and standards
3. To maximize the effectiveness of and to minimize interference to/from the system audit process.

Since the technologies are moving fast, new laws and standards come into effect each year. As a PACS professional, the administrator has the duty to make sure that the system complies with the new laws and standards.

6. Personnel Security

The objectives of this section are:

1. To reduce risks of human error, theft, fraud or misuse of facilities;

2. To ensure that users are aware of information security threats and concerns, and are equipped to support the hospital security policy in the course of their normal work;
3. To minimize the damage from security incidents and malfunctions and learn from such incidents.

In the design of a PACS, there are a lot of automatic features such as PACS Broker and barcode systems for minimizing the manual input of data. Using the above automatic data inputting systems, most of the human errors can be eliminated.

7. Security Organization

The objectives of this section are:

1. To manage information security within the Company;
2. To maintain the security of organizational information processing facilities and information assets accessed by third parties.
3. To maintain the security of information when the responsibility for information processing has been outsourced to another organization.

This section addresses the security management as part of the PACS business. All parties including administrators, end users, and management are held responsible for the security of the organization.

8. Computer and Operations Management

The objectives of this section are:

1. To ensure the correct and secure operation of information processing facilities;
2. To minimize the risk of systems failures;
3. To protect the integrity of software and information;
4. To maintain the integrity and availability of information processing and communication;
5. To ensure the safeguarding of information in networks and the protection of the supporting infrastructure;
6. To prevent damage to assets and interruptions to business activities;
7. To prevent loss, modification or misuse of information exchanged between organizations.

Figure 1.

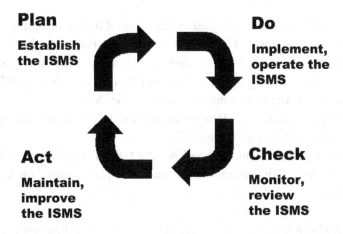

This section describes the involvement of all front line staff including clinicians, radiographers, administrators, and nurses in computer and operations management. In a filmless hospital, all staff involved are required to work together for a new workflow design, change of operation procedures for security purposes.

9. Asset Classification and Control

The objectives of this section are: To maintain appropriate protection of hospital assets and to ensure that information assets receive an appropriate level of protection.

In PACS, the asset classification and control cover and include the archiving servers, database servers, Web servers, manuals, staff, system configuration files, system log, activity log, firewall configuration, preventive maintenance reports, and audit reports. Each type of asset is protected with appropriate control according to its class.

10. Security Policy

The objectives of this section are: To provide management direction and support for information security.

All staff involving in PACS business from senior management to front line workers should be made aware of the security policy.

Plan-Do-Check-Act Model

As Figure 1 shows, the cycle begins at the point of determining the scope of the ISMS. An important aspect of ISO 27000 is that of the Plan-Do-Check-Act (PDCA) model, which can be applied to the ISMS. This is an approach for developing, implementing and improving the effectiveness of an organization's ISMS. Figure 1 (below) shows how the PDCA model applies to the ISMS.

The full cycle, from consideration of the standard's merits through to actual implementation, is depicted in Figure 2.

The cycle depicted in Figure 2 outlines the typical stages that can be followed when adopting ISO 27000 as an internal standard. These stages are detailed in the points below:

- The merits of the standard are considered, such as enhancing the security of the hospital, as well as the confidence of new/existing users and partners.
- A decision is made by hospital management to implement ISO 27000. It may be the case that the healthcare organization wishes to simply become compliant by adhering to the standard, or it may mean that certification is sought.

Figure 2.

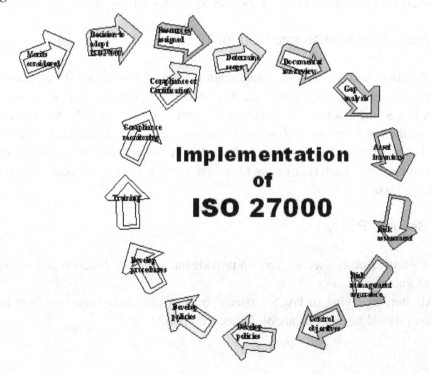

- Resources in terms of people and time are allocated for the project. Assistance may be sought from an experienced ISO 27000 consultant at this stage.
- The scope of the ISMS is determined. This means that the area/s of the health-care organization to be measured against the standard are selected. This should be a reasonable representation of the organization's activities.
- A review of existing documentation takes place to assess the extent of measures already in place, such as the ISO 9000 quality manual and security policies.
- A gap analysis is undertaken to identify the gaps between existing and required controls, processes and procedures.
- An inventory is taken of all relevant information assets.
- A risk assessment (ISO/IEC 13335-3, 1998) is carried out in order to deter-mine the extent of risk to the ISMS, often comparing impact of risks with the likelihood of these risks actually occurring. A Risk Assessment document is the resulting deliverable.
- Once risks have been identified and established in the Risk Assessment document, the healthcare organization must decide how such risks are to be managed. From these decisions, responsibilities for managing these risks are determined and documented.
- Appropriate controls and objectives to be implemented are selected, either from the standard, or not, as the case may be. The standard does not contain an exhaustive list, and additional controls and objectives may be selected. A Statement of Applicability (SoA) is the resulting deliverable following selec-tion of controls.
- Policies are created based on the SoA.
- Relevant procedures based on the policy definitions and guidelines are created and documented.
- A training programme is undertaken to educate all employees to ensure that good practice for Information Security is adopted throughout the business.
- A programme of compliance monitoring is implemented. This is to ensure that the good work achieved to date is maintained.
- Once compliance has been achieved, certification may be optionally sought from an accredited body. This requires an audit, which will examine the healthcare organization's adherence to the standard. A successful audit result will mean that the healthcare organization will gain certification.

REFERENCES

Calder, A. (2006). *Information Security Based on ISO 27001/ISO 17799: A Manage-ment Guide*. Van Haren Publishing, First Edition. ISBN-10: 9077212701.

ISO/IEC TR 13335-3 (1998). *Information technology — Guidelines for the management of IT Security — Part 3: Techniques for the management of IT Security.* American National Standards Institute. First edition.

ISO/IEC 17799 (2005). *Information technology - Security techniques - Code of practice for information security management.* ISO/IEC/JTC 1/SC 27 Distributed through American National Standards Institute (ANSI) (23 Aug 2007); ASIN: B000Y2TUKU.

ISO/IEC 27001 (2005). *Information Technology - Security Techniques - Information security management systems - Requirements (Information Technology).* British Standards Institution (2005); ISBN-10: 0580467813; ISBN-13: 978-0580467813.

Tong, C. K. S., Chan, K. K., & Huang, H. Y. H. (2004). *The Application of ISO 17799 and BS 7799 Information Security Management in Picture Archiving and Communication System.* RSNA 2004.

Tong, C. K. S., Fung, K. H., Huang, H. Y. H., & Chan, K. K. (2003, June). Implementation of ISO 17799 and BS 7799 in picture archiving and communication system: Local experience in implementation of BS 7799 standard. CARS 2003. Computer Assisted Radiology and Surgery. *Proceedings of the 17th International Congress and Exhibition, 1256,* 311-318.

Chapter III
High Availability
Technologies for PACS

INTRODUCTION

PACS disasters can, and do, appear in a variety of forms including storage hard disk failure, file corruption, network breakdown, and server malfunction. The PACS disasters are commonly classified into hardware, environmental and physical, network, database system, and server failures. A single point of hardware failure in PACS is at the PACS controller, or the main archive server. When it occurs, it renders the entire PACS inoperable and crippled, until the problem is diagnosed and resolved. Recently, various techniques were developed for the prevention of PACS disasters caused by the actual loss and inaccessibility of data. All those techniques are commonly called "High Availability (HA) Technologies" (Marcus, Stern, 2003). The objective of this chapter is to discuss various HA technologies for the prevention of PACS disasters.

HIGH AVAILABLE TECHNOLOGIES

Network

Nevertheless, all of the PACS devices still need to be connected to the network (Marcus, Stern, 2003). In order to maximize system reliability, a PACS network should be built with redundancy. To build a redundant network, two parallel gigabit optical fibres are connected between the PACS and the hospital networks forming two network segments using four Ethernet switches. The Ethernet switches are configured in such a way that one of the network segments is in active mode while the other is in standby mode. If the active network segment fails, the standby network segment will become active within less than 300 ms to allow the system to keep running continuously.

Server Clustering

The advantage of clustering computers (Marcus, Stern, 2003) (Huang, 2004) for high availability is seen if one of the computers fails; another computer in the cluster can then assume the workload of the failed computer (Thomas, 2007) at a pre-specified time interval. Users of the system see no interruption of access. The advantages of clustering DICOM Web servers for scalability include increased application performance and the support of a greater number of users for image distribution.

   Clustering (Nesbitt, Schultz, and Dasilva, 2005) can be implemented at different levels of the system, including hardware, operating systems, middleware, systems management and applications. The more layers that incorporate clustering technology, the more complex the whole system is to manage. To implement a successful clustering solution, specialists in all the technologies (i.e. hardware, networking, and software) are required. For clustering the Web servers, we can connect all Web servers using a load balancing switch. This method has the advantages of low server overhead and requiring no computer processor power.

Database Cluster

Since the hearts of many medical information systems (Lou, 1997) such as PACS, HIS, and RIS (Smith, 2005) (Huang, 2004) are their databases, protection of the databases is an essential task during the design of a filmless hospital project. Database clustering is one of the most efficient for protection and load balancing of database service. It is a technique to connect several computer servers to provide a high available database service. The advantages of database cluster include:

- **High availability:** Able to deliver 99.99% availability using parallel server architecture with no single point of failure.
- **Dynamic scalability:** Incrementally scale-out the applications as hospital needs grow.
- **High-Performance:** Deliver the performance and throughput required to meet the most demanding hospital applications.
- **No data synchronization:** A single database is used without any data synchronization.

Storage

A storage area network (SAN) is a high speed, special purpose network (or sub-network) that interconnects different kinds of data storage devices with associated data servers on behalf of a larger network of users. Typically, a storage area network is part of the entire hospital network of computing resources. The advanced features of SAN are its supporting of high speed data transfer, disk mirroring, backup and restore, archival and retrieval of archived data, data migration from one storage device to another, and the sharing of data among different servers in a network. SANs can also incorporate sub-networks with network attached storage (NAS) systems.

Redundant Array of Inexpensive Disks (RAID)

In PACS, redundant array of inexpensive disks (RAID) technology can provide protection on the availability of the data in the server. In RAID level 5, no data is lost even during the failure of a single hard disk within a RAID group. This is essential for a patient care information system. Extra protection can be obtained by using additional global spare hard disks for automatic protection of data during the malfunctioning of more than one hard disk. Today, most storage area network (SAN) designed for high capacity storage are built on RAID technology.

Web Technology

Since the Web technology (Dreyer, 2005) (Huang, 2004) can provide a reliable platform for the distribution of various kinds of information including medical images and that it makes low demand on the Web client, it is selected as a tool for major medical image distribution. Hence, any computer running on common platforms such as Windows or Mac can access the Web server for image viewing using Internet Explorer or Netscape. Any clinical user can carry out his duty anytime and anywhere within a hospital.

Fault Tolerance

Fault tolerant describes what happens to a computer system or a component designed so that, in the event that a component fails, a backup component or procedure can immediately take its place with no loss of service. Fault tolerance can be provided by software, or embedded in hardware, or provided by some combination. In the software implementation, the operating system provides an interface that allows a programmer to "checkpoint" critical data at pre-determined points within a transaction. In the hardware implementation (for example, with Stratus and its VOS operating system), the programmer does not need to be aware of the fault tolerant capabilities of the machine. At a hardware level, fault tolerance is achieved by duplexing each hardware component. Disks are mirrored. Multiple processors are "lock-stepped" together and their outputs are compared for correctness. When an anomaly occurs, the faulty component is determined and taken out of service, but the machine continues to function as usual.

QUALITY MANAGEMENT OF PACS

Quality Control

One side effect of installing a clinical PACS is that users become dependent upon the technology and in some cases it can be very difficult to revert back to a film based system if components fail. The nature of system failures range from slow deterioration of function as seen in the loss of monitor luminance through sudden catastrophic loss of the entire PACS network. Therefore, it is important to have a Quality Control (QC) program for a PACS. The scopes of QC are including the maintaining the quality, quantity, and integrity of acquired radiological image data in the PACS. A daily PACS QC programs are described in Figure 1 for PACS with a department scale. In Figure 1, all radiological images are temporary stored in the QC workstations where the image quality and quantity are checked by duty radiographers/technologists. After image checked, the radiographers/technologists can archive the images to the PACS which automatically routed a set of data in the Web servers. The duty radiographers/technologists are able to browse the archived images through the Web browsers in the QC workstations. In a filmless hospital, the radiological images are distributed to various clinical departments through hospital or enterprise Web servers. The PACS QC is described as in Figure 2 which also includes the QC of the hospital or enterprise Web servers.

In the QC workstation, routine quality control is practised on all aspects of PACS, from acquisition, through network routing, through display, and including

Figure 1. Quality control program for a PACS and imaging modalities

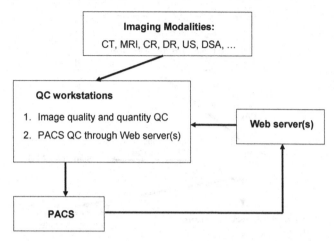

Figure 2. Quality control program for a hospital or enterprise PACS

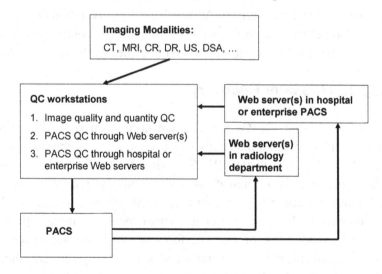

archiving. Whenever possible, the system components perform self and between platform checks for active processes, file system status, errors in log files, and system uptime. When an error is detected or an exception occurs, a message will be sent to departmental manager or PACS manager manually or electronically. Daily quality control is performed to ensure that studies can be moved from each acquisition

Figure 3. Normal operation of a high available PACS with a standby system

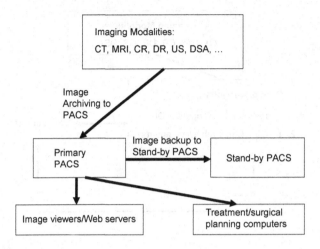

device to a workstation through the PACS and that the workstation display is correct. Regular monitor checks are performed for luminance and contrast adjustment. The results of selected quality control reports will be checked by PACS manager.

Backup and Disaster Recovery

A single point of failure in PACS during a disaster scenario is the main archive storage and server. When a major disaster occurs, it is possible to lose an entire hospital's PACS data. Few current PACS archives feature for disaster recovery, but the design is limited at best. These drawbacks include the frequency with which the backup is physically removed to an offsite facility, the operational costs associated to maintain the backup (Lou, 1997), the ease of use to perform the backup consistently and efficiently, and the ease of use to perform the PACS image data recovery.

In a high available PACS, a primary and a standby system are implemented in the hospital network. The basic duties of primary PACS are including image archiving, distribution to image viewers, Web servers, treatment and surgical planning computers. Besides, all incoming image data of a primary PACS are synchronized to its standby system under normal operation as shown in Figure 3. During the breakdown of the primary PACS, the standby system can picked up the above basic duties of the primary PACS while responsible to restore image data to the recovered primary PACS if necessary as shown in Figure 4.

Figure 4. Under abnormal operation, the standby PACS picked up the loading of the primary PACS while restoring the data to primary system

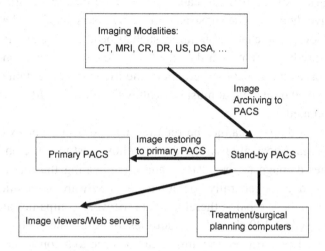

Data Recovery

Data recovery (Marcus, Stern, 2003) (Lou, 1997) is the process of salvaging data from damaged, failed, wrecked or inaccessible primary storage media when it cannot be accessed normally. Often the data is being salvaged from storage media formats such as hard disk drive, storage tapes, CDs, DVDs, RAID, and other electronics. This can be due to physical damage to the storage device or logical damage to the file system that prevents it from being mounted by the host operating system. Although there is some confusion as to the term, data recovery can also be the process of recovering deleted information from a storage media for forensic purposes.

Physical Damage

When data is to be deleted from a storage media, a variety of methods are commonly used including deletion, formatting and overwriting. If data has been accidentally deleted there are normally ways to recover it. When a file is deleted from an operating system such as Windows and, if applicable, removed from the recycle bin, the data is not gone. The operating system simply removes the pointer to the file in question and does not touch the actual data. The space allocated for the file is then made available as free space, and as the computer is used, new data may be written to that same space. Before this is done, the data is still intact and can be recovered by a variety of different data recovery software that moves beyond the operating systems file indexing scheme.

A wide variety of failures can cause physical damage to storage media. CD-ROMs can have their metallic substrate or dye layer scratched off; hard disks can suffer any of several mechanical failures, such as head crashes and failed motors; tapes can simply break. Physical damage always causes at least some data loss, and in many cases the logical structures of the file system are damaged as well. This causes logical damage that must be dealt with before any files can be rescued from the failed media.

Most physical damage cannot be repaired by end users. For example, opening a hard disk in a normal environment can allow dust to settle on the surface, causing further damage to the platters and complicating the recovery process. Furthermore, end users generally do not have the hardware or technical expertise required to make these repairs; therefore, data recovery companies are consulted. These firms use Class 100 clean room facilities to protect the media while repairs are being made. The extracted raw image can be used to reconstruct useable data after any logical damage has been repaired. Once that is complete, the files may be in useable form.

Although physical damage does cause severe data loss, in many cases, the loss can be minimized. For example, if the police was raiding a house, and the user shot his/her HDD in several places, much of the data is actually untouched. The police would then take the HDD, and slice the platters into several pieces. They then take those platters and read the data off of them, then reassemble the new data into a "virtual HDD". This process takes a lot of time, so it is usually only used in criminal cases where it is essential that the data be recovered. Data recovery can even be accomplished for alternate digital media such as Flash cards for digital cameras, old tape drives, etc.

Logical Damage

Far more common than physical damage is logical damage to a file system. Logical damage is primarily caused by power outages that prevent file system structures from being completely written to the storage medium, but problems with hardware (especially RAID controllers) and drivers, as well as system crashes, can have the same effect. The result is that the file system is left in an inconsistent state. This can cause a variety of problems, such as strange behavior (e.g., infinitely recurring directories, drives reporting negative amounts of free space), system crashes, or an actual loss of data. Various programs exist to correct these inconsistencies, and most operating systems come with at least a rudimentary repair tool for their native file systems. Linux, for instance, comes with the fsck utility, Mac OS X has

Disk Utility and Microsoft Windows provides chkdsk. Third-party utilities are also available, and some can produce superior results by recovering data even when the disk cannot be recognized by the operating system's repair utility.

Two main techniques are used by these repair programs. The first, consistency checking, involves scanning the logical structure of the disk and checking to make sure that it is consistent with its specification. For instance, in most file systems, a directory must have at least two entries: a dot (.) entry that points to itself and a dot-dot (..) entry those points to its parent. A file system repair program can read each directory and make sure that these entries exist and point to the correct directories. If they do not, an error message can be printed and the problem corrected. Both chkdsk and fsck work in this fashion. This strategy suffers from a major problem, however; if the file system is sufficiently damaged, the consistency check can fail completely. In this case, the repair program may crash trying to deal with the mangled input, or it may not recognize the drive as having a valid file system at all.

The second technique for file system repair is to assume very little about the state of the file system to be analyzed, and using any hints that any undamaged file system structures might provide, rebuild the file system from scratch. This strategy involves scanning the entire drive and making note of all file system structures and possible file boundaries, then trying to match what was located to the specifications of a working file system. Some third-party programs use this technique, which is notably slower than consistency checking. It can, however, recover data even when the logical structures are almost completely destroyed. This technique generally does not repair the underlying file system, but merely allows for data to be extracted from it to another storage device.

While most logical damage can be either repaired or worked around using these two techniques, data recovery software can never guarantee that no data loss will occur. For instance, in the FAT file system, when two files claim to share the same allocation unit ("cross-linked"), data loss for one of the files is essentially guaranteed.

The increased use of journaling file systems, such as NTFS 5.0, ext3, and XFS, is likely to reduce the incidence of logical damage. These file systems can always be "rolled back" to a consistent state, which means that the only data likely to be lost is what was in the drive's cache at the time of the system failure. However, regular system maintenance should still include the use of a consistency checker. This can protect both against bugs in the file system software and latent incompatibilities in the design of the storage hardware. One such incompatibility is the result of the disk controller reporting that file system structures have been saved to the disk when it has not actually occurred. This can often occur if the drive stores data in its write cache, then claims it has been written to the disk. If power is lost, and this data contains file system structures, the file system may be left in an inconsistent state such that the journal itself is damaged or incomplete. One solution to this problem is to use hardware that does not report data as written until it actually is written. Another is using disk controllers equipped with a battery backup so that the waiting data can be written when power is restored. Finally, the entire system can be equipped with a battery backup (see UPS) that may make it possible to keep the system on in such situations, or at least to give enough time to shut down properly.

Some kinds of logical damage can be mistakenly attributed to physical damage. For instance, when a hard drive's read/write head begins to click, most end-users will associate this with internal physical damage. This is not always the case, however. Often, either the firmware on the platters or the controller card will instead need to be rebuilt. Once the firmware on either of these two devices is restored, the drive will be back in shape and the data accessible.

One Time Two Factor Password (OTTFP)

OTTFP tokens generate new PIN numbers every 30 to 60 seconds and can be used in addition to static user IDs and passwords to log on to a Web site. The idea is that if the static credentials are stolen, say, in a punishing attack, the malicious user would still have to guess the PIN to gain access. But since the time window is short to guess the PIN, it would be nearly impossible to break in.

CONCLUSION

During the planning of a PACS, the level of availability of the system achieved should be defined clearly. In general, four levels of availability can be found in various PACS designs. Level one availability is the most basic level of system with essentially no protection at all. Level two availability is not significantly different from level one except that it includes online data protection such as Redundant Array of Independent (or Inexpensive) Disks (RAID). Level three is called High Availability in which at least two servers are configured as a cluster for providing a non-stop service. The level four availability is Disaster Recovery which involves a recovery of PACS service from a backup server at a remote site. These four levels of availability have different level of requirements on servers, network, application, storage, and management. Today, many PACS do not have a high available design or adequate backup system for the main archive server due to several issues including cost. Several large scale PACSs utilize the Fault Tolerance, resilient, or cluster design but have not been critically tested for their usefulness of their high availability. An information security management system is required on the top of technology for the management of a PACS. The implementation of such system will be discussed the following chapters.

REFERENCES

Dreyer, K. J. (2005). Computer fundamentals. In Dreyer K. J., Mehta A., Thrall J. H. (Eds.), *PACS: A Guide to the Digital Revolution,* (pp. 173-182). 2nd ed., Springer Verlag. ISBN: 0387260102; ISBN-13: 9780387260105.

Dreyer, K. J. (2005). Web distribution. In Dreyer K. J., Mehta A., Thrall J. H.. (Eds.), *PACS: A Guide to the Digital Revolution,* (pp. 373-382). 2nd ed., Springer Verlag. ISBN: 0387260102; ISBN-13: 9780387260105.

Huang, H. K. (2004). PACS Controller and Image Archive Server. In Huang, H. K., (Ed.), *PACS – Basic Principles and Applications,* (pp. 255-276). New York: John Wiley & Sons. ISBN: 0471251232; ISBN-13: 9780471251231.

Huang, H. K. (2004). Display Workstation. *In Huang, H.K., PACS – Basic Principles and Applications,* (pp. 277-306). New York: John Wiley & Sons. ISBN: 0471251232; ISBN-13: 9780471251231.

Huang, H. K. (2004). Integration of HIS, RIS, PACS, and ePR. *In Huang, H.K., PACS – Basic Principles and Applications,* (pp. 307-330). New York: John Wiley & Sons. ISBN: 0471251232; ISBN-13: 9780471251231.

Huang, H. K. (2004). PACS Data Management and Web-Based Image Distribution. *In Huang, H.K., PACS – Basic Principles and Applications*, (pp. 333-352). New York: John Wiley & Sons. ISBN: 0471251232; ISBN-13: 9780471251231.

Lemke, H. U., Niederlag, W., Heuser, H., & Pollack, T. (*2001). PACS Planning and Evaluation using Quality Function Deployment*. Retrieved 16 January 2008 from http://www.uniklinikum-giessen.de/kis-ris-pacs/archiv/2001/di1015.pdf

Levine, L. A. (2005). PACS strategic plan and needs assessment. In Dreyer K. J., Mehta A., Thrall J. H. (Eds.), *PACS: A Guide to the Digital Revolution,* (pp. 27-44). 2nd ed., Springer Verlag. ISBN: 0387260102; ISBN-13: 9780387260105

Lou, S. L. (1997). An automated PACS image acquisition and recovery scheme for image integrity based on the DICOM standard. *Computerized Medical Imaging and Graphics, 21*(4), 209-218.

Marcus, E., & Stern H. (2003). Blueprints for High Availability. Wiley. 2nd edition. ISBN-13: 978-0471430261.

Nagy, P. G., & Schultz T. F. (2005). Storage and enterprise archiving In Dreyer K J., Mehta A., Thrall J. H. (Eds.), *PACS: A Guide to the Digital Revolution,* (pp. 319-346). 2nd Edition, Springer Verlag. ISBN: 0387260102; ISBN-13: 9780387260105.

National Electrical Manufacturers Association (2008). *Digital Imaging and Communications in Medicine (DICOM) Part 14: Grayscale Standard Display Function.* DICOM PS 3.14-2008.

Nesbitt, K. M., Schultz, T. F., & Dasilva, R. (2005). PACS architecture. In Dreyer K. J., Mehta A., Thrall J. H. (Eds.), *PACS: A Guide to the Digital Revolution,* (pp.249-268). 2nd edition, Springer Verlag. ISBN: 0387260102; ISBN-13: 9780387260105.

Smith, G. (2005). Introduction to RIS and PACS. In Dreyer K. J., Mehta A., Thrall J. H. (Eds.), *PACS: A Guide to the Digital Revolution,* (pp. 9-26). 2nd ed., Springer Verlag. ISBN: 0387260102; ISBN-13: 9780387260105.

Thomas, J. (2007). *Business Continuity Planning - PACS Version 3.0.* Retrieved 15 October 2007 from http://www.dilysjones.co.uk/IG4U/Business%20Continuity%20Planning.pdf

Chapter IV
Implementation of Information Security Management System (ISMS)

INTRODUCTION

Fundamental to ISO 27000 (ISO/IEC 27001:2005, 2005) is the concept of an information security management system (ISMS). The information security management system (ISMS) is the part of the overall management system, which is based on a business risk approach, to establish, implement, operate, monitor, maintain, and improve information security. The management system includes organization, structure and policies, planning activities, responsibilities, practices, procedures, processes, and resources. For the management of information security, its scope, administration and resources will depend on the size of the healthcare organization and information resources in question. The ISMS should be effective if it is to be useful to the organization. Information security should be an integral part of the healthcare organization's operating and business culture. Information security is primarily a management issue, rather than a technical issue, although one should not ignore the technical problems especially given the widespread dependence on the use of IT. Information security management is not a one-off exercise, but should be seen as an ongoing activity of continual improvement. Well-managed information security is a business enabler. No organization can operate success-fully in today's world without information security. A well chosen management system of controls for information security, properly implemented and used, will make a positive contribution to the success of the healthcare organization, not just a cost against the bottom line.

IMPLEMENTATION OF ISO 27000 IN PACS

Implementation of ISO 27000 (Calder, 2006) (ISO/IEC 27001:2005, 2005) using the Plan-Do-Check-Act (PDCA) model, provides an approach to developing, im-plementing and improving the effectiveness of an healthcare organization's ISMS. Details are discussed in the following sections.

Plan Phase

a.   **Study the benefits and merits of the standard** to the healthcare organization, hospital, medical centre, or clinic. It should include the quality and quality management improvements, legal, and regulatory compliance, and customer satisfactory.
b.   **A decision should be made by hospital management** to implement the standard
c.   **Allocation of resources** in terms of money, people and time
d.   **Define the scope of the ISMS** in terms of the characteristics of the healthcare business, the organization, its location, assets and technology. The scope of the ISMS may be a limited part of the healthcare organization and independ-ently defined, or the scope may be defined to be the whole organization. The ISMS scope needs to be well defined and complete. The scope needs to take into account of the interfaces with other systems, organizations, third party suppliers, and it also needs to take into account of any dependencies, e.g. security requirements that need to be satisfied by the ISMS.
e.   **Define a ISMS policy** in terms of the characteristics of the healthcare business, the organization, its location, assets, technology and take into account of any legal and regulatory requirements, and contractual or third party obligations or dependencies. The ISMS policy has to be approved by management. This policy shall include a framework for setting objectives, giving management direction and action, establishing the risk management context and criteria against which risk will be evaluated.
f.   **Define a systematic approach to risk assessment** this should be an approach that is best suited to the ISMS. The healthcare organization needs to include

criteria for accepting risks and the identification of acceptable levels of risk. The method of risk assessment that an organization adopts is entirely the decision of the management of the organization. It is important to note that whatever method is used it needs to deal with management systems covering all the control areas of the ISO 27000; this method needs to cover the risks related to organizational aspects, personnel controls, business processes, operational and maintenance processes and procedures, legal, regulatory and contractual matters, and information processing facilities.

Risk assessment is a mandatory requirement. The complexity of the risk assessment method and approach will depend on the complexity of the ISMS under review. The techniques employed should be consistent with the complexity and the levels of assurance required by the organization.

g.   **Identify the risks** to the assets taking into account the threats and vulnerabilities associated with these assets and the impacts that the losses of confidentiality, integrity and availability may have on the assets. Again the risks need to relate to all the control areas as indicated in f) above.

h.   **Assess the risks** based on the information processed in g) above, taking care to include all the control areas. This will involve the healthcare organization assessing the harm to its operation as result from a security failure and the likelihood of such a failure happening. The organization needs also to estimate the level of risk and to determine whether the risks are acceptable or required treatment within its own operation context.

i.   **Identify and evaluate options for the treatment of risks.** Once the healthcare organization has identified, assessed and understood the impact that risks might have on its operation it can take various actions to manage and treat these risks appropriately within its operational context. The actions the organization could consider include applying appropriate controls to reduce the risks, avoiding the risks through non-engagement of a risk related activity, transferring the risk (wholly or parity) to another party such as an insurer, or knowingly and objectively accepting the risk.

j.   **Select control objectives and controls for the treatment of risks.** If the healthcare organization decides to apply controls to manage and treat risks, then it first needs to select a system of controls that is suitable for this purpose. The controls an organization can select from are contained in Annex A of ISO 27001. The organization may also need to select additional controls not included in Annex A. As discussed, the selected controls should be cost effective, i.e. the cost of their implementation should not exceed the financial impact of the risks they are intended to reduce. Of course, some impacts will be non-financial. Account should also be taken of those impacts related to safety, personal information, legal and regulatory obligations, image and reputation.

k. **Prepare a Statement of Applicability** The SoA (Statement of Applicability) is a mandatory requirement for those healthcare organizations that are seeking certification to ISO 27001. The SoA is a document, which presents the control objectives, and controls that have been selected, and this selection shall be linked to the results of the risk assessment and risk treatment processes. This linkage should indicate the justification and rationale for the selection of control objectives and controls. A listing of the control objectives and controls **does not alone** constitute a valid SoA.

l. **Relevant procedures** based on the policy definitions and guidelines are created and documented.

m. **A training programme** is undertaken to educate all hospital staff to ensure that good practice for Information Security is adopted throughout the hospital.

n. **A programme of compliance monitoring** is implemented. This is to ensure that the good work achieved to date is maintained.

Once compliance has been achieved, certification may be optionally sought from an accredited body. This requires an audit, which will examine the organization's adherence to the standard. A successful audit result will mean that the healthcare organization will gain certification.

Do Phase

The **Do phase** is designed to ensure that the healthcare organization has an appropriate set of processes in place to implement and use the ISMS they have established in the Plan phase. This includes producing a risk treatment plan for managing the information security risks the organization has identified and assessed. This plan should outline what management actions need to be invoked, the responsibilities of those involved in the process of managing the information security risks and those involved in any security relevant to user/manager activity related to the ISMS.

The healthcare organization should have a set of processes in place for the implementation of the risk treatment plan and the system of selected controls, taking into account the funding for the ISMS, allocation of roles and responsibilities, the roll out of an appropriate awareness and training programme, management of resources and operations, and deployment and use of procedures for managing information security incidents.

Effectiveness is the by-word when implementing the selected controls. Controls should be effective in their management of the security risk(s) for which they have been selected. Their cost effectiveness should also be considered — there may be many degrees of implementation for a given control. The degree (for instance, how much training, recording or reporting) of implementation should be finely judged to avoid wasted resource. Over implementation can lead to frustration among staff affected by the control, often resulting in a reduction in the effectiveness of overall control. Security and control will always impinge on the lives and working practices of people but it should never become a burden.

It is also important to remember that security is not there to prevent staff from doing what they are employed to do rather; it should enable them to do it with managed and effective control. It should enable them to demonstrate their fulfilled accountabilities; establish their trustworthiness without leaving a trail of doubts. Staff will soon see well-implemented security as a benefit, rather than as an inconvenience.

Check Phase

Check phase is designed to ensure that the healthcare organization has an appropriate set of processes in place to monitor and review the ISMS they have implemented in the **Do phase.** For the ISMS to be effective in managing the information security risks it is important to monitor and keep track of any changes that might affect the ISMS. These changes might be the threats, vulnerabilities or impacts in turn due to changes in:

- The hospital environment or context: new business partners, new or different supply chains, new, different or modified customer base, expansion into different markets, market conditions, third party arrangements, outsourcing arrangements, home working;
- Hospital policy or objectives;
- The organizational structure, workforce, operational environment;
- The use and deployment of technology: new systems and applications, upgrades, expanding networks, greater diversity of system platforms, greater use of remote working, greater third party access, more outsourcing arrangements;
- The legal and regulatory environment.

These examples of changes can all have an effect on the risks and impact on a hospital operation. A re-assessment of the risks, level of residual risk and level of acceptable risk is necessary to ensure the ISMS remain effective.

During the **Check Phase** the healthcare organization needs to undertake reviews and re-assessments of its ISMS:

1. is the scope still valid,
2. the system of controls still valid and effective,

3.   are the procedures still valid and being used correctly in the current operational context,
4.   are the allocated roles and responsibilities still valid and
5.   are the assigned security activities being performed as expected,
6.   is the security incident handling processes still appropriate,
7.   have the results of the security incident handling processes been dealt with correctly and
8.   is the business continuity plan still appropriate.

During the **Check Phase** the results of management reviews, security audits, system tests, security incident reports, feedback and suggestions from information system owners, managers and users should all be taken in account to ensure that the ISMS is still appropriate for the hospital and is still managing the information security risks to the level of acceptable risk.

Act Phase

The **Act phase** is designed to ensure that the healthcare organization has an appropriate set of processes in place to maintain and improve the ISMS following the processes implemented on the **Check phase.** The monitoring and review processes in the **Check phase** may have identified changes that require improvements to the ISMS to ensure that the information security risks are being properly managed.

Risk is constantly changing, being influenced by internal and external conditions. It is therefore necessary to manage it proactively with reviews being made in response to changes identified in the **Check** phase. Incidents demonstrate risks realized and may require escalation procedures to ensure they are responded to promptly and effectively. Risk should be monitored with regular reviews of threats, the system of controls in place and their effectiveness, and audits.

In ISO 27001 there is a requirement that the healthcare organization shall have a set of processes in place to be able to continually improve the effectiveness of the ISMS. This will involve the use of information security policy, security objectives, results from audits and reviews, analysis of monitoring activities, and corrective and preventive actions.

The **Act phase** will need to have process in place to implement any identified ISMS improvements and to take corrective and preventive actions with the ISO 27001 standard. The healthcare organization shall identify non-conformities of the implementation and operation of the ISMS, determine the causes of these non-conformities, evaluate the need for actions to eliminate the causes of the non-conformities, and take corrective actions to prevent their recurrence. In addition, the organization shall identify any potential non-conformities and their causes, and determine preventive actions needed. An important aspect is making sure that all actions, corrective and preventive are recorded and that appropriate communication channels are in place to convey the results of the ISMS improvements to the right people in the organization and that implementation of actions actually takes place as a result of this communication. The organization shall ensure that the implemented improvements meet the desired requirements and achieve their intended objectives. This includes reviewing the corrective and preventive actions that have taken place.

SYSTEM OF DOCUMENTATION

Requirements

It is important that the ISMS is a documented management system complying with the requirements of ISO 27001. The ISMS documentation shall include:

- Statements of security policy in accordance with the mandatory requirement in ISO 27001;
- The ISMS scope in accordance with the mandatory requirement in ISO 27001;
- Procedures and controls to support the ISMS;
- A risk assessment report in accordance with the mandatory requirements given in ISO 27001;
- A risk treatment plan in accordance with the mandatory requirement in ISO 27001;
- Procedures needed to ensure the effective planning, operational and control of the information security processes in accordance with the mandatory requirement in ISO 27001;
- Records providing evidence of conformity to requirements and effective operation of the ISMS;
- Statement of Applicability in accordance with the mandatory certification requirement in ISO 27001.

Control of Documentation and Records

ISO 27001 defines a set of mandatory requirements for the control of documents and records to ensure that the ISMS documents are adequately protected and controlled. These requirements shall be satisfied by an appropriate set of procedures and processes to ensure the documents and records are protected and controlled. This is an important part of the risk management process alongside the other controls for information security.

Records play an especially important part in the world of information security management. When an information security incident occurs it is important that the incident is dealt with to degree of timeliness and priority commensurate with its severity. In most cases evidence is required to be able to deal with the incident in the most appropriate manner: where and when did it happen, what were the circumstances, who/what did it, what was the outcome and so on. Good, accurate record keeping can provide this evidence. Of course, there are legal requirements for the collection and presentation of evidence in the case of a criminal incident. Therefore it is not only important to keep records, but also that these records are protected and their integrity, availability and confidentiality are ensured.

In ISO 27001, the control requirements for documentation and records have been harmonized with the requirements specified in other management system standards, e.g. ISO 9001. This offers several benefits to a healthcare organization, including the opportunity to have combined/integrated audits, economize on the resources needed to manage and maintain the system of documentation and records; it can provide better control of the business assets and smoother, more integrated management.

Management Responsibility

It is important that the management shall provide evidence of its commitment processes and activities that are involved in the establishment, implementation, operation, monitoring and review, maintenance and improvement of the ISMS in accordance with the ISO 27001 standard. From establishing information security policy, setting objectives, allocating roles and responsibilities, communication of the importance of information security management to the business, provision of resources for the ISMS, deciding upon the acceptable level of risk through to conducting management reviews there needs to positive, visible, real support and commitment from management.

The healthcare organization shall ensure that it provides adequate resources to implement the requirements and processes identified in the ISO 27001 standard, this includes all requirements defined in clauses 4 through 7 inclusive. It also shall ensure that these resources are managed appropriately according to clause 5.2 of the standard. Users, staff, managers, and where necessary contractors, should be given training commensurate with their job role and function and their specific information security responsibilities. The organization shall ensure that they provide appropriate awareness to all users, staff, managers to ensure that the ISMS is effective and that information security is marketed as an important day to day aspect of business.

The healthcare organization should as part of its general training and awareness programme include information security management, and it needs to ensure it has allocated the right roles and responsibilities to those that have been trained, and that those are competent in dealing with information security management issues. This can range from a simple level of understanding and competency that all staff should have, e.g. handling passwords, basics of physical security, proper use of email, virus protection and so on, through to more involved levels which not all staff would be expected to be competent in, e.g. configuring a firewall, managing the information security incident handling process.

Management Review of the ISMS

It is important that the management shall review the healthcare organization's ISMS according to an established plan and review programme in accordance with clause 6 of the ISO 27001 standard. Review of the ISMS enables the organization to judge and assess whether improvements and changes are needed to the ISMS. The **Check Phase** stresses the importance of monitoring and reviewing changes to the business and operational environment of the ISMS to identify and evaluate whether the ISMS is still valid and provides effective information security. After reviewing the situation it may mean that some policies and procedures need to be added/changed/improved, some technical controls need to be added/changed/improved and so on. Without reviewing and auditing the ISMS on a regular basis the ISMS can become out of date, ineffective and inefficient in managing the risks the organization faces, and so eventually the organization is investing in an ISMS that is no longer useful or relevant.

There are various types of audit and review that an organization may need to consider: a first party audit and review (e.g. an internal ISMS audit), a second party audit and review (e.g. as might be a requirement of a customer requirement or contractual arrangement) or a third party audit and review (e.g. a ISO 27000 certification carried out by an independent third party certification body).

ISO 27001 defines specific requirements for the input and output of management reviews. It is important that organizations make sure that sufficient and accurate information is input into the review proves to enable the right decisions can be made and appropriate actions can be taken. If organizations are to go to the effort of having management reviews then it is important that sufficient information is available to make these right decisions to avoid wasting time and resource.

It is important that the healthcare organization carries out an internal ISMS audit in accordance with the mandatory requirement given in the ISO 27001 standard. On the other hand, whether or not the organization goes for third party certification is a management decision but is not mandatory. However all the requirements specified in clauses 1 to 7 of the ISO 27001 standard are mandatory for certification.

RISK ASSESSMENT

Security risk analysis (ISO/IEC TR 13335-3, 1998), otherwise known as risk assessment, is fundamental to the security of any organization. It is essential in ensuring that controls and expenditure are fully commensurate with the risks to which the organization is exposed. However, many conventional methods for performing security risk analysis are becoming more and more untenable in terms of usability, flexibility, and critically... in terms of what they produce for the user. This section is intended to explore the basic elements of risk, and to introduce a security risk assessment methodology and tool which is now used by many of the world's major corporations. It also embraces the use of the same product to help ensure compliance with security policies, external standards (such as ISO 27000) and with legislation (such as Data Protection legislation).

Introduction to Risk Analysis

Security in any system should be commensurate with its risks. However, the process to determine which security controls are appropriate and cost effective, is quite often a complex and sometimes a subjective matter. One of the prime functions of security risk analysis is to put this process onto a more objective basis. There are a number of distinct approaches to risk analysis. However, these essentially break down into two types: quantitative and qualitative.

Quantitative Risk Analysis

This approach employs two fundamental elements; the probability of an event occurring and the likely loss should it occur. Quantitative risk analysis makes use of a single figure produced from these elements. The problems with this type of risk analysis are usually associated with the unreliability and inaccuracy of the data. Probability can rarely be precise and can, in some cases, promote complacency. In addition, controls and countermeasures often tackle a number of potential events and the events themselves are frequently interrelated. Not with standing the drawbacks, a number of organizations have successfully adopted quantitative risk analysis.

Qualitative Risk Analysis

This is by far the most widely used approach to risk analysis. Probability data is not required and only estimated potential loss is used. Most qualitative risk analysis methodologies make use of a number of interrelated elements:

- **Threats:** These are things that can go wrong or that can 'attack' the system. Examples might include fire or fraud. Threats are ever present for every system.
- **Vulnerabilities:** These make a system more prone to attack by a threat or make an attack more likely to have some success or impact. For example, for fire a vulnerability would be the presence of inflammable materials (e.g. paper).
- **Controls:** These are the countermeasures for vulnerabilities. There are four types: Deterrent controls reduce the likelihood of a deliberate attack Preventative controls protect vulnerabilities and make an attack unsuccessful or reduce its impact Corrective controls reduce the effect of an attack Detective controls discover attacks and trigger preventative or corrective controls. These elements can be illustrated by a simple relational model:

Procedures

Identification of Processes

From the Scope of the ISMS, the business processes are identified. These are the core processes that directly deliver product/services to clients and the supporting processes that enable them.

Identification of Assets

Each process owner conducts a survey of the processes for which they have responsibility and identifies the information assets and other assets relevant to information security management. The assets are grouped under the headings listed below. The only purposes of these headings are to stimulate thought and provide a convenient method of cataloguing.

Information Assets

e.g. databases, data files, system documentation, user manuals, training material, operational and support procedures, intellectual property, business continuity plans, fall back arrangements.

Paper Documents

e.g. contracts, guidelines, company documentation, business results, HR records, purchase documents, invoices.

Software Assets

e.g. application, system, development tools, utilities.

Physical Assets

e.g. computers, servers, routers, hubs, firewalls, communication equipment, magnetic media, other equipment, cabinets, safes, rooms.

People

e.g. personnel, customers, subscribers, contractors, cleaners, security.

Services

e.g. computing, telecommunications, heating, lighting, gas, water, air conditioning, intruder alarms, fire control, generators, UPS.

Company Image and Reputation

e.g. adverse publicity, failure to deliver.

An Asset Template is available to facilitate the above.

Valuation of Assets (and Potential Impacts)

In order to identify the appropriate protection for assets, it is necessary to assess their values in terms of their importance to the business or their potential values given certain opportunities. These values are usually expressed in terms of the potential business impacts of unwanted incidents such as loss of **Confidentiality, Integrity, Availability and Legality**.

- **Confidentiality:** Ensuring that information is accessible only to those authorized to have access.
- **Integrity:** Safeguarding the accuracy and completeness of information and processing methods.

- **Availability:** Ensuring that authorized users have access to information and associated assets when required.
- **Legality:** Ensuring that the asset within the scope is legal.

The process owner defines the value of each asset identified, in terms of his or her perception of the impact on the process, or on the hospital generally, or to the client in the event of loss, theft, unavailability, corruption or other security breach. The perceived value is rated as:

- High (3)
- Medium (2)
- Low (1)

Impact Rating		
L(1)	M(2)	H(3)

Impact corresponding to Confidentiality			Impact corresponding to Integrity			Impact corresponding to Availability			Impact corresponding to Legality		
L(1)	M(2)	H(3)	L(1)	M(2)	H(3)	L(1)	M(2)	H(3)	L(1)	M(2)	H(3)

Asset Value of Confidentiality Impact Rating = 1, 2, 3
Asset Value of Integrity Impact Rating = 1, 2, 3
Asset Value of Availability Impact Rating = 1, 2, 3
Asset Value of Legality Impact Rating = 1, 2, 3

The assets identified from each survey are summarized onto a single document.

Risk Measures Matrix

RISK = Impact Rating x THREAT x VULNERABILITY/Number of machines

Where:
Impact Rating is the **loss consequence**. For each individual asset, identify undesirable events and the effect that the loss, damage, or destruction of that asset would have on the organization.

Impact Rating (0= not much loss, 1 = loss less than HKD1,000 or minimum down time, 2 = loss more than HKD1,000 or larger than 1 hour downtime, or loss in organization reputation)		
L(1)	M(2)	H(3)

Threat is the capability and intention of an adversary to undertake actions that are detrimental to an organization's interests. Threat is a function of the adversary only; the owner or user of the asset cannot typically control it. However, the adversary's intention to exploit his capability may be encouraged by vulnerability in an asset or discouraged by an owner's countermeasures.

In order to assess whether an adversary poses a threat the analyst or security specialist must determine if they have the intent and capability to cause an unwanted event and their **history** of attacks against the types of assets.

Threat value (History of occurrence, 0 = never happen in any site, 1 = happened before in other site(s) but never happen in the same city, 2 = happened before in the same city, 3 = happened once before in the site, 4 = happened frequently in the site)				
L(0)	M(1)	M(2)	M(3)	H(4)

Vulnerability is any weakness in an asset or countermeasure that can be exploited by an adversary or competitor to cause damage to an organization's interests. The level of vulnerability, and hence level of risk, can be reduced by implementing appropriate security countermeasures. Therefore whether **appropriate security countermeasures exist** will count for the value of vulnerability here.

Vulnerability value (a measure of vulnerability and the effectiveness of existing countermeasure, 1 = asset with strong control, 2 = asset with control, 3 = non secure asset without control or with ineffective control)	
L(1)	H(3)M(2)

In the previous formula the "threat × vulnerability" segment represents the probability of the unwanted event occurring, and the "loss effect" represents the consequence of the loss of the asset to the organization.

Probability Rating = THREAT × VULNERABILITY

Probability Rating								
L(0)	L(1)	L(2)	M(3)	M(4)	M(6)	H(8)	H(9)	H(12)

Corresponding Risk Index	Impact Rating corresponding to Confidentiality			Impact Rating corresponding to Integrity			Impact Rating corresponding to Availability			Impact Rating corresponding to Legal		
Probability Rating	L(1)	M(2)	H(3)	L(1)	M(2)	H(3)	L(1)	M(2)	H(3)	L(1)	M(2)	H(3)
0	0	0	0	0	0	0	0	0	0	0	0	0
1	1	2	3	1	2	3	1	2	3	1	2	3
2	2	4	6	2	4	6	2	4	6	2	4	6
3	3	6	9	3	6	9	3	6	9	3	6	9
4	4	8	12	4	8	12	4	8	12	4	8	12
6	6	12	18	6	12	18	6	12	18	6	12	18
8	8	16	24	8	16	24	8	16	24	8	16	24
9	9	18	27	9	18	27	9	18	27	9	18	27
12	12	24	36	12	24	36	12	24	36	12	24	36

Acceptable Risk Index

The acceptable risk index is defined as the risk at worst situation with the strongest control.

Acceptable Risk Index = MAX(Impact Rating)× MIN(VULNERABILITY) x MAX(THREAT)

$$= 3 \times 1 \times 4$$
$$= 12$$

Effectiveness of Control

All security controls can be classified into preventive and corrective types. The incidence rate of preventive controls can show the effectiveness of the control. A preventive control with high incidence rate (5 times in a year) indicates ineffective

Figure 1. Methodology of enhancing effectiveness of controls

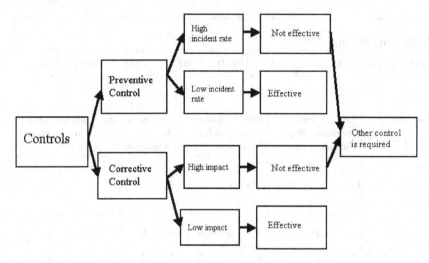

of the control. Other control is required. A low incidence rate shows effective of the control applied.

For corrective control, the impact of the incidence is the indicator of the effectiveness of the control. A high impact (more than HK$1,000) shows an ineffective of the applied control while a low impact (less or equal to HK$1,000) indicates an effective control. Any identified ineffective control requires a replaced of other stronger control.

Continuous Assessment

This model is a continuous process. The PACS team will constantly monitor any changes in their assets, the threat, and their vulnerabilities, as well as the larger infrastructure of which the organization is an element. As changes appear, then we will return to the model, enter the changes, possibly arrive at a new risk assessment, and recommend new countermeasure options. The continuous nature of risk assessment allows us to develop a risk-aware culture that understands, validates, and implements the decisions of the risk acceptance authority and the resulting countermeasures.

Identification of Control Objectives, Controls and Countermeasures

For each threat listed, relevant control objectives* and controls* from ISO/IEC27001:2005 are identified.

*A catalogue of vulnerabilities, threats and controls is available.

As the control objectives and controls are duplicated across the listed assets, a summary document 'Controls Identified from Risk Assessment' is produced to provide the ISO/IEC27001 elements for the Statement of Applicability.

Report to Security Forum

A summary report is provided for the Security Forum.

This report summarises the occasions that process owners have identified particular assets under the defined 'value' categories. From this, the Management Forum can identify clearly assets that are considered to have most value to the hospital and its clients and hence require most attention and degree of assurance from control objectives, controls and countermeasures. The remaining assets can be considered as having lower value and the degree of assurance required is reflected in the policies and procedures adopted to manage the associated risks. Risk index value greater than 12 for any asset is not acceptable and will be reported to the security forum for further action.

Monitoring and Review

The responsibility for the upkeep of the asset identification and perceived valuation remains with the process owners who review the situation regularly and especially when any significant changes are made to the business processes.

Changes in hospital organizational structure may result in changes to process ownership. Handover of responsibilities includes acceptance of the risk assessment procedure for any inherited processes.

This chain of sub-procedures provides the auditable path demonstrating the justification for the control objectives, controls and countermeasures selected for the management framework.

REFERENCES

Calder, A. (2006). *Information Security Based on ISO 27001/ISO 17799: A Management Guide*. Van Haren Publishing. First Edition ISBN-10: 9077212701.

ISO/IEC TR 13335-3 (1998). *Information technology — Guidelines for the management of IT Security — Part 3: Techniques for the management of IT Security*. American National Standards Institute. First edition.

ISO/IEC 17799 (2005). *Information technology - Security techniques - Code of practice for information security management.* ISO/IEC/JTC 1/SC 27 Distributed through American National Standards Institute (ANSI) (23 Aug 2007). ASIN: B000Y2TUKU.

ISO/IEC 27001 (2005). *Information Technology - Security Techniques - Information security management systems - Requirements (Information Technology).* British Standards Institution ISBN-10: 0580467813; ISBN-13: 978-0580467813.

ISO 27799 (2006). *Health informatics – Security management in health using ISO/IEC 17799* (draft). International Organization for Standardization.

Tong, C. K. S., Chan, K. K., & Huang H. Y. H. (2004). *The Application of ISO 17799 and BS 7799 Information Security Management in Picture Archiving and Communication System.* RSNA 2004

Tong, C. K. S., & Wong, E. T. T. (2005). *The Application of ISO 17799/BS 7799 Information Security Management in Picture Archiving and Communication System for Healthcare Industry.* Encyclopedia of Multimedia Technology and Networking. Idea Group Publishing (June 1, 2005). ISBN-10: 1591405610; ISBN-13: 978-1591405610.

Section II
Implementation of Filmless Hospital

Chapter V
Planning for a Filmless Hospital

INTRODUCTION

Filmless hospital is transforming at an unprecedented rate. Physicians, nurses, clinicians, pharmacists, radiologists, emergency departments, local doctor's offices, operating rooms, intensive care units, and insurance offices all must have instantaneous access to information from CT, MR, and X-ray images to treat their patients. Considering that these individuals could be on different floors of a hospital, across a campus, or scattered over several states, connecting them in real-time and in a cost-effective manner to the information they need is a monumental IT challenge. Detail planning is important in a filmless hospital project.

PLANNINGS

In most of filmless hospital projects, the following plans can be identified. They are capacity plan, cost control, backup plan, emergency response plan, and workflow plan.

Capacity Planning

Like other information technology (IT) service, speed, around-the-clock availability, and security are the most common indicators of quality of service of a PACS. Since the design of a PACS varies from a clinic to a hospital, many possible alternative architecture can implement a PACS service. In order to minimize the risk of systems failures, advance planning and preparation are required to ensure the availability of adequate capacity (Dugmore, Lacy, 2006) and resources to deliver the required system performance. Projections of future capacity requirements should be made, to reduce the risk of system overload. The operational requirements of new systems should be established, documented, and tested prior to their acceptance and use.

Item	Modalities	Size of an image (Mbyte)	Number of studies per year (a)	Number of images per study (b)	Size of storage required (Tbyte) (axb)
1.	CT	0.5			
2.	MRI	0.25			
3.	CR	8			
4.	DR	10			
5.	Mammo	15			
6.	US	0.25			
7.	SXR	1			
8.	DSA	1			
9.	OT	unknown			
Total volume of storage required per year					

Capacity Planning is the determination of the overall size, performance and resilience of a computer or system. It shall be monitored, tuned, and estimated for future capacity requirements to ensure the required system performance. The detailed components of a Capacity Planning initiative will vary, depending upon the proposed usage of the system, but the following should always be considered:-

1. Identification of the total volume of various image data
    The total volume of input data should include:

2.   Identification of the computing power of image archive servers (IAS)

Servers	Loading measured at peak hours
TKOAS01	<80%
TKOAS02	<80%
TKONWG01	<80%

3.   Identification of the database server loading (DS)

Servers	Loading measured at peak hours
TKODB01	<80%

4.   Identification of the image storage (IS)

Source	Image Capacity
SAN	<90%
Tape	Half a year capacity
MOD	Half a year capacity

5.   Identification of the Web servers loading (WSL)

Source	Web servers loading
Web servers CPU	<90%
Storage Capacity	<90%
Memory	<80%

6.   Identification of the network bandwidth loading (NBL)

Source	Network Bandwidth Loading
Switches	<90%

7.   Identification of the image loading requirement (IL)

Source	Image Loading requirement at peak hours
Web servers	First image should be arrived and displayed within 3 seconds
Image viewing stations	First image should be arrived and displayed within 3 seconds

8.   Identification of the image prefetching requirement (IP)

Source	Image Prefetching requirement at peak hours
Web servers	All image should arrive within 30 minutes
Image viewing stations	All image should arrive within 20 minutes

9.   Identification of the broker loading (BL)

Source	Broker Loading
Switches	<90%

10. Evaluation of PACS requirement (EPACS)

Source	Estimation of the configuration of PACS component by vendor
PACS requirement	Vol, IL, IP, IS
Configuration of PACS component	ISA, DS, IS, WSL, NBL, BL

11. Regular review of PACS performance
     PACS vendor should submit half year performance report of the system.

12. Regular capacity planning
     Yearly capacity planning should be performed based on the previous performance report of the system. The capacity plan will be submitted to management for discussion.

Cost Control

Cost control is an important task (Lemke, Niederlag , Heuser, & Pollack, 2001) (Levine, 2005) for hospital administrators, PACS managers, and radiologists during their management of a PACS project (Nagy, Schultz, 2005). There are many operational costs that should be considered when trying to utilize a cost savings analysis. The followings are the most common and easiest to quantify:

Hard Costs

•   Breakdown costs of a PACS:

PACS System

costs may vary by:
No. of procedures per year
No. of modalities connectivity
No. of concurrent users
Special Features (3D, Flythrough, template)

Primary System

Hardware / Software (base license for large Hospital)

Hardware / Software (base license for medium Hospital)

Online capacity (TB)

Disk base nearline capacity (TB)

Tape library

Additional license

Resilience System

Hardware / Software (base license for large Hospital)

Hardware / Software (base license for medium Hospital)

Online capacity (TB)

Disk base nearline capacity (TB)

Backup / offsite capacity (TB)

PACS Broker (HL7/DICOM for RIS integration)

PACS Network

PACS Workstations

Dual Colour LCD (2M)

Dual Mono LCD (3M)

Dual Mono LCD (5M)

Web review workstations

Single Colour LCD (1M)

Dual Colour LCD (1M)

Web Server for Radiology PACS only

Hardware / Software (or license only)

Additional license

Service for migration, installation ..

Others (such as server room, HA network)

- **Operational or variable costs:**
  - ° Salaries associated with file room.
  - ° Film for copies and image storage.
  - ° Collateral materials needed to support hard copy image storage.
  - ° Processor maintenance and chemicals.
  - ° Water and sewage along with the decrease in environmental hazard liability.
  - ° Time inefficiencies, retrieving films, searching for lost films, hanging films and copying films.
  - ° Purging and storing films.
- **Space:**
  - ° Dark room space.
  - ° File room space.
  - ° Storage for film supplies in both radiology and materials management.

Soft Costs

Costs are realized by determining the benefits outside of radiology. Once determined some of the benefits could be measured prior to installation. To date only assumptions can be made on most benefits as there are not enough PACS installed that fully integrated to hospital operations to quantify.

- **Increased efficiencies for Physicians:**
  - ° Highly efficient consults can take place without either party leaving their location. This translates into less time wasted for physicians to either meet physically or have the patient schedule visits for consults while transporting images.
  - ° Physicians can possibly see more patients as they could easily review patient records from the office.
  - ° An integrated PACS could also create patient schedules customized according to the radiologist schedule, as all radiologists do not perform exactly alike.

Decreased Operational Costs

- Full PACS integration allows true centralized schedules with physicians and sometimes even patients scheduling their own exams.
- Conflict scheduling is immediately available because the PACS/RIS interface allows resource management as well as physician management.

- Results reporting goes hand in hand with image transfer creating less delay in patient treatment therefore potential savings on hospital stays. This translates into a higher competitive edge for contracts with HMOs etc.
- Faster treatment allows for a healthier patient population which will essentially help curb the rising medical costs.
- With full integration patients physically access the medical system at a reduced rate since a higher degree of information is available remotely. Patients don't have to drive, park and seek directions to find departments for medical information.
- With decreased physical contact less ancillary staffing is needed as patient population grows allowing for growth in revenue generating positions.

Revenue Enhancement

Cost occurs as services outside the normal geographic boundaries are provided. Hospitals can partner with the radiologists and staff physicians, to the benefit of both, while extending patient care to remote areas.

- **Add revenue through remote patient care:**
  - ° Provide imaging services to remote areas without radiology service.
  - ° Perform over reads for smaller hospitals and Emergency interpretation services for rural facilities.
- **Increase the hospital profile through increased physician expertise:**
  - ° PACS integration allows Hospitals to attract and market specific physician specialists and experts.
  - ° Not everyone likes to live in a metropolitan area. This is an opportunity for rural hospitals to compete with larger facilities.
- **Hospitals can strategically place services:**
  - ° Merge with other hospitals to strengthen community position and create a hospital services network.
  - ° Decrease costly duplicate services through merging.
- **Managed Care and Capitated Care need not decrease Hospital revenue:**
  - ° An integrated PACS allows hospitals to compete for contracts with a better understanding of cost of services.

Backup Plan

The purpose of backup (ISO/IEC 17799:2005, 2005) (ISO 27799, 2006) is to maintain the integrity and availability of information and information processing facilities. Back-up copies of image data, system information and software shall be taken and tested regularly in accordance with the agreed backup policy.

Information Backup Planning

Information Asset Description	Backup Period	Backup Methods	Backup Tools	No. of Copies	Backup Location	Responsible Person
DDS Tape [inside Broker Autoloader]	Daily	Auto	Veritas	1	PACS Rm	PACS Team
DDS Tape [for PACS Database Backup]	Daily	Manual	Tar	1	PACS Rm	PACS Team
M.O. Disk [for image backup]	On demand	Auto	PACS Function	1	PACS Rm	PACS Team
DLT [for image backup]	On demand	Auto	PACS Function	1	PACS Rm	PACS Team
CD-RW [for PACS activity logs backup]	Daily	Auto	PACS Function	1	PACS Loading Area	PACS Team
Floppy disk [for smart card user accounts and access log backup]	Monthly	Manual	Server Function	1	PACS Rm	PACS Team

Emergency Response Plan

The objective of emergency response plan is to ensure a consistent and effective approach applied to the management of emergency information security incidents in PACS. Responsibilities and procedures of emergency responses shall be established and managed to ensure a quick, effective, and orderly response to those information security incidents. There shall be mechanisms in place to enable the types, volumes, and costs of information security incidents to be quantified and monitored. In this section, a list of suggested strategies in the event of failure of the PACS system or related components is described including:

- A simplified list of potential failure scenarios
- A summary of resources in place to ensure service recovery in the event of failure
- An estimation (where possible) of the likely time the service may be unavailable
- A description of the potential impact on the service due to the failure
- A list of emergency responses during the outage

Potential Failure Scenarios

Below is a simplified list of potential failure scenarios. This list is broken down into major common groups as follows:

Network

- Local network failure affecting connectivity to the computer room
- Loss of connectivity from the computer room to the entire trust
- Loss of connectivity to PACS cluster data store
- Loss of connectivity to modality clusters
- Full network connectivity failure

Electricity Supply

- Loss of electricity affecting the computer room—Essential power supply triggered
- Loss of electricity affecting the computer room—Does not trigger essential power supply
- Local loss of electricity to PACS enabled area
- Total loss of electricity supply to the Trust

PACS Server Cluster

- PACS Server Cluster Component Failure (e.g. Connectivity Manager / Workflow Manager)
- Loss of entire PACS Server Cluster (full scale disaster)

RIS / Connection to RIS

- Loss of automatic transfer of demographic information to modalities
- Loss of automatic transfer of demographic information and accession numbers to PACS
- Limitation or loss of reporting facility
- Pre-fetch failure

PACS / RIS Interface

- Loss of PACS or PACS/RIS interface

Workstations

- Workstation failure
- Monitor failure

Modalities

- Modality failure
- Modality workstation failure
- Modality networking failure

Cluster Data Store

- Cluster Data Store failure

Emergency Response Plan

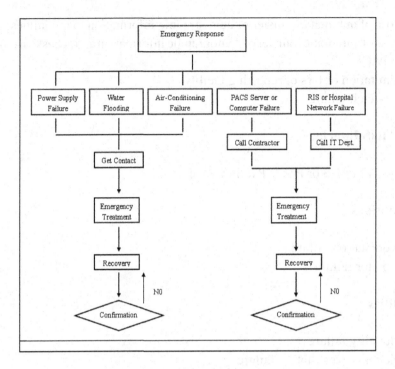

Sample Policy for Emergency Response

1.0 Objective

In the PACS system, for the failure or downtime or electrical supply, air conditioning etc., perform incident response according to predefined schedule or plan, to prevent extension of downtime.

2.0 Scope

- applicable to PACS system power supply, air conditioning, fire distinguisher etc.,
- applicable to PACS team as well as other staff in the whole hospital

3.0 Procedure

I.   Power Supply Failure, Water Flooding and Air Condition Failure

3.1 Get Contact

- **Standard**
  Clarify downtime and reason
  - ○ **Content**
    Any non-planned power / water flooding / Air Condition downtime
  - ○ **Preparation**
    Call EMSD
  - ○ **Procedure**
    Call the phone support
  - ○ **Critical Point**
    Information should be exact and concise
  - ○ **Time Limit**
    5 minutes
  - ○ **Responsible Person**
    All relevant staff in PACS
  - ○ **Consideration**
    Mis-communication would affect the incident response procedure

3.2 Emergency Treatment

- **Standard**
  To minimize the loss
  - ○ **Content**
    Take the emergency procedure
  - ○ **Preparation**
    All emergency/backup light in good condition, backup power generator and UPS in good condition
  - ○ **Procedure**
    1. Power supply
       a. Check backup power generator and UPS is working properly
       b. Inform senior management
       c. Shut down the power supply main source, make sure the UPS is working properly. If backup power generator and UPS is running out, shut down all relevant PACS system.
       d. Evacuate all PACS staff in case if necessary

2.   Water flooding
   a.   Inform senior management
   b.   If it affects the PACS operation for a long time, should shut down the PACS system first.
3.   Air conditioning
   a.   Inform senior management
   b.   If it affects the PACS operation for a long time, should shut down the PACS system first.

○   **Critical Point**
All relevant backup equipment (e.g. lighting, backup power generator, UPS) should be in good condition and test regularly

○   **Time Limit**
5 minutes

○   **Responsible Person**
All relevant staff in PACS

○   **Consideration**
Improper deployment of the incident response procedure will result in equipment failure

3.3 Recovery

• **Standard**
Power supply 220V, proper water supply

○   **Content**
Recover power supply and water supply

○   **Preparation**
Monitor the recovery of power and water supply

○   **Procedure**
1.   close power supply main source
2.   inform all relevant department/team member about the recovery, inform them to re-open the equipment

○   **Critical Point**
Should not re-open the equipment before power is back

○   **Time Limit**
1 hour

○   **Responsible Person**
All relevant staff in PACS

○   **Consideration**
Re-open equipment before power supply is back would result in equipment failure

3.4 Confirmation

- **Standard**
  Equipment is working properly
  - ° **Content**
    Normal operation
  - ° **Preparation**
    N/A
  - ° **Procedure**
    Should check all machine condition
  - ° **Critical Point**
    All machine should be operated without overloading
  - ° **Time Limit**
    20 minutes
  - ° **Responsible Person**
    All relevant staff in PACS
  - ° **Consideration**
    If overloading found during re-open of equipment, shut down and check the faulty machine

II. PACS Server / Computer / Radiology Information System (RIS) / Hospital Network Failure

3.5 Call PACS Contractor or IT Department

- **Standard**
  Clarify downtime and reason
  - ° **Content**
    Any PACS Server / Computer / RIS / Hospital network downtime
  - ° **Preparation**
    Call PACS maintenance contractor
  - ° **Procedure**
    Call the phone support
  - ° **Critical Point**
    Information should be exact and concise
  - ° **Time Limit**
    5 minutes
  - ° **Responsible Person**
    All relevant staff in PACS
  - ° **Consideration**
    Mis-communication would affect the incident response procedure

3.6 Emergency Treatment

- **Standard**
  Fast, efficient and recover in one time
  - ○ **Content**
    Check and fix
  - ○ **Preparation**
    N/A
  - ○ **Procedure**
    Check with the contractor or IT department
  - ○ **Critical Point**
    Vendor should arrive to fix the problem within 1 hour
  - ○ **Time Limit**
    4 hours
  - ○ **Responsible Person**
    All relevant staff in PACS
  - ○ **Consideration**
    Delay of recover will affect the operation of machine or overheat

3.7 Confirmation

- **Standard**
  Machine and PACS system working properly
  - ○ **Content**
    Test that the machine and PACS system working properly
  - ○ **Preparation**
    N/A
  - ○ **Procedure**
    Check whether machine and PACS system are working as expected
  - ○ **Critical Point**
    No unexpected behaviour of the machine and PACS system
  - ○ **Time Limit**
    1 hour
  - ○ **Responsible Person**
    All relevant staff in PACS
  - ○ **Consideration**
    If the machine and PACS system do not work properly for once, it will affect the integrity of the system

4.0 Related Record

- **Standard**
  The information should be correct
    - ° **Content**
      Equipment maintenance form and LOG
    - ° **Preparation**
      N/A
    - ° **Procedure**
      N/A
    - ° **Critical Point**
      N/A
    - ° **Time Limit**
      N/A
    - ° **Responsible Person**
      All relevant staff in PACS responsible for maintenance
    - ° **Consideration**
      The failure to LOG down the failure reason will affect future mainte-
      nance of PACS

Workflow Plan

The purpose of workflow plan (Reiner, Siegal, 2005) (Siegal, Reiner, Knight, 2005) is to establish a workflow blueprint that addresses the accurate and efficient access of the data. Basically it means that there should be only one data entry point for all patient information with connectivity to as many portals as needed. This allows retrieval of that same information thus enabling patient data searches, image acquisition, image interpretation and archiving. This also avoids the errors during re-enter of the same data. This should indicate to everyone the importance of full HIS/RIS integration to PACS with the **RIS** being the **prime enabler** between the HIS and the PACS. There are three major areas of integration: **HOSPITAL, RA-DIOLOGY, and ENTERPRISE WIDE**.

ORDER/ENTRY

The integration of hospital and radiology begins with **ORDER/ENTRY**. Remote order entry capability should be available for the clinicians who need to request a radiological service for both in-patients and out-patients. Remote capabilities will greatly enhance efficiencies. Since radiology is a demanding service and there is nothing better than knowing ahead of time what the demand is. The remote capabilities can be point to point dial-up services or through networked computers.

At the point of order entry many things should occur:

- Upon the physician placing the order/request, the system should prompt for a diagnosis,
  ° No diagnosis - no order.
- The diagnosis, once entered, should perform a keyword search of the appropriateness criteria database,
  ° The order cannot be placed/accepted without a direct correlation between physician order, diagnosis and appropriateness criteria.
- The system should verify the acceptance of the order immediately if it is considered a non-scheduled exam and gives an estimated time of the appointment. Should the exam need to be scheduled:
  ° The system should prompt for any special patient needs or room needs and ask about patient mobility as well as other equipment to be transported with the patient.
    ➢ Depending upon the special needs and the items checked the system will allocate the time needed for the exam.
  ° The order entry system should then search for available times,
    ➢ Before giving an appointment the system should calculate the time needed for proper patient preparation, and also check for any prerequisite testing to be done, IE blood work, BUN etc .
    ➢ The system should also check for exam appropriateness - evaluate whether another exam should be done instead, At this point the system should check if appropriate other exams have been performed and if no history exists ask for previous exam results.
- Once the order has been accepted and a slot reserved,
  ° The system alerts radiology of the pending exam (places it on the schedule),
  ° Places a flag in the patient chart for nursing,
  ° Prints a dietary restriction, if needed, to both nursing and the dietician,
    ➢ The dietary department must sign off on this.
  ° Prints a patient prep, if needed, sheet for nursing,
    ➢ Nursing must sign off on this at each shift change.

HOSPITAL RECEPTION (HIS/RIS)

Upon entering the hospital the patient proceeds to the registration desk where all pertinent insurance and patient information is gathered/verified and the proper exam(s) are ordered/verified. The information is then collectively verified with the patient. The information is then processed through to the RIS (because a Radiology Exam has been ordered) (Smith, 2005) (Huang, 2004). The RIS then filters the information and posts the patient in the queue of exams to be done and assigns the patient to the proper modality or modalities. The exams are performed according to a rules-set of exam sequence that has been preset by the facility thus allowing the exams to be done in the proper order. The information is then ready for concerned modality to download the patient data into the units acquisition screen.

RADIOLOGY RECEPTION (RIS/PACS/HIS)

The patient then proceeds to radiology for the exam and notifies the receptionist. The receptionist has the patient review the information on the scheduling monitor to verify validity and makes any changes that are necessary. Any changes are then reflected back to the HIS. The patient then waits for the technologist to perform the exam.

The technologist calls the patient, verifies that the information about the exam and patient are correct and then downloads that information to the acquisition screen of the modality and performs the exam. Upon exam completion a quality control technologist reviews the information and either request repeats or releases the exam to be read. At this point the exam is identified by the technologist performing the exam as well as the QA technologist.

The radiologist then either requests additional views or interprets the exam as is, the radiologist also at this point has access to pertinent patient information regarding previous Lab work, old exams etc. etc. Once read the system simultaneously archives the exam and releases it to the facility pending proper medical information release authority as well as notifying the physician of exam completion.

ENTERPRISE WIDE (RIS/PACS/HIS)

Once the examination is released to the hospital every physician with proper authorization may view the image and report. Depending upon the extent of the hospital the physicians could have access from within their office. The requesting physician would be able to view the report through HIS in his office.

Also at this point the exam can be billed. All the previous information gathered at the order entry point and patient registration is then applied to the bill. This assures that the bill will be paid correctly but not timely.

REFERENCES

Dugmore, J., & Lacy, S. (2006). Achieving ISO/IEC 20000 - Capacity Management. *BSI Standards* (January 13, 2006); ISBN-10: 0580446417; ISBN-13: 978-0580446412.

Huang, H. K. (2004). Industrial Standards (HL7 and DICOM) and Work Flow Protocols (IHE). In Huang, H. K. (Ed.), *PACS – Basic Principles and Applications*, (pp. 171-194). New York: John Wiley & Sons. ISBN: 0471251232; ISBN-13: 9780471251231.

Huang, H. K. (2004). Integration of HIS, RIS, PACS, and ePR. In Huang, H. K. (Ed.), *PACS – Basic Principles and Applications*, (pp. 307-330). New York: John Wiley & Sons. ISBN: 0471251232; ISBN-13: 9780471251231.

ISO/IEC 17799 (2005). *Information technology - Security techniques - Code of practice for information security management.* ISO/IEC/JTC 1/SC 27 Distributed through American National Standards Institute (ANSI) (23 Aug 2007); ASIN: B000Y2TUKU.

ISO 27799 (2006). *Health informatics – Security management in health using ISO/IEC 17799 (draft).* International Organization for Standardization.

Lemke, H. U., Niederlag, W., Heuser, H., & Pollack, T. (2001). *PACS Planning and Evaluation using Quality Function Deployment.* Retrieved 16 January 2008 from http://www.uniklinikum-giessen.de/kis-ris-pacs/archiv/2001/di1015.pdf

Levine, L. A. (2005). PACS strategic plan and needs assessment. In Dreyer, K. J., Mehta, A., Thrall, J. H. (Eds.), *PACS: A Guide to the Digital Revolution*, (pp. 27-44). 2nd ed., Springer Verlag. ISBN: 0387260102; ISBN-13: 9780387260105.

Nagy, P. G., & Schultz, T. F. (2005). Storage and enterprise archiving In Dreyer, K. J., Mehta, A., Thrall, J. H. (Eds.), *PACS: A Guide to the Digital Revolution*, (pp. 319-346). 2nd ed., Springer Verlag. ISBN: 0387260102; ISBN-13: 9780387260105.

Nesbitt, K. M., Schultz, T. F., & Dasilva, R. (2005). PACS architecture. In Dreyer, K. J., Mehta, A., Thrall, J. H. (Eds.), *PACS: A Guide to the Digital Revolution*, (pp. 249-268). 2nd ed., Springer Verlag. ISBN: 0387260102; ISBN-13: 9780387260105.

Reilly, S. R., & Avrin, D. (2005) Financial modeling. In Dreyer, K. J., Mehta, A., Thrall, J. H. (Eds.), *PACS: A Guide to the Digital Revolution,* (pp. 125-144). 2nd ed., Springer Verlag. ISBN: 0387260102; ISBN-13: 9780387260105.

Smith, G. (2005). Introduction to RIS and PACS. In Dreyer, K. J., Mehta, A., Thrall, J. H. (Eds.), *PACS: A Guide to the Digital Revolution,* (pp. 9-26). 2nd ed., Springer Verlag. ISBN: 0387260102; ISBN-13: 9780387260105.

Siegal, E. L., Reiner, B. L., & Knight, N. (2005). Reengineering workflow: The radiologist's perspective. In Dreyer, K. J., Mehta, A., Thrall, J. H. (Eds.), *PACS: A Guide to the Digital Revolution,* (pp. 97-124). 2nd ed., Springer Verlag. ISBN: 0387260102; ISBN-13: 9780387260105.

Thomas, J. (2007). *Business Continuity Planning - PACS Version 3.0.* Retrieved 15 October 2007 from http://www.dilysjones.co.uk/IG4U/Business%20Continuity%20Planning.pdf

Chapter VI
Design of a Filmless Hospital

INTRODUCTION

More rapidly than any technological advance in medical history, filmless hospital is changing the clinical and business aspects of radiology practice by delivering substantial cost savings, improved efficiency and quality, and greater access in an era of high demand and severely constrained resources. Systems are available in many variations, from mini-PACS to hospital-wide or enterprise-wide PACS. However, among the variations, the basic structure of a PACS is similar as shown in Figure 1.

DESIGN OF A FILMLESS HOSPITAL

Computer Network Within A Hospital (Local Area Network)

In most cases the local area network (LAN) for image transfer is better to be isolated from the hospital network. This is not saying that there is no inter-communication because there must be a bridge between the two. The radiology imaging network must function independently of all other networks. The image network can't af-

Figure 1. Schematic diagram of a filmless hospital

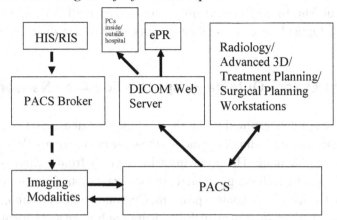

Where HIS is Hospital Information System,
 RIS is Radiology Information System,
 ePR is electronic Patient Record,
 DICOM Web Server is a Web server for distribution of medical images in Digital Imaging and
 Communication in Medicine (DICOM) format,
 ➤ is the flow of image data,
 ➤ is the flow of patient demographic data

ford to compete for space on any other information network that will not only slow down but could shut down.

Today, three types of computer network are used in a hospital for PACS. They are fast Ethernet, gigabit Ethernet, and optical fibre.

Fast Ethernet is a collective term for a number of Ethernet standards that carry traffic at the nominal rate of 100 Mbit/s, against the original Ethernet speed of 10 Mbit/s. Of the 100 megabit Ethernet standards 100baseTX is by far the most common and is supported by the vast majority of Ethernet hardware currently produced. Full duplex fast Ethernet is sometimes referred to as "200 Mbit/s" though this is somewhat misleading as that level of improvement will only be achieved if traffic patterns are symmetrical. Fast Ethernet was introduced in 1995 and remained the fastest version of Ethernet for three years before being superseded by gigabit Ethernet.

Gigabit Ethernet is a term describing various technologies for transmitting Ethernet frames at a rate of a gigabit per second, as defined by the IEEE 802.3-2005 standard. Half duplex gigabit links connected through hubs are allowed by the specification but in the marketplace full duplex with switches is the norm.

Optical fibre uses a near-infrared (NIR) light wavelength transmitted via two strands of Multi-mode optical fibre, one for receive(RX) and the other for transmit(TX). Optical fibre is specified to work over a long distance of up to 20 km.

Computer Network Outside Hospital (Wide Area Network)

The largest area of concern will be for those hospitals that are part of a system or have affiliations. In this realm of operations the wide area network (WAN) is going to be the most problematic. The problems arise not only from technology but also area availability. The technology is there, in most cases, but for those facilities in remote areas service will become a problem. Communications technology can be segregated into distinct areas of availability, Rural, Suburban and City. All technology has a price; speed costs money.

The following are a few of the more common services provided by the telecommunications companies that go beyond normal telephone line for medical image distribution.

ISDN—Integrated Services Digital Network

- Utilizes existing copper phone wires and has capabilities, at a basic rate, of 128 Kilobits/second. Most modems have a speed of 28.8 or 56 Kilobits. ISDN is becoming available on a fairly widespread basis.
  - ° It is great for Tele-commuting, video conferencing and on call applications for radiologists.
  - ° Biggest benefit - it allows direct connections to a hospital network allowing archive access (technologist will not have to send old exams).

T1—T3

- Utilizes a network connection and consists of a leased line which utilizes a point to point connection. Speed range commonly starts @ 56 Kbs and well into the Mbs range. It is offered by all communications companies but can be very expensive.
  - ° Cost is derived from usage and the distance between points of contact.
  - ° The biggest benefit seen is speed yet is best utilized if one or two sites need to be connected.

Asynchronous Transfer Mode (ATM)

Asynchronous Transfer Mode, instead of sending information in a continuous stream it sends it in cell packets. Packets allow faster information transfer because less information is sent for error correction purposes. Error correction occurs at the receiving end.

- Allows speed of 155 Mbs.
- This service is usually not available on a wide spread basis.

Others

Satellite and Radio-wave communications are additional methods and can transfer tremendous amounts of data. A satellite is usually way beyond the financial capabilities of most institutions but Radio is usually not. Radio-wave communications can offer significant advantages over leased line. There are some limiting features and requirements but overall the benefits outweigh the negative aspects. The points of connection must be in a viewable line of site, there can be no physical obstruction between sites and are somewhat distance limited. There are big benefits derived from having this ability.

- One time start up cost. The start up cost is comparable to setting up an SMDS or T1 line. No monthly service bills other than a maintenance contract for equipment.
- Additional sites can be added as needed at a known cost.
- Unlimited use and multiple functions. Can be used for teleconferencing as well as general information exchange.
- Annual savings over conventional leased lines can pay for the start up cost in the first year.

RIS

RIS is the heart of any PACS. All of the above, except hard copy film integration, can be handled with the integration of the RIS. This is argument enough to have a RIS. Choosing a RIS is just as important as choosing the PACS vendor. Both must communicate and both must have an upgrade path. Do not fall for the sale of one system doing it all. Assuredly the system will end up doing both poorly.

Let each do what they do best. A RIS is built to handle massive amounts of information and handle it in very short period of time. Utilize the RIS to eliminate spelling mistakes, set schedules for the modalities, route and pre-fetching the co-coordinated exams, keep track of images, integrate to the HIS for physician communication, produce imaging and modality reports, and to set maintenance schedules that are incorporated into the examination load.

PACS Broker

A RIS/Modality interface is a must. The interface must be bidirectional. A bidirectional interface offers the means for the modality to accept information from the RIS for patient demographics etc and allows the modality the path to send information back to the RIS for validation. The information provided would consist of exam start and completion along with total images and where the images are located. Exam location is critical to retrieval speed. When an exam is requested from a workstation other than the original destination, why retrieve from the archive when retrieving from a local station is faster, a RIS is built to handle this logic function with great speed and resource efficiency.

The bi-directional interface of the RIS to modality will work wonders for scheduling and image retrieval. It will eliminate common spelling errors that can occur with printed patient requests, this feature alone can prevent costly time of editing patient files because the data is validated without any manual typing. Without this feature, think of the time it will take to correct normal errors in typing patient names for image capture. Without a validation feature, examinations performed on the same patient have a high risk of winding up in separate files.

Image Distribution

The RIS, if instituted properly, can provide an interface to the HIS allowing image access utilizing low cost terminals. The common HIS terminals will need upgraded monitors specifications. They would allow image viewing on the nursing units at a cost lower than the conventional clinical review unit sold by most PACS vendors. Additionally these same terminals can be used for normal patient record retrieval.

Picture Archiving and Communication System (PACS)

In a typical design of a PACS, a number of services are involved within the system during archiving including data registration, receiving, compression, and storage. The services involved during retrieving are data query, retrieving, decompression, and delivery. In a PACS of small scale, all the above services are installed in a computer server. Each service is handled by a computer processor.

In a PACS of larger scale, two designs can be used for handling of the services. The first design is using separate computer server for each service. This type of design is called "Multiple Computer Single Processor" (MCSP) PACS. The second design is using a single computer with multiple processors and multiple tasking computer operating system for handling all procedures. This type of systems is called "Single Computer Multiple Processor" (SCMP) PACS. These two types of PACS are as shown in the following figure.

In a MCSP PACS, during image archiving, the new in-coming images are firstly registered in the database computer and received in another computer. After the images received, they are compressed and stored in the archive. During image query, user sends a query request to the database computer. The PACS can retrieve the required images according to the request. The retrieved images are decompressed and then delivered to the client computer.

In a MCSP PACS, all PACS services including registration, query, image receiving, compression, decompression, store, and retrieval are handled by different processors in a time-sharing multi-task computer. During image archiving, the new in-coming images are in the database through a registration service. The images are then received, compressed and then stored in the archive by different processors within the same computer. During image query and retrieval, the request is handled by a database service. After the location of the images is searched, the retrieved images are decompressed and delivered to the user.

The features of MCSP and SCMP PACS designs are compared and listed in the following table.

Figure 2. Service diagram of a PACS

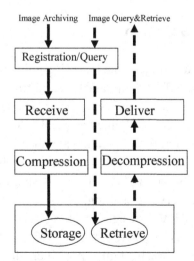

Figure 3. Comparison of MCSP and SCMP PACS designs

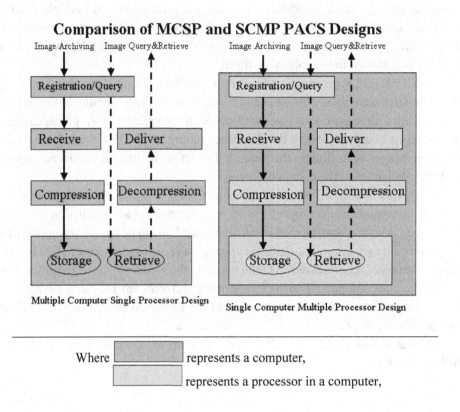

High Available PACS Design

During the design of a PACS project, the following guidelines can be found useful: Simplicity, Expandability, Affordability, and Reliability (SEAR). With simple design and operation, the system should be user understandable and fully automatic. It can minimize the labouring cost and time for trouble-shooting. Expandable design can extend the life of a system from outdating and increase the capacity and speed of the PACS. All initial, operation, and upgrade costs should be affordable and accountable. Reliability can be improved by the design of high available or fault tolerance systems such as server clustering.

A high available MCSP PACS design is making use of two groups of computers for providing the PACS services: active MCSP PACS and standby MCSP PACS. The design is shown as the following figure. A resilient linkage is installed between the active and standby PACSs. This linkage is used to communicate between the

Table 1. Comparison of MCSP and SCMP PACS designs

MCSP	SCMP
Multiple less-powerful computers	Single powerful computer
Independent resource for archiving and retrieving jobs	Required for time sharing operating system
Higher power consumption and heat dissipation	Common resource for archiving and retrieving jobs
Occupy more space	Occupy less space
Required for network between each process	No network required between each process

two PACS about the status of the systems. In the normal status, the active PACS can provide all the radiology services to the users and report its normal status to the standby PACS. Any change of the status or malfunctioning of the active PACS, the standby PACS will takeover the PACS services until the recovery of the active PACS. Since in a MCSP PACS, this resilient linkage may involve several computer, its efficiency and overhead maybe a problem in the design.

In a high available SCMP PACS design, two powerful computers are used for providing all the PACS services: active SCMP PACS and standby SCMP PACS. A resilient linkage is installed between the active and standby PACS computers. This linkage is just between two computers and relatively manageable. The design is shown as the following figure.

A comparison of high available MCSP and SCMP PACS is as shown in the following table.

Archive

Archives are actually very simple to configure. It is much the same as a film library, yet there is one obvious difference; it is now electronic. The same decisions must be made regarding how much space is needed and how fast an access is needed. Physical space is not the limiting factor of an electronic archive. Physically a digital archive can hold approximately 10 years of images in a 12 X 12 room, dependant upon environmental conditions. The limiting factor for digital archives is retrieval needs. The archive configuration can be broken into two pieces - Size and Configuration and Design.

Archive Size

To size the archive is very simple - convert the current examinations into digital data size formats. All equipment vendors can provide their users with the actual

Figure 4. High available MCSP PACS design

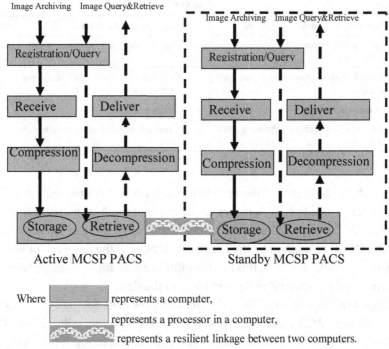

Where [ ] represents a computer,

[ ] represents a processor in a computer,

[ ] represents a resilient linkage between two computers.

Table 2. Comparison of high available MCSP and SCMP PACS

High Available MCSP	High Available SCMP
Requirement of a network of ten computers	Start with two computers
Complicated network design	Simple design
Multiple points of failure	No single point of failure

size of the images in DICOM format that are produced. Break the archive volumes down by modalities such as CT, MRI, US, NM, Angiography, Fluoroscopy, Diagnostic etc.. Follow the following exercise, the annual and total archive needs can be calculated:

- Calculate the average number of Images per Exam (A),
- From modality vendor get the DICOM image size, this will be in Bytes, (B),
- Multiply A x B to get average exam size, in Bytes (C),

Figure 5. High available SCMP PACS design

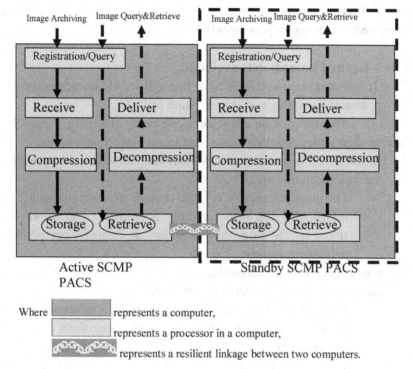

Where [ ] represents a computer,

[ ] represents a processor in a computer,

[ ] represents a resilient linkage between two computers.

- Multiply C times the Modality Volume which will give the annual data needs (D),
- Add up all the Modalities to get a total annual archive need (E), most likely will come out in Giga or Tera-Bytes,
- Multiply E times the retention statute which will give total archive size needs, excluding growth factors.

Every facility should take into account the average experienced/projected growth. Facilities with high Paediatric usage are going to need a much larger archive because of the longer retention statute. Some users may want to separate Paediatrics out like any other modality and add that in as a permanent fixture to the archive needs.

Archiving is another issue that should be examined closely. The archive must have the functional ability to store all images for a predetermined length of time, most likely for the full file retention statute. There are many solutions to image storage. It is better to have the forethought in choosing which technology is the best now and in the future.

As with most technologies archive structure and formats change with time. Currently archive needs can be placed into three categories, live (short term), intermediary and long term (or permanent).

- **Live—fast and immediately available:**
  - ° Information is stored in SCSI or faster disks and located at the point of interaction, on the workstation being utilized.
    - ➢ The information available is constantly changing or volatile.
- **Intermediary (Secondary)—slow and immediately accessible:**
  - ° Information is stored in SATA disks and located on the network as an accessible on line archive.
    - ➢ The storage capacity is large enough to not significantly hinder information retrieval for daily operations. The information is stored for the purpose of providing an intermediary point before permanent storage.
- **Permanent (Tertiary)—accessible:**
  - ° Information is still available for retrieval.
    - ➢ The capacity is configured to store enough information to fit the business needs of the client. This could range from one year to 10 or more years depending upon the industry standards.
    - ➢ This could also incorporate data back up and disaster recovery solutions.

Types of Media Used In Archive

Archive media plays the most important role in PACS. As much as the PACS/RIS/MODALITY interface is a significant part of PACS, the archive is what makes it all happen. Without storage media, who knows what information is available. When any information is produced how is it transferred to another for use. Currently archive media falls into three categories, disk, optical and tape.

- **DISK**—Exactly the same as what is on a PC—can be constructed as a Hard Drive or a Redundant Array of Inexpensive Disks (RAID) Drive.
  - ° Hard Drive usually holds operating system and serves as short term storage.
    - ➢ Configured up to 100 Giga Bytes probably more in the near future.
    - ➢ Very fast data transfer with access times in milliseconds.
    - ➢ Inexpensive.
    - ➢ Should be considered as live storage.

- ○ RAID Drive is usually for information storage. Depending on the configuration, it can be used as system backup. In this case it is used expressly for speed.
  - ➤ Configured in excess of 1,000 Giga Bytes.
  - ➤ Very fast data transfer with access times still in the millisecond range.
  - ➤ Relatively inexpensive depending on size.
  - ➤ Should be considered as live.
- • **OPTICAL**—Two technology types—Optical Disk (OD) or Compact Disk ROM (CD). I do not know the difference between OD and CD other than I must assume it is different writing technology. CD currently does not have the capacity of OD. OD technology has two types Write Once Read Many, meaning single use, (WORM) and Re-Writeable usually meaning magneto-optical.
  - ○ WORM
    - ➤ Storage capacity varies with disk size. Some disks are 12 inches or greater.
    - ➤ Single use only.
    - ➤ Provides longer image life, no degradation, than magnetic tape.
    - ➤ Easy to use and fairly inexpensive.
    - ➤ Storage of multiple disks can become a problem.
  - ○ Re-Writeable OD
    - ➤ Each disk holds approximately 2.4 Giga Bytes.
    - ➤ Gives tremendous storage capacity when set up in a Juke Box configuration; greater than 100 disks on-line.
    - ➤ Data access and transfer and rate is relatively fast but slower than Disk.
    - ➤ Relatively expensive and can be very expensive if it is used as permanent storage.
    - ➤ Should be utilized as intermediary storage.
- • **TAPE**—many types—tape media is changing, not only are access times decreasing but capacity and longevity are also increasing. Tape comes with a variety of sizes and recording methods, LTO, DAT and Optical Tape. All tape storage should be considered a long term or permanent archive solution.
  - ○ LTO tape (Linear Tape-Open)—LTO is a tape standard developed by HP, IBM, and Seagate. LTO tape stores data in 384 data tracks which are divided into four data bands of 96 tracks each. The four data bands are bordered by bands of servo information which are written during tape manufacture. Data bands are filled one-at-a-time, in a linear fashion. LTO tapes contain 4KB of non-volatile memory which can be read

through a non-contacting passive Radio-Frequency (RF) interface. This storage space contains data about the tape and can be read without the time required to read the magnetic tape itself.

- ➢   Large capacity in some cases more than 800 Giga Bytes per tape.
- ➢   Can be set up in Juke Box configuration allowing storage capacity in the Tera byte range.
- ➢   Access time is long because data is stored sequentially although the file method is changing. Time should not be considered a minus because data transfer is still faster than the manual method. Additionally this becomes seamless with IT integration.
- ➢   Offers an economical storage.
- ➢   Best utilized as permanent storage.

Configuration and Design

The RAID archive should be located onsite but the TAPE archive could be stored off-site for Disaster Recovery purpose.

Displays

Liquid Crystals Displays

LCDs rely on the fundamental electro-optical characteristics of liquid crystals (LCs) to form an image. When the molecular orientation within an LC is altered by the application of an external electric field, the optical characteristics of the material change. This electro-optical effect is used in LCDs to modulate light transmission. An LCD is composed of a large array of LC cells (each representing a pixel of the image), polarizer filters, and a backlight. The height and volume of the LC cells are controlled by spacers.

Light is generated by the backlight and directed to the front through a first polarizing filter, the LC cell, and an exit polarizing filter. The amount of the transmitted light intensity is primarily controlled by the change in polarization induced by the voltage applied to the LC cell in relation to the polarization orientation of the first and second polarizer. The maximum amount of transmitted light (i.e., the maximum luminance of the display) is determined by the intensity of the backlight, the nature of the polarizers, the transmission of the LC cell in its full "on" state, the transmission characteristics of additional colour filters (for colour displays), and the aperture ratio (the fraction of the pixel area that is transparent). The minimum luminance of the display is primarily determined by the opaqueness of the LC cell in its full "off" state. In an AMLCD, the switch between on and off states is controlled through voltage changes produced by a thin-film transistor (TFT) array. Displays can be characterized as being normally white or normally black, depending upon the relation of the pair of polarizers relative to the intrinsic "twist" in the LC material. For example, if a pair of crossed polarizers is used, with LC material having no intrinsic twist, all light is linearly polarized after passing through the first of the polarizing filters. When no voltage is applied, all light will be fully blocked by striking the second (crossed) polarizer, and this display is characterized as normally black. Alternatively, the pair of polarizers may be collinear, so that light that passes through the first polarizer is transmitted through the second polarizer in the absence of voltages. This display is characterized as normally white. It is somewhat more straightforward for normally white displays to provide a higher maximum luminance Lmax, since the twist is not needed to achieve the maximum luminance. However, for a normally white display it is difficult to achieve a low Lmin value, since the opaqueness of the display depends upon the efficiency of the LC material in providing the twist. A unique aspect of LCD devices is that the light emission is non-Lambertian. This is due to two major reasons: first, the optical anisotropy of the LC cell, which depends upon the manufacturing design and the applied voltage, and second, the effect of polarized light being transmitted and viewed in a direction collinear with the polarizing filter (termed a sine squared effect since it varies as $\sin \theta$, where θ is the viewing angle). These two effects result in a potentially severe angular dependence of the luminance. The angular dependency affects the contrast as well as luminance of the presented image as a function of the viewing angle. More advanced LCD designs have aimed to minimize this angular dependence by (1) varying molecular alignments in subregions (domains) within individual pixels (Nam et al. 1997), (2) modifying the orientation of the LC molecules to remain in the plane of the display (in-plane switching) (Wakemoto et al. 1997), or (3) adding a negative birefringence plate to compensate for the optical anisotropy (Hoke et al. 1997). It is common for the first two methods to also include the third. Using hydrogenated amorphous silicon (a-Si:H) TFT technology, AMLCDs have achieved very high information content and colour pixel resolution. Monochrome 2560 × 2048 (5 megapixels) workstation quality and colour 3840 × 2400 (9.22 megapixels) AMLCDs have recently been introduced commercially. On the market, different designs of LCD monitors with different features are available. A comparision of the features of LCD Guideline from Royal College of Radiologist and some commerical medical and general purpose are shown in Table 3.

Table 3. Comparison of LCD Guideline of Royal College of Radiologists

	Minimum	Recommended	Dicom Part-14 LCD	General purpose LCD	Medical grade LCD
Screen resolution	>=1280x1024	>=1500x2000	1280x1024	1280x1024	1600x1200
Screen size	>=42 (17"~)	>=50 (20")	48.1	48.1	54
Maxi luminance	>=170cd/m^2	>=500cd/m^2	280cd/m^2	280cd/m^2	500cd/m^2
Contrast ratio	>=250:1	>=500:1	1000:1	1000:1	700:1
Greyscale calibration	~10% GSDF	Calibrated	NA	NA	Calibrated
Greyscale bit depth	8bit-greyscale /24bit color	>=10bit grey scale	24-bit color	24-bit color	8-bit Gray
Interface	Digital-analogue	DVI	Analogue/DVI	RGB /DVI	DVI
Pixel defects ISO13406-2	Class 2 2 per million	Class1 0 defects	NA	NA	NA
Other tools			Tools for user calibrate to Dicom Part-14	NA	AAPM TG18

Diagnostic Workstation

* Configuring a radiology workstation must take into account the radiologist's preferences, functions and the type of image to be viewed. Any design configuration decision must provide a cost benefit solution. Designing a workstation is going to vary with each site and is dependent upon both individual preference and physician function. Not every diagnostic station has to be 2K, if a radiologist only interprets small matrix images there is no need of the more expensive 2K units. There is also no need of greater than eight monitors for any one unit yet four or six will usually do.
  ○ Particular attention must be given to lighting and placement of the workstation.
    ➢ Lighting should be reflected (indirect), and controllable. There must be no chance of direct light applied to the monitor and the ambient room brightness is adjusted to the radiologist's preference. A good way to do this is by using wall sconces or ceiling to wall reflected light.
    ➢ Placement of workstations is critical. Workstations should be placed so that no two have a direct opposite placement. Proper placement

Figure 6. Design of a PACS for filmless hospital

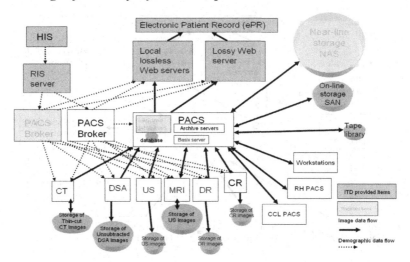

reduces the reflection from one workstation onto another. Workstations should be placed, if possible, in a semi circular format with the room entrance facing the radiologist, preventing outside reflection and reducing intermittent shadows created by hallway traffic.

Clinical Workstation

Clinical workstations fall into two categories, Clinical-Diagnostic and Clinical-Reference, each having the same basic configuration yet differing in patient care level application. The first category, Clinical-Diagnostic, is defined by the specific uses of the Critical Care and Emergency Departments. Both have a higher level viewing need than the nursing unit which is where a Clinical-Reference is indicated. Commonly the CCU and ED workstation directly relates to how the patient will be treated while the Clinical Reference is used more as a report to image correlation.

Restricting the placement of workstations relevant to clinical application will save a tremendous amount of money. Typically the Clinical-Diagnostic station should be purchased from a PACS vendor while the Clinical-Reference can be an integrated workstation provided by the HIS vendor. This is dependent upon the HIS vendor having a true HIS-RIS-PACS interface.

Figure 7. Business flow chart of a PACS

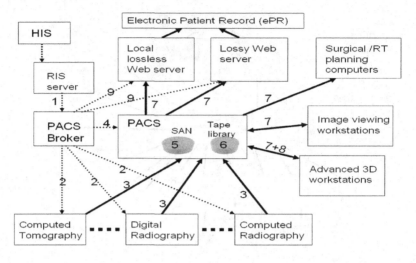

Figure 8. Processes in a PACS

Process No	Sub-Process	Process Location
1.	Patient demographic data retrieval	PACS Broker
2.	Modalities receiving worklist	Modalities
3.	Image receiving	PACS Servers
4.	Image verification	PACS Servers
5.	Image on-line storage	PACS Server, SAN
6.	Image archiving to tape library	Tape Library
7.	Image distribution to clinicians directly or through ePR	Web servers/ 3D workstations
8.	Archive of secondary captured images	Advanced 3D workstations
9.	Image verification	Web servers

CONCLUSION

The challenge of handling large volumes of patient-related data and images has now outgrown traditional ways of dealing with such information. Sharing, retrieving, saving, and viewing high-resolution medical images (MRIs, X-rays, etc) in conjunction with corresponding patient information accurately and reliably every time demand technology like Picture Archive Communication System (PACS).

PACS serves as a constantly growing and evolving repository for medical images and patient information. Medical information can easily be stored, recalled, displayed, manipulated and printed digitally, greatly improving the efficiency of imaging departments. However, like most other applications designed for such specific purposes, PACS needs to be implemented effectively. Patient information requirements, such as storage, security, and retrieval should be determined in advance and matched with the most appropriate storage methods. Thus, health professionals have had electronic storage and access to medical diagnostic images, but the sheer volume of image data, in terms of generated images and size of image files, has always overloaded the capabilities of PACS. Not enough space and slow access has especially been a problem in long-term, large storage of images.

Archive Design

The price and capacity of archive media change almost as quickly as the time of day. The archive design should obviously incorporate the current as well as future needs. The following recommendations should be considered:

- Size of the archive should be able to accommodate the existing image files and future expansion. For PACS with large volume, it is better to be divided into separate archives by function.
- The live archive should have capacity of at least six months since most patient follow-up care occurs within the first six months of treatment.
- The secondary archive should have a capacity of up to 5 years for minimizing the pre-fetching of images from tape library.
- The long term archive should have a capacity of a month for backup and recovery of the archive only.
- Offsite digital archives should be considered for backup and disaster recovery. Most disaster recovery plans require an offsite location for backup data.
- A third party offsite archive can be considered. This could help to absorb some cost of a large archive by sharing it with others through the vendor.
    - This puts the burden on the vendor to keep up with the following:
        - Changes in technology,
        - Changes in the DICOM standard,
        - Equipment investment,
        - Maintenance,
        - Providing a true disaster plan for the facility.

REFERENCES

Dreyer, K. J. (2005). Computer fundamentals. In Dreyer, K. J., Mehta, A., Thrall, J. H. (Eds.), *PACS: A Guide to the Digital Revolution,* (pp. 173-182). 2nd ed., Springer Verlag. ISBN: 0387260102; ISBN-13: 9780387260105

Dreyer, K. J. (2005). Web distribution. In Dreyer, K. J., Mehta, A., Thrall, J. H. (Eds.), *PACS: A Guide to the Digital Revolution,* (pp. 373-382). 2nd ed., Springer Verlag. ISBN: 0387260102; ISBN-13: 9780387260105

Hirschorn, D. S. (2005). Image displays. In Dreyer, K. J., Mehta, A., Thrall, J. H. (Eds.), *PACS: A Guide to the Digital Revolution*, (pp. 347-362). 2nd ed., Springer Verlag. ISBN: 0387260102; ISBN-13: 9780387260105

Huang, H. K. (2004). Picture Archiving and Communication System Components and Work Flow. In Huang, H. K. (Ed.), *PACS – Basic Principles and Applications,* (pp. 155-170). New York: John Wiley & Sons. ISBN: 0471251232; ISBN-13: 9780471251231

Huang, H. K. (2004). PACS Controller and Image Archive Server. In Huang, H. K. (Ed.), *PACS – Basic Principles and Applications,* (pp. 255-276). New York: John Wiley & Sons. ISBN: 0471251232; ISBN-13: 9780471251231

Huang, H. K. (2004). Display Workstation. In Huang, H. K. (Ed.), *PACS – Basic Principles and Applications.* (pp. 277-306). New York: John Wiley & Sons. ISBN: 0471251232; ISBN-13: 9780471251231

Huang, H. K. (2004). Integration of HIS, RIS, PACS, and ePR. In Huang, H. K. (Ed.), *PACS – Basic Principles and Applications,* (pp. 307-330). New York: John Wiley & Sons; ISBN: 0471251232; ISBN-13: 9780471251231

Huang, H. K. (2004). PACS Data Management and Web-Based Image Distribution. In Huang, H. K. (Ed.), *PACS – Basic Principles and Applications,* (pp. 333-352). New York: John Wiley & Sons; ISBN: 0471251232; ISBN-13: 9780471251231

Lemke, H. U., Niederlag, W., Heuser, H., & Pollack, T. (2001). *PACS Planning and Evaluation using Quality Function Deployment.* Retrieved 16 January 2008 from http://www.uniklinikum-giessen.de/kis-ris-pacs/archiv/2001/di1015.pdf

Levine, L. A. (2005). PACS strategic plan and needs assessment. In Dreyer, K. J., Mehta, A., Thrall, J. H. (Eds.), *PACS: A Guide to the Digital Revolution,* (pp. 27-44). 2nd ed., Springer Verlag. ISBN: 0387260102; ISBN-13: 9780387260105

Nagy, P. G., & Schultz, T. F. (2005). Storage and enterprise archiving In Dreyer,

K. J., Mehta, A., Thrall, J. H. (Eds.), *PACS: A Guide to the Digital Revolution,* (pp. 319-346). 2nd ed., Springer Verlag; ISBN: 0387260102; ISBN-13: 9780387260105

National Electrical Manufacturers Association (2008). *Digital Imaging and Communications in Medicine (DICOM) Part 10: Media Storage and File Format for Media Interchange*

National Electrical Manufacturers Association (2008). *Digital Imaging and Communications in Medicine (DICOM) Part 12: Media Formats and Physical Media for Media Interchange*

National Electrical Manufacturers Association (2008). *Digital Imaging and Communications in Medicine (DICOM) Part 14: Grayscale Standard Display Function.*

Nesbitt, K. M., Schultz, T. F., & Dasilva, R.. (2005). PACS architecture. In Dreyer, K. J., Mehta, A., Thrall, J. H. (Eds.), *PACS: A Guide to the Digital Revolution,* (pp.249-268). 2nd ed., Springer Verlag. ISBN: 0387260102; ISBN-13: 9780387260105

Pizer, S. M. (1981). Intensity mappings to linearize display devices. *Computer Graphics and image Processing, 17*(3), 262 -268.

Reiner, B. L., & Siegal, E. L. (2005). Reengineering workflow: A focus on personnel and process In Dreyer, K. J., Mehta, A., Thrall, J. H. (Eds.), *PACS: A Guide to the Digital Revolution,* (pp. 73-96). 2nd ed., Springer Verlag. ISBN: 0387260102; ISBN-13: 9780387260105

The Royal College of Radiologists (2008). *Picture Archiving and communication Systems (PACS) and guidelines on diagnostic display devices.*

Samei, E., Badano, A., Chakraborty, D., Compton, K., Cornelius, C., Corrigan, K., Flynn, M. J., Hemminger, B., Hangiandreou, N., Johnson, J., Moxley, M., Pavlicek, W., Roehrig, H., Rutz, L., Shepard, J., Uzenoff, R., Wang, J., & Willis, C. (2005). *Assessment of Display Performance for Medical Imaging Systems.* Report of the American Association of Physicists in Medicine (AAPM) Task Group 18, Medical Physics Publishing, Madison, WI, AAPM On-Line Report No. 03, April 2005.

Smith, G. (2005). Introduction to RIS and PACS. In Dreyer, K. J., Mehta, A., Thrall, J. H. (Eds.), *PACS: A Guide to the Digital Revolution,* (pp. 9-26). 2nd ed., Springer Verlag. ISBN: 0387260102; ISBN-13: 9780387260105

Siegal, E. L., Reiner, B. L., & Knight, N. (2005). Reengineering workflow: The radiologist's perspective. In Dreyer, K. J., Mehta, A., Thrall, J. H. (Eds.), *PACS: A Guide to the Digital Revolution,* (pp. 97-124). 2nd ed., Springer Verlag. ISBN: 0387260102; ISBN-13: 9780387260105

Thomas, J. (2007). *Business Continuity Planning - PACS Version 3.0*. Retrieved 15 October 2007 from http://www.dilysjones.co.uk/IG4U/Business%20Continuity%20Planning.pdf

Chapter VII
Implementation of Filmless Hospital

INTRODUCTION

A PACS has tremendous benefits (Bryan, Weatherburn, Watkins, Buxton, 1999) and values outside of radiology as well as internally. The biggest benefit derived from a PACS is breaking the physical as well as time barrier for information exchange. The other benefit from PACS implementation is not the decreased operating cost in Radiology. The radiology cost benefit, while significant, does not compare with the system wide benefits of networking images throughout the hospital and physician offices.

All PACS implementations should start with a business plan. This is the summation of many small plans and also summarizes the global goal. The plan should be segmented into smaller separate plans for cost justification, risk assessment, capacity planning, and the last consisting of an implementation plan.

THE BUSINESS PLAN

A business plan (Lemke, Niederlag, Heuser, & Pollack, 2001) for setting up a filmless hospital is required for a successful project. The first thing in the plan is to define a clear objective for the project which is fully understandable by the whole healthcare organization from front line staff to senior management. The detail business plan should include the followings:

Cost Justification

This covers the area of hard and soft cost reductions and revenue enhancement (Reilly, Avrin, 2005).

- Hard cost reduction should include low skill labour costs in the darkrooms, film libraries, film management, and film cost. However, in real situation, the Full Time Equivalent (FTE) of the labour costs may be reduced but the net cost associated with this will most likely be offset by the higher paying job of a PACS network administrator either within radiology or Information Systems.
- Soft cost reduction will include decreased film waiting time for clinicians, no film transportation is required, improved infection control as less physical interaction is needed, and thus leads to increased productivity of staff.
- Revenue enhancement can be experienced by setting up new services for the radiologists and clinician as a profit sharing venture. This can be realized because there is no longer the physical boundary of geographic location. Services such as providing remote medical consultation for small hospitals are now possible.

Risk Assessment

This includes an inventory checking and assessment relating to the risk of filmless hospital operation.

- Evaluate medical equipment or imaging modality that need integration including their upgradability.
- Evaluate personnel needs and technology education level of all users.
- Compile a list of imaging equipment, computer equipment, network equipment, vendors, and training capabilities.
- Check with local networking and internet service providers regarding services available in the area.

Capacity Planning

- Set up a methodology to evaluate the needs and resource requirement.

- Assess and evaluate the existing resources and if they can meet the current needs.
- Determine what current resources can be utilized.
- Assess the future needs.
- Integrate available resources, present a plan that incorporates future resource needs.

Implementation Plan

Communications Plan

A successful PACS implementation (Levine, 2005) necessitates strong collaboration between unlikely and possibly heretofore unrelated departments and operational areas. Key constituents include referring physicians and their offices, radiologists, frontline radiology staff, the hospital information technology (IT) department, and all other hospital staff, as well as patients. The best way to ensure that communications are clearly conveyed to all constituents in an appropriate, timely manner is to have communications as part of the PACS project plan.

- Selling the concept and benefits to the radiology department is important.
- Clinicians are key personnel who must not only buy into the theory but the real benefit as well. They are the first to realize manual film handling is time wasting for them and their patients due to film availability and transport.

Implement PACS in Phases

- Phased implementations allow the process to stop at any point for adjustments.
- The completion of one phase does not mean that the next must follow immediately. Phases may be months or even years apart.
- Each phase, upon completion, allows the next phase to be implemented with a lessons learned approach. No two phases, like institutions, are alike. Every phase incorporates new people and services that are likely to have different needs than others

Organizational Structure

- To prepare for PACS, critically access existing staff resources to determine what skill sets are on hand, which are needed, and who will be responsible for each aspect of the new technology and operations in a PACS environment. Furthermore, PACS will blur the lines of responsibility between information technology (IT) and radiology, calling for more creative reporting relationships than may currently characterize an organization.

• A PACS implementation team is required to have primary responsibility for the rollout. All constituents need representation in the PACS implementation team. Some constituents, such as referring physicians, will serve temporarily as advisors to the team during phases critical to their interests. Others, such as the IT department, will have ongoing participation as core members of the team. The project plan will reflect involvement of all constituents, as tasks cross over operational areas and are assigned to multiple team members for completion.

• A PACS administrator is required for managing and co-ordinating all the PACS related service in the hospital. Whether that person resides in radiology or in the IT department will depend on an institution's unique situation. Depending on the size of the institution and time frame for implementation, other positions may need to be created for PACS support, such as those for training, quality assurance, and user support.

• Skills in information technology, project management, information security management, and more sophisticated operational management/tracking will be required for many PACS related tasks in the department.

Training Prior to Implementation

• Training prior to implementation of PACS includes both knowledge-based training on the vendor's system as well as more generic training in computers (some staff may need to learn how to operate a mouse and navigate Windows-based software programs). Each position, both existing and new, needs to be evaluated and the skill sets required must be identified. Then, each staff member should be assessed for training needs. Radiologists and key referring physicians need to be included in this training assessment. Some knowledge/skill deficits can wait until after initial implementation; most cannot.

Vendor(s) Communications

• PACS administrator should know the duties of the vendors.
• The PACS installation will require coordination among multiple vendors and specialists within the institution. Communication among vendors is also one

of the duties of PACS team. The PACS vendor needs to have a clear plan for who is accountable and how coordination takes place. Areas in which multiple vendors and site specialists may find themselves cooperating to bring PACS live include:

i	**PACS Installation:** Involves PACS vendor, on-site network specialist
ii	**RIS/PACS Integration:** Involves RIS vendor, PACS vendor, RIS applications manager
iii	**Modality Integration:** Involves modality vendor, PACS vendor, network specialist
iv	**CR/DR Integration:** Involves computed radiography/digital radiography vendor, PACS vendor, network specialist

Contingency Plan

A well-developed contingency plan (Thomas, 2007) will mitigate disruptions to the hospital in the event of technology failure. The following points should be addressed in the plan:

i	Carefully define potential problems and their symptoms
ii	Identify the point of detection and responsibility. Typically this would be the person most likely to notice the problem first.
iii	Where possible, the systems should include self-monitoring tools that can examine system loads, delays, and other problems that might affect performance. These features are typically found in the vendor's response to the Request for Proposal.
iv	Protocols to disseminate the nature of the problem to the end users should be developed in advance. The responsible person for problem detection should be trained on how to execute the protocol. Leveraging pager systems, email, and intranet broadcast messages is an effective way to get the message out. The communication should include performance expectations during the disruption.
v	Everyone who interacts with the system should understand their roles and actions in the event that a contingency plan is executed. This includes technologists, radiologists, and supporting staff.

Handle All Modality Integration Issues Prior to Implementation

i	Prior to PACS implementation, all modalities that are not already DICOM compliant need to be upgraded. DICOM compliance includes DICOM Store, DICOM Modality Worklist Management, DICOM Perform Procedure Step, and DICOM Print. DICOM Store is a requirement for PACS. A Modality Worklist Management and Perform Procedure Step are important for accurate data entry and the realization of the potential for technologist productivity improvement.

ii	PACS implementation requires that all imaging modalities and associated equipment (eg, workstations and DICOM printers) be connected to the hospital network infrastructure. If this is not already in place, it can be a significant project in and of itself and should be undertaken prior to PACS implementation.
iii	Planning for integration of imaging modalities needs to occur at both times, when bringing existing equipment online with PACS and when purchasing and installing new equipment. In either case, the modality vendor, PACS vendor, and on-site network specialist will need to cooperate extensively
iv	All newly purchased equipment after PACS implementation must be integrated with the PACS. Alert the modality vendor of this need, and have the vendor take ownership for testing and documenting compatibility prior to any signed purchase agreement. In addition, have the radiologists and technologists who work in that modality review and sign off on the compatibility documentation

Quality Control (QC) Program

To maximize the effectiveness of the PACS, it is important to be confident that every examination performed and completed in the RIS is received and archived in PACS. After a study has entered the PACS, it must appear on the radiologist's worklist to be interpreted in a timely manner. Rigorous QC measures are needed for each modality.

Develop Film-Printing Protocols

- The need to print film in a digital department will diminish but not disappear. To accelerate the transition to a film-limited environment, develop printing protocols and printing guidelines and place them in a readily accessible manual.
- Limiting the demand for printed film sometimes requires limiting the circumstances under which film can be printed for a digital examination. The radiologists will therefore also guide technologists and image librarians on the guidelines for printing. The radiologists are providing a tool by which the technologists and image librarians, as image gatekeepers, can enforce the move to a digital department.

Workflow Analysis

Prior to the implementation of the system, a workflow analysis (Reiner, Siegal, 2005) (Siegal, Reiner, Knight, 2005) is required inside and outside the radiology and clinical departments to determine which processes would change with the introduction of the electronic system and how to accomplish the changes.

Implementation Summary

A PACS project typically takes 90–120 days for implementation. This time frame is very short and will require an intense period of preparation for the facility and medical community. Key activities in the implementation include:

- determining the location and handling the installation of all the network drops and power outlets;
- building and testing the interface/integration of RIS to PACS;
- testing and certifying modality DICOM readiness;
- creating current workflow documentation and post-PACS redesign;
- and communicating to the radiology staff, hospital staff, referring community, and power users of film about the upcoming change in radiology.

Trainings

- The training of technologists, radiologists, clinicians, and support staff should begin before the filmless operation of the hospital.
- A few administrators and radiologists can attend off-site system administration classes at the vendor's training centre.
- Application specialists come to the site and work directly with the technologists, radiologists, and support staff as well as conduct "train the trainer" classes. The "trainers" then go on to teach other members of the department and the clinicians.
- The technologists are instructed in the differences between the film screen approach and that of digital radiology (DR) and computed radiography (CR). They also learn how to use the electronic workstations to review, evaluate, and prepare their images.
- The clerical staff, which have been responsible for matching studies and hanging the films on the alternator, are now trained to use the digitizer, the dry laser printer, and the electronic workstation to send the current and previous images to the radiologists for interpretation.
- The radiologists were instructed on the use of the reading station to view the images. They spent considerable time with an application specialist and a system administrator deciding on display modes, hanging (display) protocols, and selecting which electronic tools would be most useful to them. The reading stations were configured to suit the radiologists' preferences.
- At least one administrator should be trained for ISO 27000 lead/internal auditor. Security awareness training should be provided for all users regularly.

Obstacles to Being Filmless

The requests of film printing mainly fall into three categories: concerns about image quality, the accuracy of measurements obtained on the electronic workstations, and non-availability of image viewing stations. The transition from film screen to computed radiography presents some challenges. Some studies are more difficult for the radiographers/technologists to do using C-arm (e.g. C-spine, swimmer's view). The varying density of the body part caused problems that are not experienced in film screen methods. Special efforts may be required to resolve these problems.

Deploy the Filmless Hospital Service

The greatest threat to the success of filmless facility would be the lack of adequate image viewing stations. Therefore, a number of clinical review stations should be installed on all clinical departments, wards, and in the clinics; The detail configuration and design should be discussed and agreed with the clinical users. Some issues about deploying filmless hospital service are as follows:

i	**Single or dual LCD monitors**
	Dual monitor is the recommended and preferred configuration. The dual monitor removes limitations that are created when more than one image needs to be displayed at one time. A single monitor with a split screen for image display will not provide a film equivalent or improvement in efficiency, thereby causing the potential end-user to push back for film or creating a slower adaptation to soft-copy utilization.
	Single monitor configuration is the option if budget or space is limited.
ii	**Medical grade or general purpose LCD monitors**
	Since medical grade are ten times more expensive than general purpose LCD monitors. Most new general purpose LCD monitors are good enough for reviewing clinical studies but their performance degrades with time due to aging. Quality control is important for maintaining the quality of the monitors.
	Medical grade LCD monitors are essential for primary clinical diagnosis and act as a reference
iii	**Radiology reports**
	The amount of radiology reporting should be agreed between radiology and clinical departments.
iv	**Replacing light boxes with LCD monitors**
	Many facilities mount all monitors on the wall where the light boxes previously have been. Some clinical departments have mobile carts for PC- and monitor-mounting configurations for image viewing purpose.
v	**Deploying by phases**
	Considering service deploying by phases

Customer Service

The extensive distribution network would only be useful if people could actually use the system. The image viewing stations should be user friendly so that the users feel comfortable viewing their images on the PACS. However, some basic customer services may still be required as follows:

i	Provide "train the trainer" classes for the "super users" from each area of the hospital.
ii	Training classes for the new system.
iii	Computer-Based Training loaded on the review stations or any other PC. This tutorial would walk a user through all the important parts of the software and is available on every shift.
iv	PACS help desk for any PACS-related problem.

No Film Policies

After installation of adequate image viewing system, electronic solutions will provide the major radiology service for the wards, operation theatres, A&E, conference rooms, teaching files, and presentations. There are few acceptable reasons to print. Film is only printed when the patient is going to be transferred to another hospital without PACS. If someone wants film for any other reason, they must request an exception from the head of radiology department.

CONCLUSION

PACS implementation planning is a complicated and challenging business in many ways. The above PACS implementation planning approach provides a guideline to tackle this problem.

REFERENCES

Bryan, S., Weatherburn, G. C., Watkins, J. R., & Buxton, M. J. (1999). The benefits of hospital-wide picture archiving and communication systems: a survey of clinical users of radiology services. *Br J Radiol, 72*(857), 469–78. PMID 10505012

Lemke, H. U., Niederlag, W., Heuser, H., & Pollack, T. (2001). *PACS Planning and Evaluation using Quality Function Deployment*. Retrieved 16 January 2008 from http://www.uniklinikum-giessen.de/kis-ris-pacs/archiv/2001/dil015.pdf

Levine, L. A. (2005). PACS strategic plan and needs assessment. In Dreyer, K. J., Mehta, A., Thrall, J. H. (Eds.), *PACS: A Guide to the Digital Revolution*, (pp. 27-44). 2nd ed., Springer Verlag. ISBN: 0387260102; ISBN-13: 9780387260105

Reiner, B. L., & Siegal, E. L. (2005). Reengineering workflow: A focus on personnel and process In Dreyer, K. J., Mehta, A., Thrall, J. H. (Eds.), *PACS: A Guide to the Digital Revolution,* (pp. 73-96). 2nd ed., Springer Verlag; ISBN: 0387260102; ISBN-13: 9780387260105

Reilly, S .R., & Avrin, D. (2005). Financial modeling. In Dreyer, K. J., Mehta, A., Thrall, J. H. (Eds.), *PACS: A Guide to the Digital Revolution*, (pp. 125-144). 2nd ed., Springer Verlag. ISBN: 0387260102; ISBN-13: 9780387260105

Siegal, E. L., Reiner, B. L., & Knight, N. (2005). Reengineering workflow: The radiologist's perspective. In Dreyer, K. J., Mehta, A., Thrall, J. H. (Eds.), *PACS: A Guide to the Digital Revolution*, (pp. 97-124). 2nd ed., Springer Verlag. ISBN: 0387260102; ISBN-13: 9780387260105

Chapter VIII
Quality Control, Quality Assurance, and Business Continuity Plan in PACS

INTRODUCTION

As PACS gains widespread use, the importance of Quality Control (QC), Quality Assurance (QA), and Business Continuity Plan (BCP) in PACS is rising. The purpose of QC/QA is to measure the quality and performance of a PACS for minimizing the chance of getting any avoidable risk. However, in the real world, there is still some risk in any complicated system. Therefore, BCP is used to reduce the impact and downtime of hospital PACS system operation due to changes or failures in the company operation procedure. The purpose of BCP is to make sure that the critical part of PACS system operation is not affected by critical failure or disaster.

PACS BUSINESS

PACS has become an essential element in a filmless hospital (Bryan, Weatherburn, Watkins, Buxton, 1999). Before the planning for QA and BCP, the business model of PACS in a hospital can be presented as follow in Figure 1.

In the business model, the key assets include film scanners, digital imaging modalities (CT, MR, CR, DR, US, etc.), image viewing workstations, database

Figure 1. PACS business model

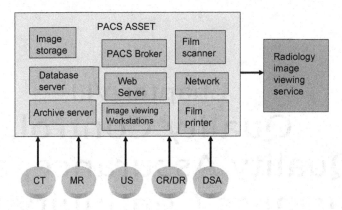

server, image storage, archive server, PACS broker, film printer, and web server. All the above equipments are utilized for providing a radiology image viewing service for the clinical departments in the hospital under a service level agreement. The agreement usually includes the storage period for the images, the quality of the images in the archive, the speed of the image retrieval, the level of customer service, and contingency of the service. The radiology image viewing service may include image viewing in ward area, holding filmless conferences, radiology image reporting, image viewing in out patient clinics, supporting of image distribution network for referring physicians and surgeons, film printing on demand for patients and referring physicians.

QUALITY CONTROL IN PACS

Quality Control (QC) is a system of routine technical activities used to measure and control the quality of the inventory as it is being developed. There are two types of quality control activities: QC in operational procedures and QC in emergency procedures.

Quality Control in Operational Procedures

Data Transfer Verification

In radiology department, hundreds of radiology procedures are performed daily. It is the responsibility of radiographers or technologists for checking each study that is sent and received by the PACS server. In PACS server, DICOM compliant storage class users and providers will eventually be able to use DICOM Verify to ensure that all data are transferred satisfactorily. Even though, there is no guarantee that the image received contains no error. In some sites, the PACS are configured to route all successfully received images to a Web server. The radiographers can browse all the routed images in the Web server and ensure that the images stored in the PACS server to be error-free.

HIS/RIS Interface Oversight and Worklist Management Supervision

A person is designated in PACS team to oversee daily operation of this system. This person is responsible for reviewing all changes to demographics which occur automatically and change demographics on those cases which cannot be determined automatically. However, this job can be replaced by a PACS Broker supervised by an administrator. PACS Broker is responsible for verifying that order entry records submitted after study completion are correctly matched to the study and updating the information of patient status in the PACS.

Continuous System Monitoring

All PACS is expected to provide a 7x24 service in a filmless hospital. PACS administrator should be available 7x24, using pagers and a rotating call coverage schedule. Automated monitoring should be performed at all times, with pager notification of problems. Simple Network Management Protocol (SNMP) is a technique used in network management systems to monitor network-attached devices for conditions that warrant administrative attention. This SNMP management technique should be considered if possible.

During the system monitoring, the following items should be noticed as a minimum:

- Network connectivity
- Workstations, servers and PACS Broker
- Enough free disk space on all systems
- Tape library operation, and queue status
- Printer operation and printer queue status

Repair and Maintenance

Most PACS are built with a variety of manufacturers' equipment and expected to be functional inter-operatively. At least one person in the PACS team should be responsible for calling service on all imaging equipment related to the PACS including the imaging modality. Every failure and error should be diagnosed internally first to aid in calling service and minimizing down time. There should be a clear service call list for each piece (or type) of equipment. All repairs and failures should be logged to determine common sources of problems

Quality Control in Emergency Procedures

Reading Cases During PACS Failures

The quality control activities during the normal PACS operation have been discussed as above. There are other quality control activities required in the emergency procedures during the malfunctioning of PACS. In case of emergency, the first task of the PACS administrator is to make an estimation of the cause of the failure and to determine the time required to correct the problem. According to the estimated length of the downtime, the problems can be classified into level of severity as follows:

- Up to 30 minutes
- 30 minutes to 6 hours
- More than 6 hours

Reading Cases During PACS Failures Lasting up to 30 Minutes

In case the PACS failures lasting up to 30 minutes, images can be displayed in modality consoles. The newly acquired images can by-pass the PACS and be sent directly to the Web servers so that the clinicians can read the images in their PCs connected to the Web servers. Film printing can be started for the new images if requested by users. Finally, all unread cases are pushed from the scanners to the PACS when operation is returned to normal.

Reading Cases During PACS Failures Lasting 31 Minutes to 6 Hours

When the PACS failures lasted for 31 minutes to 6 hours, the routing of all images to Web servers will have already been started. All newly acquired films can be printed until the PACS recovered. Administrator should ensure that all cases are pushed from the scanners to the PACS when operation is returned to normal.

Reading Cases During PACS Failures Lasting more than 6 Hours

In case of a major breakdown of the PACS which lasts for more than 6 hours, all newly acquired images will have by-passed the PACS and be sent directly to the Web servers so that the clinicians can read the images in their PCs connected to the Web servers. Clinicians are allowed to request film printings for all old un-dictated cases. Administrator should also have to ensure that all cases are pushed from the scanners to the PACS when operation is returned to normal

Failure of the WAN

Since remote consultation through teleradiology is a common practice today, radiologists can access their hospital through broadband network or ISDN lines. Some PACS have connection to the Wide Area Network through a Virtual Private Network technology. In the case of a failure of the WAN, then alternative communication methods are needed such as ISDN backup lines.

QUALITY ASSURANCE IN PACS

Quality Assurance (QA) is a planned system of review activities and procedures conducted by personnel not directly involved in the routine process. PACS Quality Assurance (QA) is an overarching topic that covers all aspects of system design and implementation, embracing everything from information governance to network performance. PACS QA is a core component of PACS acceptance testing, and quality of service should be maintained thereafter through regular performance monitoring.

From a clinical perspective, image quality is the major consideration for anyone using PACS for primary (diagnostic) image interpretation. PACS should support image QA through system design, and PACS training should ensure that staff can acquire and manipulate images to optimize image display. Medical physicists have an important role in the acceptance testing and monitoring of acquisition modalities and medical display devices.

Usually, PACS team is responsible for the governance of the QA activities such as reporting to departmental management about the PACS, setting up the QA criteria, holding of regular PACS QA meeting, conducting QA audit for the PACS, and management of the PACS QA activities.

PACS Team

According to ISO 27000 requirements or common practice, a security or management forum should be responsible for the information security of the healthcare organization. In PACS project, a PACS team is established. The members of PACS should include:

- PACS Manager
- Medical Physicists
- RIS/HIS/IT Department representatives
- Radiologists
- Departmental Administrators
- Radiographers
- Clinicians,
- Senior management

PACS Team QA Meetings

Any PACS project of various scales from a departmental PACS to an enterprise filmless hospital, communication is always an important part of the project. Regular meeting of the PACS team is one of the major communication channels. During installation and immediately afterward, PACS team meetings need to be held weekly s for management of the progress of the PACS implementation. Meetings can switch to monthly later after successful installation. There should be a fixed agenda including QA, security, review of the system, audit result, and a summary of PACS performance with tracking over time.

PACS QA Scope

Since QA is an indication of the performance of the system, the following measurements should be tracked as a minimum requirement:

i	Study volume • The size of studies acquired in a period of time such as number of cases, series, images, etc. • Comparison of the result with the previous year.
ii	Film consumption • The number of cases printed • Film usage • Film printing time

iii	Archive volume • Number of cases archived • Average time for archiving • Number of cases retrieved • Average time for retrieval
iv	Database volume • The size of database files • Establish benchmark queries periodically to evaluate the database speed as the database grows in size
v	Evaluate performance of service
vi	Evaluate the following • Cases wrongly identified • Images which are not displayed correctly • Cases with wrong Window/Level • Cases with wrong orientation and labelling • Cases which are incomplete ° Cases which can not be retrieved from archive
vii	Perform film printer sensitometry daily
viii	Evaluate paper and film print image quality weekly
ix	Evaluate monitor quality regularly
x	Cross-calibrate monitors and printers

LCD Monitor Quality

Since the ultimate goal of PACS is to provide a high quality medical image viewing service to clinicians, the quality of the image display LCD monitors is important. For medical images there have been several guidelines that have been developed for calibration. DICOM committee reserves Part 14 for the Grayscale Standard Display Function (GSDF). This standard defines a way to take the existing Characteristic Curve of a display system (i.e. the relationship between the Luminance Output for each Digital Driving Level, DDL, or pixel value) and modify it to the Grayscale Standard Display Function. At the heart of the Grayscale Standard Display Function is the Barten Model which is a mathematical model of the human visual response. This model takes into account the perceptivity of the human eye. Given the black and white levels of the display system, it will spread out the luminance at each of the intermediary Digital Driving Levels such as to maximize the Just Noticeable Differences (JND) between each level. A JND is the luminance difference that a standard human observer can just perceive. Calibration has the aim that each DDL will be as distinguishable as possible from neighbouring levels, throughout the luminance range, and it will be consistent with other display systems that are similarly calibrated. A part of DICOM, supplement 28, describes the GSDF. It is a formula based on human perception of luminance and is also published as a table (going up to 4000 cd/m). It also uses linear perceptions (Perceptual Linearization) and JND.

Display Gamma (Gamma)

Gamma is also called display gamma. Gamma describes the nonlinear relationship between the pixel levels in the computer and the luminance of the monitor (the light energy it emits). The equation is,
  Gamma (γ) is a power function with the form:

$$L = C \times E^\gamma + B$$

Where C is set by the monitor Contrast control.
E is the pixel level normalized to a maximum of 1. For an 8 bit monitor with pixel levels 0 - 255, value = (pixel level)/255.
B is the black level controlled by the monitor Brightness control.
The relationship is linear if $\gamma= 1$. For TFT LCD, the actual value of γ may range from about 2.2 to 2.6.

Perceptual Linearization

Since the eye doesn't respond linearly to light; it responds to *relative* brightness or luminance differences. For medical imaging, it is of great importance that information in the data is accurately mapped to brightness sensation. The fidelity of soft-copy achromatic displays was investigated before and after applying perceptual linearization. This procedure first proposed by Pizer [Computing Graphics and Image Processing 17, 262-268 (1981)], was developed to guarantee the fidelity of a display in such a way that equal steps in the input values to the display system should evoke equal steps in visual perception of the human observer. Pizer tried to realize this under the assumption that the steps are perceptually equal if they contain an equal number of just noticeable differences (JNDs). The idea of perceptual linearization was adopted by other research groups and standardization bodies, such as the American College of Radiology and the National Electrical Manufacturers Association (ACR/NEMA). The perceptual linearization of video display monitors plays a significant role in medical image presentation. First, it allows the maximum transfer of information to the human observer. Second, for an image to be perceived as similarly as possible when seen on different displays, the two displays must be standardized. Third, perceptual linearization allows us to calculate the perceived dynamic range of the display device, which allows comparison of the maximum inherent contrast resolution of different devices.

Medical vs. General Purpose Monitors

General purpose monitors have a fixed gamma of 2.3~2.6. Corrections for visual response and mappings to printers must be done in software. This reduces the number of bits that are achievable. Medical monitors have adjustments for gamma in hardware (after the D/A) and hence allow corrections without a reduction in the number of bits. Some medical monitors have corrections for ambient lighting conditions

The PACS & Teleradiology special interest group provides guideline for minimum and recommended specification for primary diagnostic display devices used for clinical image interpretation as in Table 1. This guidance applies to all workstations where CR, DR, fluoroscopy, ultrasound, CT, MR, nuclear medicine and PET images are viewed (excluding mammography).

Guidelines for Diagnostic Display Device

The UK PACS & Teleradiology special interest group provides the following guidelines for diagnostic display devices:

1. The minimum specification for diagnostic display devices is only appropriate if clinical image viewing is performed according to image viewing guidelines, making use of the application software zoom, pan, magnification, and windowing tools.

Table 1.

	Minimum	Recommended
Screen Resolution [2] (Native Pixel Array)	1280 x 1024 (~ 1.3 megapixels)	>= 1600 x 1200 [3] (~ 1.9 megapixels)
Screen Size (Viewable Diagonal)	42 cm (~17")	>= 50 cm (~ 20")
Maximum Luminance	171 cd/m2	>= 500 cd/m2
Luminance Ratio (Maximum/Minimum)	250:1	>= 500:1
Greyscale Calibration	Within 10% GSDF	Calibrated to GSDF
Grey-scale bit depth	8 bit grey-scale (24 bit colour)	>= 10 bit grey-scale
Video Display Interface	Digital-analogue	Digital video interface (DVI)

2.   LCD devices should be run at their native resolution to ensure that there is a 1:1 match between screen pixels and screen resolution, and therefore no loss of image quality due to screen interpolation. CRT displays can be run at a variety of resolutions with no loss of display quality; however care should be taken that the correct aspect ratio is maintained to avoid distortion of the image.

3.   High fidelity displays (>= 3 megapixels) are recommended in radiology and other areas where large numbers of images are reported to reduce image interpretation and reporting times, and thereby assist department workflow.

If a primary display workstation does not meet all the recommendations outlined above, then a local risk assessment should be undertaken as to whether the workstation can be used for primary diagnostic clinical interpretation. PACS workstations not suitable for diagnostic use should be clearly labeled and the rationale for imposing restrictions on clinical use should be covered in PACS training.

QA of Image Display Devices (Monitors)

All PACS display devices used for primary diagnostic clinical image viewing should undergo formal QA acceptance testing and regular performance monitoring. In the UK, guidance on these procedures is provided by IPEM, referencing guidance from the MHRA, AAPM and IEC. A summary of the 2005 IPEM guidance is given in Table 2.

Summary of Image Display Monitor Guidance from IPEM 2005 Recommended Standards for Routine Performance Testing of Diagnostic X-ray Imaging Systems, IPEM Report 91.

In addition to the 2005 IPEM guidance, it is recommended that all primary diagnostic displays meet acceptance criteria matching the minimum specification guidelines for display devices used for clinical image interpretation summarized in Table 1.

BUSINESS CONTINUITY PLAN

In all mission critical information systems, a Business Continuity Plan (BCP) is one of the essential parts in the core which is managed by middle managers and governed by senior managements. In the filmless hospital project, a significant investment is made for a modern and efficient healthcare service; however it also brings new challenges for the management of such project. There is the potential for immense disruption to the hospital if downtime, scheduled or unscheduled is

Table 2.

Physical parameter	Frequency	Remedial level
Image display monitor condition	Daily to weekly	Image display monitors should be clean, and the perceived contrast of the test pattern should be consistent between monitors connected to the same workstation. Ensure that the 5% and 95% details superimposed on the 0% and 100% squares respectively are visible
Greyscale contrast luminance ratio	3 monthly	Ratio white to black < 250
Distance and Angle	3 monthly	± 5 mm
Calibration		± 3°
Resolution	3 monthly	Grade AAPM TG18-QC resolution patterns according to the reference score (CX > 4)
Greyscale drift	6 to 12 monthly	Black baseline ± 25%
		White baseline ± 20%
DICOM greyscale calibration	6 to 12 monthly	GSDF ± 10%
Uniformity	6 to 12 monthly	U% > 30%
Variation between monitors	6 to 12 monthly	Black baseline > 30%
		White baseline > 30%
Room illumination	6 to 12 monthly	> 15 lux

not addressed fully within a BCP. This section systematically outlines the plan for the hospital to address any such disruption in service.

According to the application of ISO 27000 in a filmless hospital, the objective of BCP is to counteract interruptions to PACS activities and to protect critical PACS processes from the effects of major failures of information systems or disasters and to ensure their timely resumption.

Implementation of BCP

The best run PACS can find itself involved in a disaster or service interruption of one kind or another. Fires, floods and explosions are the main causes of disaster but these are happily, fairly rare. More common reasons for invoking the business continuity plan are viruses, unreliable data, and hardware and software failures.

Methodology

A BCP usually starts with an impact analysis which is used to identify the events that can cause interruptions to business processes, along with the probability. The study of business processes is called business analysis. The impact analysis lists all the key business processes for a filmless hospital. The impact of such interruptions and their consequences for information security are analyzed by an impact analysis. Based on the result of the risk assessment and impact analysis, business continuity plans and disaster recovery plans can be developed and implemented to maintain and restore operations. It can also ensure the availability of PACS service at the required level and in the required time scales following the interruption to, or failure of, the critical PACS processes. The priority of resource allocation for business continuity and disaster recovery are calculated based on the result of impact analysis. For better management and communication, a single framework of business continuity plans shall be maintained to ensure that all plans are consistent, information security requirements are addressed consistently, and priorities for testing and maintenance are identified.

Business Analysis

Business process can be represented by a business flow chart such as the following in Figure 2.

Figure 2. Business flow chart for a filmless hospital

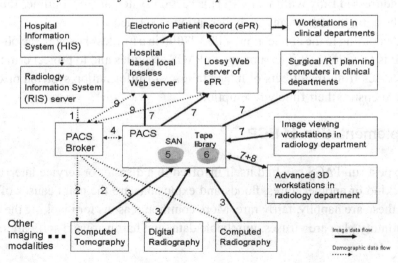

Table 3. Business analysis of a PACS

Process No	Sub-Process	Process Location
1	Patient demographic data retrieval	PACS Broker
2	Modalities receiving worklist	Modalities
3	Image receiving	PACS Servers
4	Image verification	PACS Servers
5	Image on-line storage	PACS Server, SAN
6	Image archiving to tape library	Tape Library
7	Image distribution to clinicians directly or through ePR	Web servers/ 3D workstations
8	Archive of secondary captured images	Advanced 3D workstations
9	Image verification	Web servers

Figure 3. Business continuity plan of a filmless hospital

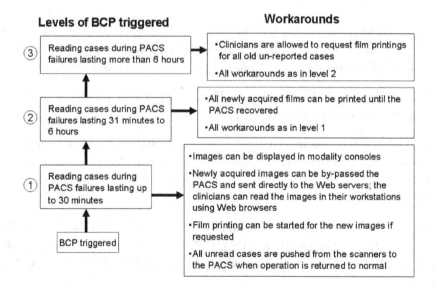

Impact Analysis

From the result of business analysis, the Process 7 is the most critical event for the filmless hospital project and agreed by management. The proposed BCP is illustrated as follow in Figure 3.

As a requirement of ISO 27000, business continuity plans have to be tested and updated regularly to ensure that they are up to date and effective.

CONCLUSION

In a filmless hospital, a managed process has to be developed and maintained for business continuity of the healthcare organization and which also addresses the information security requirements needed for the PACS. This process is usually managed by a professional team including radiologist, hospital administrators, and PACS managers. BCP is an important part of a filmless hospital project, especially for a major hospital. Regular maintenance and update of the plan is required. In conclusion, the proposed systematic BCP approach can effectively minimize the impact to the patient caring and life saving service during the break down of the PACS or network.

REFERENCES

Bryan, S., Weatherburn, G. C., Watkins, J. R., & Buxton, M. J. (1999). The benefits of hospital-wide picture archiving and communication systems: a survey of clinical users of radiology services. *Br J Radiol, 72*(857), 469–78. PMID 10505012

Hayt, D. B. (2001). Filmless in 60 days: The Impact of PACS within a large urban hospital. *Journal of Digital Imaging, 14*(2), 62-71.

Huang, H. K. (2004). Picture Archiving and Communication System Components and Work Flow. In Huang, H. K. (Ed.), *PACS – Basic Principles and Applications,* (pp. 155-170). New York: John Wiley & Sons. ISBN: 0471251232; ISBN-13: 9780471251231

Huang, H. K. (2004). Industrial Standards (HL7 and DICOM) and Work Flow Protocols (IHE). In Huang, H. K. (Ed.), *PACS – Basic Principles and Applications,* (pp. 171-194). New York: John Wiley & Sons; ISBN: 0471251232; ISBN-13: 9780471251231

Huang, H. K. (2004). Display Workstation. In Huang, H. K. (Ed.), PACS – Basic Principles and Applications, (pp. 277-306). New York: John Wiley & Sons. ISBN: 0471251232; ISBN-13: 9780471251231

Huang, H. K. (2004). Integration of HIS, RIS, PACS, and ePR. In Huang, H. K. (Ed.), PACS – Basic Principles and Applications, (pp. 307-330). New York: John Wiley & Sons. ISBN: 0471251232; ISBN-13: 9780471251231

ISO/IEC 27001 (2005). *Information Technology - Security Techniques - Information security management systems - Requirements (Information Technology)*. British Standards Institution. ISBN-10: 0580467813; ISBN-13: 978-0580467813

ISO 27799 (2006). *Health informatics – Security management in health using ISO/IEC 17799 (draft)*. International Organization for Standardization.

National Electrical Manufacturers Association (2008). *Digital Imaging and Communications in Medicine (DICOM) Part 14: Grayscale Standard Display Function*.

Nesbitt, K. M., Schultz, T. F., & Dasilva, R.. (2005). PACS architecture. In Dreyer, K. J., Mehta, A., Thrall, J. H. (Eds.), *PACS: A Guide to the Digital Revolution*, (pp.249-268). 2nd ed., Springer Verlag. ISBN: 0387260102; ISBN-13: 9780387260105

Pizer, S. M. (1981). Intensity mappings to linearize display devices. *Computer Graphics and image Processing, 17*(3), 262 -268.

Reiner, B. L., & Siegal, E. L. (2005). Reengineering workflow: a focus on personnel and process In Dreyer, K. J., Mehta, A., Thrall, J. H. (Eds.), *PACS: A Guide to the Digital Revolution,* (pp. 73-96). 2nd ed., Springer Verlag. ISBN: 0387260102; ISBN-13: 9780387260105

Reilly, S. R., & Avrin, D. (2005). Financial modeling. In Dreyer, K. J., Mehta, A., Thrall, J. H. (Eds.), *PACS: A Guide to the Digital Revolution,* (pp. 125-144). 2nd ed., Springer Verlag. ISBN: 0387260102; ISBN-13: 9780387260105

The Royal College of Radiologists (2008). *Picture Archiving and communication Systems (PACS) and guidelines on diagnostic display devices*

Samei, E., Badano, A., Chakraborty, D., Compton, K., Cornelius, C., Corrigan, K., Flynn, M. J., Hemminger, B., Hangiandreou, N., Johnson, J., Moxley, M., Pavlicek, W., Roehrig, H., Rutz, L., Shepard, J., Uzenoff, R., Wang, J., & Willis, C. (2005, April). *Assessment of Display Performance for Medical Imaging Systems*. Report of the American Association of Physicists in Medicine (AAPM) Task Group 18, Medical Physics Publishing, Madison, WI, AAPM On-Line Report No. 03.

Smith, G. (2005). Introduction to RIS and PACS. In Dreyer, K. J., Mehta, A., Thrall, J. H. (Eds.), *PACS: A Guide to the Digital Revolution*, (pp. 9-26). 2nd ed., Springer Verlag. ISBN: 0387260102; ISBN-13: 9780387260105

Siegal, E. L., Reiner, B. L., & Knight, N. (2005). Reengineering workflow: The radiologist's perspective. In Dreyer, K. J., Mehta, A., Thrall, J. H. (Eds.), *PACS: A Guide to the Digital Revolution*, (pp. 97-124). 2nd ed., Springer Verlag. ISBN: 0387260102; ISBN-13: 9780387260105

Thomas, J. (2007). *Business Continuity Planning - PACS Version 3.0.* Retrieved 15 October 2007 from http://www.dilysjones.co.uk/IG4U/Business%20Continuity%20Planning.pdf

Section III
PACS Total Quality Management

Chapter IX
PACS Quality Dimensions

BACKGROUND

A large number of studies have attempted to identify the factors that contribute to good PACS quality, such as that shown by Reiner et al (2003). Results from these studies (Bauman, 2000; Ralston, 2000) reveal that the success of PACS requires healthcare organizations and managers to adequately address various types of challenges: technological (e.g., integration with other information systems), managerial (e.g., project management), organizational (e.g., availability of resources), behavioural (e.g., change management), and political (e.g., alignment among key participants). Most investigations have considered a single, or at best, a small number of factors contributing to a fragmented view of PACS success. Broadly, these studies may be classified into those that consider the impact of PACS on radiologists' workload and productivity (Gale, 1999), those that consider its clinical implications (Hertzberg, 2000) and those associated with performance of the radiology department (Hayt, 2001).

Rather than measuring the quality of the PACS performance, other researchers have preferred to focus on the quality of the information, that the system produces, primarily in the form of images and reports. For instance, Lou et al. (1997) considered the data integrity and completeness of acquired images. Quality of images in terms of timeliness, accuracy, completeness, and so forth, was also considered to be a key success factor in several evaluative studies (Cox, 2002; Pavlicek, 1999; Pilling, 2003; Blado, 2002).

Indeed, Cox's work was part of a wider evaluation exercise undertaken to assess the impact of the introduction of a PACS on the adult intensive care unit (AICU) at the Royal Brompton NHS Trust in London. The objectives of the research were to evaluate the perceptions of PACS of the medical and ancillary staff working within AICU as well as to undertake a preliminary assessment of its impact on the workload of radiographers. Questionnaires, interviews and a process analysis were undertaken. The research findings indicate that the overall perception of staff towards the introduction of the PACS was positive. The impact of the system on the workload of radiographers was significant, reducing the time taken to obtain an image from 90 to 60 minutes. However, lessons to be learned for future PACS implementations include the need to ensure compatibility with existing IT systems and adequate IT support. In short, once this expanded, but rather fragmented view of PACS success is recognized, it is not surprising to find that there are so many different measures of PACS quality in the literature depending upon which aspect of PACS the researcher focused his or her attention.

PACS OPERATING PROBLEMS

In spite of the adherence to various PACS-QA programs and the presence of various theoretical quality frameworks for the hospital administration, operating problems are still encountered in most PACS. For instance, in the image-guided surgery environment, the problems can generally be grouped under the four categories: hardware, software, hardware/software integration and human factors.

The goal of image guided surgery is the seamless creation, visualization, manipulation and application of images in the surgical environment with fast availability, reliability, accuracy and minimal additional cost. A computer network devoted to image-guided surgery ensures fast and efficient transfer of images from the scanner to the surgical navigation workstation in the operating room. The network server also serves images to desktop PCs where pre-surgical planning can be done. The network for image-guided therapies at Hong Kong hospitals generally includes connections to all CT and magnetic resonance imaging scanners, as well as connections via a dedicated server to home and office PCs and surgical navigation workstations. This smooth workflow and the presence of a multidisciplinary team that includes surgeons, radiologists, radiation oncologists, physicists and engineers with a competent technical support staff should offer the key to good PACS quality. However, following problems were observed in two Hong Kong hospitals:

Hardware Problems

Hardware problems frequently encountered would include:

- **Complexity of controls:** Nursing staff and to a lesser extent, surgeons have difficulty using many of the workstation functions. Although many felt this to be a result of the need for more training, there was a unanimous desire for less complex, more automated controls. There was particular difficulty obtaining satisfactory window and level settings. Surgeons found adjusting these controls non-intuitive and indeed, spot checks by radiologists of images displayed on the operating room screens revealed suboptimal settings in the majority of cases.
- **Suboptimal PACS workstation design and operation:** In the operating room most surgeons and staff surveyed felt the workstation location was to some degree suboptimal. Issues raised included the distance from the operating room table, height of the monitors, and inconvenient placement of keyboard and pointing device with respect to the operating room table. Nurses in particular complained that the workstation obstructed operating room traffic flow.

Software Problems

- **Poor image quality:** Several surgeons perceived poorer image quality with intraoperative images with respect to image exposure and positioning. They expressed the opinion that this was a result of less attention to quality by technologists who believe the surgeons could use image manipulation tools to correct any deficiency caused by poor technique.
- **Need for true image aspect ratio:** Orthopedic surgeons use prosthesis templates which they lay across the image on the screen. This requires the image to be formatted 1:1 as would be the case with film. The surgeons have found that setting labeled as 1:1 is not actually 1:1 and they must manually adjust the image with the magnification controls. They have requested that the software be modified appropriately.
- **Cumbersome image navigation:** Manipulation of multiple studies/sequences: Displaying multiple studies, multipart studies or with MRI, multiple sequences were felt to be cumbersome by most surgeons and staff. Having additional monitors in the operating room was most often rejected as a solution because of space limitations. More sophisticated software has been suggested to better manage image navigation.

System Integration Problems

- **System failures:** One side effect of installing a clinical PACS is that users become dependent upon the technology and in some cases it can be very difficult to revert back to a film based system if components fail. The nature of system failures ranges from gradual deterioration of function as seen in the loss of monitor luminance through sudden catastrophic loss of the entire PACS network. While no surgery was ever postponed or canceled because of PACS failure or malfunction, fear of losing the ability to view images was expressed by many surgeons. Protection from malfunction was felt to be essential. The ability to print film as a backup was felt to be desirable.

- **Glare from ambient light:** Ambient light results in substantial glare making images difficult to see optimally. Glare is a problem for at least two reasons. The first is that the glare light will cause the pupil to constrict more than it would if there were no glare. This results in less of the information illumination getting to the retina. Secondly, the glare source can result in veiling glare within the eye itself. This results from the scattering of light by the vitreous portion of the eye, and is increased with extraneous light entering the eye.

- **Time for intraoperative examinations:** Most intraoperative images are acquired using portable x-ray machines. The imaging plate is then taken by the radiology technologist to the PACS image reader in the radiology department. There was consensus in the perception that there has been a longer period between operating room image acquisition and availability for review when compared to a film-based system. This was attributed to: (1) Lack of a film reader near the operating room. Before PACS implementation, the film processor was located near the operating room. (2) Lack of notification when images were ready for review. (3) frequent difficulty in finding images in the system.

- **Image retrieval time:** Imaging studies are kept "on-line" (in short term storage on a hard drive) for approximately two to three weeks before being archived on an optical jukebox. Images are available in less than one minute when on-line but retrieval of images from the optical storage generally takes four to fifteen minutes. The longer retrieval time for archived images is generally not considered an issue in the operating room because most images are either acquired within two to three weeks of surgery or have been retrieved from the archive prior to surgery. In the few instances where images must be fetched from optical disk, waiting time is unacceptable to the surgeons.

- **Conversion of analogue images to digital images:** For a smooth conversion of previous analogue images to digital images and to cater for the growing medical-imaging demands the hospital is required to find a medical image management system capable of fast and reliable digital archiving, retrieval and real-time access.

- **Network congestion:** The fundamental problem is that networks can be over-loaded and there is rarely quality of service. For example, when an HTML file is sent to a specialist from a Web server, the Transmission Control Protocol (TCP) program layer in that server divides the file into one or more packets, numbers the packets, and then forwards them individually to the Internet Protocol (IP) program layer. Although each packet has the same destination IP address, it may get routed differently through the network. At the other end (the client program in the specialist's computer), TCP reassembles the individual packets and waits until they have arrived to forward them to him as a single file. Current end-to-end Internet congestion control under tail-drop (TD) queue management experiences various performance degradations such as multiple packet losses, high queuing delay and low link utilization.

Human Factors

The term "human factors" has grown increasingly popular as the air transport industry has realized that human error, rather than mechanical failure, underlies most aviation accidents and incidents. Human factors involves gathering information about human abilities, limitations, and other characteristics and applying it to tools, machines, systems, tasks, jobs, and environments to produce safe, comfortable, and effective human use. In aviation, human factors is dedicated to better understanding how humans can most safely and efficiently be integrated with the technology. That understanding is then translated into design, training, policies, or procedures to help humans perform better. In view of the importance of patient safety, it is imperative that the concept should be applied in medical imaging.

- **Less than optimal window and level settings:** Image quality was rated as equivalent to film by all surgeons for all modalities except MRI. When considering the image manipulation capabilities of the workstation, most surgeons rated PACS image quality better than film. MRI images were perceived as having lower resolution than film. However, the surgeons expressing this opinion felt this may be a result of their inability to optimally adjust window and level controls rather than actual quality of the images themselves.
- **Inadequate formal PACS training for physicians:** Formal PACS training is offered on a one to one basis by appointment during working hours. It was initially offered to physicians and physician assistants only. A small number of the surgeons questioned had taken advantage of the formal training. This

might be due to the heavy workload of surgeons in Hong Kong. They learned how to use PACS from colleagues or by trial and error. They stated that time limitations and scheduling conflicts prevented attendance of training sessions. Fortunately most physician assistants took the training. Training was later offered to nurses on a voluntary basis. The initial exclusion of nursing staff was felt to be particularly detrimental in the operating room because the surgeons so often call upon the "non-scrubbed" nurses to operate the workstation. Most of the nurses interviewed had taken the training and were unanimous in their dissatisfaction with their ability to operate the workstation. A common situation described was a struggle with operation of a workstation with an impatient surgeon looking over their shoulder.

- **Trust within the organization:** Informal reports from general PACS operating and maintenance staff suggest that their limited trust of the PACS project team creates an obstacle to its widespread diffusion within the medical authority hospital network. Why should the staff cooperate with management in exploring his/her own mistakes? Unless a strong culture for open communication and assertiveness already exists in the hospital, relatively few PACS staff will voluntarily or willingly disclose what they believe to be the "true story". It is likely that cultural characteristics of staff have limited their trust in others (Wong, 2006).

SHORTCOMINGS OF EXISTING PACS QA

An analysis of these PACS operational problems would reveal shortcomings of the existing quality assurance approaches, viz. the imminent need of:

- A method of analyzing customer wants and needs for the purpose of providing appropriate functional services,
- A practical approach to predicting hardware and software failures,
- A method of determining PACS failure modes, causes and the risk involved,
- A method to minimize communication congestion caused by PACS servers,
- an evaluation of the organization culture, and
- A plan of monitoring PACS performance.

   The approaches that have been used by the authors to deal with the above-noted problems include:

Approaches to Hardware Problems

- **Complexity of controls:** The hospital administrators have kept an eye for PACS designs offering user friendly and more automated controls.
- **System failures:** For this issue the hospital concerned used the cause-and-effect diagram in the identification of PACS component failure causes. Recently, the administration has begun to consider using reliability modeling (RM), failure mode and effects analysis (FMEA) and condition monitoring technique to deal with this kind of problem.
- **Suboptimal PACS workstation design and operation:** Solutions considered include placing the monitors on articulated arms attached to the operating room ceiling allowing variable positioning including the ability to bring the monitors to the operating room table at eye level. Use of a transmitting keyboard pointing device (with a sterile covering) located at the operating table and the use of a foot pedal was suggested.

Approaches to Software Problems

- To deal with the problems of poor image quality, inaccurate image aspect ratio and cumbersome image navigation, the hospital administration is in the process of seeking advanced image management system which, besides providing solutions to the problems noted, would help develop a secure Internet-based medical image viewing system.
- The rise of the Internet and the ubiquity of the Web browser open up a wide range of new possibilities for distributing and accessing these images. The Internet allows people to collect information distributed across many geographically separated data sources, while the Web browser provides a common environment from where programs can be launched. The PACS software is expected to free physicians from being tied to specific workstations within a hospital and allows them to view information from almost any computer around the world in an expeditious manner. It would also allow the administration to bring together PACS information that is stored at geographically distributed sites and present it to the user in one uniform view.

Approaches to System Integration Problems

- **Glare from ambient light:** Non-glare monitors and the ability to dim the lights with a foot pedal were suggested. In the operating room environment, bringing monitors closer to the operating table would make glare less of a problem.

- **Time for intraoperative examinations:** Suggestions for improvement included placing a film reader near the operating room and having the technologist return to the operating room and display the images. The workstation could feature an audible or visible alarm when images are ready. Also, automatic image display was suggested.
- **Image retrieval time:** Solutions offered included a larger on-line capacity, resulting in a longer period until archiving, faster hardware/software, and the ability of operating room personnel to have an emergency fetch which would place needed images first in the retrieval queue.
- **Conversion of analogue images:** An image management system (IMS) is a database dedicated to working with images and their associated Metadata. It will provide a visual interface to the file structure that allows the images to be both viewed singularly and also browsed in groups. An IMS at its simplest will be able to:
  - Store images
  - Store image Metadata
  - Provide a search facility within image Metadata
  - Provide a means of visually inspecting and browsing images

However some of the most recent IMS are now providing a much wider range of additional functionality useful to the digitization of analogue images (slides, prints and negatives) and image collection. This means that recent versions of some IMS might also able to:

- Control and audit (recording all work undertaken) the complete image work-flow from capture through processing to delivery
- Capture a image, name it and enter it into the IMS all in one action
- Optimize, compress and rename image files, both individually and using a batch system to work on a whole folder of images at once
- Provide advanced features of file management, such as adding consecutive numbered suffixes to all files within a folder
- Create surrogate images
- Deliver those surrogate images both by creating static Web pages and also by dynamically creating HTML pages showing the images
- Network queue management and congestion avoidance

For the purposes of reducing network congestion delays, recently active queue management (AQM) algorithms have been proposed for supporting end-to-end transmission control protocol (TCP) congestion control. AQM is a technique of preventing congestion in packet-switched networks. An internet router typically maintains a set of queues, one per interface, that hold packets scheduled to go out on that interface. Historically, such queues use a drop-tail discipline: a packet is put onto the queue if the queue is shorter than its maximum size (measured in packets or in bytes), and dropped otherwise. Active queue disciplines drop or mark packets before the queue is full. Typically, they operate by maintaining one or more drop/mark probabilities, and probabilistically dropping or marking packets even when the queue is short.

Approaches to Human Factors

- **Quality and availability of PACS images:** This problem can be mitigated through the selection of an appropriate image management system.
- **PACS training:** Solutions to training issues which were offered included making training sessions more convenient and accessible, possibly with the use of self learning modules. It has been suggested that the self-learning modules be made available on all PACS workstations. There was consensus that training should be site-specific with more in-depth teaching of functions typically used in the operating room. Training personnel could visit various departments on a regular basis to provide guidance on-site and answer questions as they come up. Certain staff could be more highly trained and act as a resource for other staff.
- **Trust within the organization:** In order to develop a strong PACS quality and safety culture, the administration must first recognize its own organizational and occupational culture, and it must appreciate the interplay between these two with the effects of national culture of its individual members. Perhaps one could borrow the experience from the aviation industry. Since the beginning of this century, maintenance training courses are being seen as more than mere coping skills for individual maintenance professionals, or awareness training – the latest generation of maintenance resource management courses has been aimed to increase trust among licensed aircraft maintenance engineers, their managers, and the regulators so that they are able to learn from present behaviors in order to improve future quality and efficiency. The focus of contemporary maintenance programs is now moving toward active error reduction through structured communication (Patankar & Taylor, 2003).

CONCLUDING REMARK

Quality improvement in industry has a long history in the United States and around the world. Quality improvement gurus like W. Edwards Deming, Walter Shewhart, and J.M. Juran have introduced the concepts of quality improvement to American industry over the past fifty years, and largely, were responsible for renewing the competitiveness of American industry. These quality improvement tools help reduce problems in the production and distribution of manufactured goods, but they have also been applied to companies that supply services. These service applications have led to the present use of quality improvement in healthcare (Lighter, 1999).

Ever since Shewhart, quality engineers have used innumerable tools to achieve process and outcome measurement. Although these tools have been applied in industry for decades, they have only recently found application in healthcare. Part of the reason for their increasing adoption by healthcare managers is the reliance on statistical thinking rather than rigorous statistical analysis. Statistical thinking is the approach of quality engineers that utilizes descriptive statistics to validate quality evaluations, without elaborate mathematical analysis. Descriptive statistics includes mean, variance, and standard deviation to evaluate quality improvement opportunities. Quality engineers have several frequently used tools available for quality improvement, e.g. Pareto charts, fishbone diagrams, histograms, run charts, check sheets, flowcharts, etc.

Quality improvement is based on the science of improvement that pursues knowledge of general truths or operation of general laws, especially those obtained and tested through the scientific method. To create improvement then, one needs knowledge relevant to the particular problem at hand. The science of improvement is concerned with how knowledge of a specific subject matter is applied in diverse situations. Based on real-life operating experience, both authors are of the view that, besides these seven basic tools, effective quality management of PACS can be improved via following scientific tools and their practical applications in the PACS environment will be illustrated in the following chapters:

a. **Quality Function Deployment (QFD):** To deal with the tasks of defining and analyzing PACS user wants and needs for the purpose of developing functional requirements. With QFD, Voice of PACS customers (VOPC) data is reduced into a set of critical customer needs using techniques such as affinity diagrams, function analysis, etc., defined and documented in customer needs data dictionary, and prioritized. This VOPC effort is also the opportunity to recognize unfulfilled needs that can provide, at a minimum, competitive advantage, and, potentially, a break-through product or true value innovation.

b. **Hardware and Software Reliability Modeling:** To estimate hardware and software reliability in an objective and practical manner. In today's technological world nearly everyone depends upon the continued functioning of a wide array of complex machinery and equipment for their everyday health, safety, mobility and economic welfare. We expect our PACS equipment to function whenever we need them - day after day, year after year. When they fail the results can be catastrophic: loss of life and/or costly lawsuits can occur. More often, repeated failure leads to annoyance, inconvenience and a lasting customer dissatisfaction that can cause confusion in the provision of radiological service. Failure characteristics would also provide the data needed for effective PACS risk evaluation and system development.

c.   **Failure Mode and Effects Analysis (FMEA):** For PACS risk analysis. It is a procedure that helps to identify every possible failure mode of a process or product, to determine its effect on other components and on the required function of the product or process. The FMEA is also used to rank and prioritize the possible causes of failures as well as develop and implement preventative actions, with responsible persons assigned to carry out these actions.

d.   **Internet Flow Control:** This is the process of managing the rate of data transmission between two nodes to prevent a fast sender from over running a slow receiver. Flow control mechanisms can be classified by whether or not the receiving node sends feedback to the sending node. Flow control is important because it is possible for a sending computer to transmit information at a faster rate than the destination computer can receive and process them. This can happen if the receiving computers have a heavy traffic load in comparison to the sending computer, or if the receiving computer has less processing power than the sending computer.

e.   **Human Factor Engineering (HFE):** To consider the impact of human factors. In the PACS environment, human factor engineering focuses on how people interact with tasks, PACS machines (or workstations), and the environment with the consideration that humans have limitations and capabilities. PACS technologists should evaluate "Human to Human," "Human to Group," "Human to Organizational," and "Human to PACS Machine " interactions to better understand these interactions and to develop a framework for evaluation. The goal of HFE is to maximize the ability of an individual or a PACS team to operate and maintain the system at required levels by eliminating design-induced difficulty and error.

For readers who are interested in advanced use of these tools, they may refer to the following references:

Six Sigma, Reliability and Human Factor Tools	Recommended further reading	Trial/Free/ Demo software templates/ download

QFD	(1) ISO 9126 standard (ISO/ IEC 9126: Information Technology - Software Product Evaluation - Quality characteristics and guidelines for their use - 1991) (2) QFD papers on healthcare (QFD Institute). Retrievable from http://www.qfdi.org/books/healthcare.htm	(1) Traditional and Extended QFD templates: http://www.qfdonline.com (2) Request For Proposal (RFP) templates: http://rfp.technologyevaluation.com/store.asp
Hardware & Software Reliability	(1) Reliability Growth and Repairable System Data Analysis Online Reference: http://www.weibull.com/relgrowthwebcontents.htm (2) Pham, H. (2006). System Software Reliability, Springer-Verlag.	(1) Life data analysis (Weibull analysis): http://www.reliasoft.com/products.htm#weibull (2) Reliability growth and repairable systems analysis: http://rg.reliasoft.com/
FMEA	Pyzdek, T. (2003). The Six Sigma Handbook, Revised and Expanded. McGraw-Hill.	Free FMEA tools from: http://www.fmeainfocentre.com/tools.htm
Internet Flow Control	Internetworking with TCP/IP, (By D.E. Comer, 2006, Prentice Hall: Upper Saddle River, NJ)	
Human Factors	(1) ElBardissi, A.W., Wiegmann, D.A., Dearani, J.A. Daly, R.C. & Sundt, T.M. Application of the human factors analysis and classification system methodology to the cardiovascular surgery operating room. Ann Thorac Surg. 83(4):1412-8, 2007. (2) Molloy, G.J., O'Boyle, C.A. The SHEL model: a useful tool for analyzing and teaching the contribution of Human Factors to medical error. Acad Med. 80(2):152-5, 2005. (3) Human Factors and Aviation Medicine home page: http://www.flightsafety.org/hfam_home.html	

REFERENCES

Bauman, R. A., & Gell, G. (2000). The Reality of PACS: A Survey. *Journal of Digital Imaging, 13*(4), 157-169.

Blado, M. W., & Tomlinson, A. B. (2002). Monitoring the Accuracy of a PACS Image Database. *Journal of Digital Imaging, 15*(supplement 1), 87-95.

Cox, B., & Dawe, N. (2002). Evaluation of a PACS System on an Intensive Care Unit. *Journal of Management in Medicine, 16*(2 & 3), 199-205.

DeLone, W. H., & McLean, E. R. (2003). The DeLone and McLean Model of Information Systems Success: A Tenyear Update. *Journal of MIS, 19*(4), 9-30.

Emery, F., & Trist, E. (1965). The causal texture of organizational environments. *Human Relations*, 18, 21-31.

Gale, D. R., et al. (2000). An Automated PACS Workstation Interface: A Timesaving Enhancement. *American Journal of Radiology, 174*, 33-36.

Gené-Badia, J., Jodar-Solà, G., Peguero-Rodríguez, E., Contel-Segura, J. C., & Moliner-Molins, C. (2001). The EFQM excellence model is useful for primary healthcare teams. *Family Practice, 18*, 407–409.

Hayt, D. B. (2001). Filmless in 60 days: The Impact of PACS within a large urban hospital. *Journal of Digital Imaging, 14*(2), 62-71.

Hertzberg, B. S. et al. (1999). PACS in Sonography: Accuracy of interpretation using film compared with monitor display. *American Journal of Radiology, 173*, 1175-1179.

Huang, H. K. (1999). *PACS – Basic Principles and Applications*. New York: John Wiley & Sons.

Lighter, D. E. (1999). Continuous Quality Improvement-What every physician leader needs to know. In Stahl, M. J. & Dean, P. J.(Eds), *The Physician's Essential MBA*. (pp.265-268). Gaithersburg, Maryland: Aspen Publications.

Lou, S. L. (1997). An automated PACS image acquisition and recovery scheme for image integrity based on the DICOM standard. *Computerized Medical Imaging and Graphics, 21*(4), 209-218.

Morgan, G (1980) Paradigms, metaphors and puzzle solving in organization theory *Administrative Science Quarterly,* 25, 605-622.

Osborn, A. F. (1963) *Applied imagination: Principles and procedures of creative problem solving* (Third Edition). NY: Charles Scribner's Sons.

Patankar, M. S., & Taylor, J. C. (2003). *Risk Management and Error Reduction in Aviation Maintenance.* London: Ashgate.

Pavlicek, W. et al. (1999). Quality of Service Improvement from Coupling a Digital Chest Unit with Integrated Speech Recognition, Information, and PACS. *Journal of Digital Imaging, 12*(4), 191-197.

Périard, M. A., & Chaloner, P. (1996) Diagnostic X-Ray Imaging Quality Assurance: An Overview. *Canadian Journal of Medical Radiation Technology, 27*(4), 171-177.

Pilling, J. R. (2003). Picture Archiving and Communication Systems: The Users' View. *British Journal of Radiology, 76*(908), 519-524.

Ralston, M. D., & Coleman, R. (2000). Sharing of a single arching and communications system among disparate institutions: Barriers to success. *Journal of Digital Imaging, 15*(supplement 1), 3-6.

Reiner, B. I., Siegel, E. L., & Sidiqqui, K. (2003). Evolution of the Digital Revolution: A Radiologist Perspective. *Journal of Digital Imaging, 16*(4), 324-330.

Susman, G. (1990). Work groups: Autonomy, technology, and choice. In P.S. Goodman & L.S. Sproull(Eds), *Assoc. Technology and Organizations* (pp.87-108). San Francisco: Jossey-Bass.

Trist, E. (1981). *The evolution of socio-technical systems.* Occasional Paper #2 Toronto: Ontario Quality of Working Life Centre.

Weick, K. (1979). *The social psychology of organizing.* (2nd ed.). Reading, Mass: Addison-Wesley.

Wong, T. T. (2006). The Human Side of Quality. In Shenzhen, P.R. (Ed.), *Proceedings of the First Pan Pearl River Delta Quality Forum.* China, October 25-27, 2006, 97-106.

Chapter X
Customer Oriented PACS

BACKGROUND

During the early development phase of PACS, its implementation was mainly a matter of the radiology department. This is changing rapidly, and PACS planning is increasingly seen in the context of a hospital-wide or regional approach. With increased networking among healthcare institutions and the growing relevance of teleradiology scenarios, PACS strategies must take not only local but also regional and global factors into consideration.

For hospitals and healthcare institutions, quality function deployment (QFD) is a helpful tool for developing new systems or services. QFD was originally developed by Yoji Akao in 1966 when the author combined his work in quality assurance and quality control points with function deployment used in Value Engineering. QFD has been described as "a method to transform user demands into design quality, to deploy the functions forming quality, and to deploy methods for achieving the design quality into subsystems and component parts, and ultimately to specific elements of the manufacturing process" (Mizuno & Akao, 1994). QFD is designed to help planners focus on characteristics of a new or existing product or service from the viewpoints of market segments, company, or technology-development needs. The technique yields graphs and matrices. It is widely accepted that benefits of using QFD in the healthcare industry include:

- Increased customer satisfaction
- Improved quality
- Time efficiency
- Multidiscilplinary teamwork orientation
- Documentation orientation

The QFD method has been successfully applied to many industrial and manufacturing processes in order to ensure that quality is built into products at the outset rather than tested for after their production. However, this method has rarely been applied in the healthcare industry.

Moores (2005) presents a study of the potential for applying the QFD method to the analysis of the framework for safety management contained in the Ionizing Radiation (Medical Exposure) Regulations (IRMER) of 2000. In his chapter, the term quality is used to describe the degree to which the needs and requirements of the customer are fulfilled. In the case of diagnostic radiology, it was noted that safety management must not only be concerned with radiation protection but, more importantly, with the accuracy and consistency of any diagnostic outcome. According to Moores, both should be treated as important patient needs. A first stage analysis of IRMER 2000 was presented and assessed how patients' needs had been expressed by the individual IRMER components of justification, optimization, clinical audit, expert advice, equipment, and training. The analysis involved a QFD assessment by four radiation protection experts with over 100 man-years of experience. A second stage analysis assessed how the individual IRMER components had been engineered into a safety management framework through specific requirements embodied in IRMER 2000. The results of this assessment were discussed in terms of clinical, human, operational management, and equipment related aspects of the radiological process. The study highlights how the QFD approach may be applied to engineer specific aspects of radiological practice that play a key role in ensuring that patients' needs are fully met. As an example, clinical audit requirements were analyzed by means of the QFD method to indicate the design requirements of information and knowledge based systems that could provide the necessary information for this type of key management activity.

Due to recent reforms in Sweden, the demands on the people working in community-oriented healthcare service are increasing. The individual providers need professional knowledge and skills to perform their tasks quickly and safely. The individuals are also confronted with new tasks and situations of which they lack experience. At the same time, the resources for education and development are decreasing. Some work was done to describe the implementation of a prototype computer network service to support occupational therapists in their daily work (Hallberg et al, 1999). A customized QFD model, including participatory design elements, was used for: (a) identification of the occupational therapists' needs, and (b) for the transformation of these needs to prioritized design attributes. The main purpose of the prototype was to improve the visualization of the design attributes that were found to support the occupational therapists. An additional purpose was to be able to evaluate the design attributes and further improve them. The specific aim of this article is to describe the initial prototype with respect both to the tools and the information content.

Quality function deployment (QFD) was used in a healthcare system to deploy the voices of the customers in understanding their requirements and to include them for continuous improvement of quality in services provided (Radharamanan, & Godoy, 1996). The results have been analyzed as a function of: patients' reception when they arrive at hospital, the room environment where they are hospitalized when treatment is needed with specialized professional assistance, the meals quality, and the assistance from the nurse ward. These four types of benefits that are obtained with the house of quality identify opportunities for future improvements and encourage programs for improving service quality in the healthcare systems.

With regard to the understanding of the necessities of the patients, the results obtained show that there exists really a lack of information, principally in admitting patients in the hospital. Other problem that appears is the lime spent by the patient in the "waiting room", before attended by the doctor. There are many critics made about the waiting time in the doctor's consulting room in the hospital. With regard to the room the complaints are about the presence of insects principally during the warm seasons. Other information obtained was about the meals, many times served cold, but quantity served is sufficient. There were no complaints about the nurses. They are always in contact with the patients and try to transmit the information clearly about the treatment.

After two decades of operation, PACS in Europe is now moving toward a more strategic, rather than situational solution-seeking approach (Lemke, 2001). This is best exemplified by the preparation of a Request For Proposal through QFD in a reference project in Saxony, Germany. The QFD approach to PACS planning was tried in SaxTeleMed, a regional PACS project involving seven groups of hospitals throughout Saxony in Germany, and at University Hospital Zurich in Switzerland. This project will be discussed in detail later in this chapter.

As indicated in the Minutes of DICOM WG24 meeting (#3) held in November 2005 at Chicago, USA, it was agreed that a formal method should be employed to specify surgical PACS functions and to serve as a basis for definitions of DICOM objects and services. And the general chair agreed to introduce concepts and tools of QFD for specifications of surgical PACS functions in the following meeting (DI-COM, 2005). Indeed Korb et al (2005) reported the use of QFD in the development of a surgical picture acquisition and communication System (S-PACS), according to the systems engineering cycle. The first two steps (concept and specification) for the engineering of the S-PACS are discussed. A method for the systematic integration of the users needs', the quality function deployment (QFD), is presented. The properties of QFD for the underlying problem and first results are also discussed. Finally, this leads to a first definition of an S-PACS system.

THE QFD PROCESS

The QFD process comprises following steps:

1. **Product planning:** Acquiring voice of the customer, priorities and weight the voice of customer.
2. **Benchmarking:** Competitive evaluation.
3. **Design planning:** Matching engineering capabilities to customer needs and deciding trade-offs for design process.
4. **Process planning:** Target process identification from House of Quality (HOQ) matrix.
5. **Production:** Process planning provides the basis for production.

House of Quality

The house of quality (HOQ) matrix is an assembly of PACS requirements, viz. voice of customers (VOC) (the customer in a PACS project may be the patient, physician, nursing staff, administration, department manager or other stakeholder, depending on the process being reviewed), clinical requirements, patient perceptions, inter-relationships and target services. The VOC is a process used to capture the requirements/feedback from the customer (internal or external) to provide the customers with the best in PACS service quality. This process is all about being proactive and constantly innovative to capture the changing requirements of the customers with time.

The VOC is the term used to describe the stated and unstated needs or requirements of the customer. The voice of the customer can be captured in a variety of ways: Direct discussion or personal interviews, surveys, focus groups, customer specifications, observation, warranty data, field reports, complaint logs, etc. This data is used to identify the quality attributes needed for a supplied component or software to incorporate in the PACS process or product. Figure 1 shows a PACS

Figure 1. A PACS house of quality

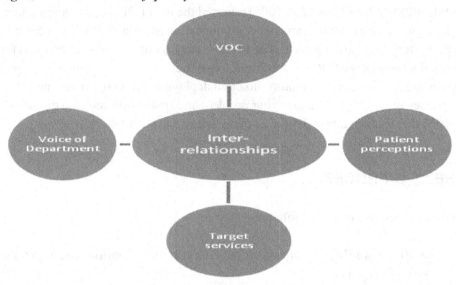

HOQ, readers may refer to Akao's (1990) monograph on Quality Function Deployment for detailed construction procedure of a HOQ. There are many ways to plan, implement and manage a PACS. Huang (1999) provides a valuable reference on basic principles and applications of PACS. In addition, there are numerous journals and conference proceedings which may be consulted to develop an understanding of the complexity of PACS and possible solution strategies for implementations. This chapter focuses on planning aspects for introducing a PACS in a hospital environment. Starting with objectives and possible methodological approaches, emphasis is given to a request for proposal (RFP) and the evaluation of corresponding tenders.

PACS Request for Proposal

Starting with a vision and specifically with some healthcare objectives for a hospital setting, a suitable plan should be worked out for the organization. The clinical and/or cost-benefit justification should be clearly stated. Typical clinical justifications may focus on objectives for improving:

- Patient management and bed occupancy.
- Patient outcome and satisfaction.
- Communication between healthcare personnel.

A highly connected radiology department with a workflow supporting real-time services can support these objectives. In addition, a cost-benefit justification may be pursued with objectives such as:

- Efficient utilization of human and material resources.
- Effective controlling of the number and cost of procedures per year.
- Improving the tangible and intangible benefits.
- Reducing running costs of services, maintenance and upgrades.

It can be assumed that the falling cost of information technology for realizing a filmless radiological department and hospital will support these cost-benefit objectives. Based on the above justifications, a more detailed project planning phase could be initiated with the following steps (Marshall, 1999):

1. Establish the mechanisms for information collection, and evaluation.
2. Establish the medical, technical, structural, and organizational aims.
3. Identify the users and their work patterns.
4. Define a project team.
5. Define the achievable deadlines for each state of the project.
6. Define the systems requirements.

A major result of the project planning phase is an effective RFP. One part of the RFP describes the institution for which the PACS is planned for and the general, administrative and legal requirements the vendors with their tenders have to fulfill. In the other part of the RFP, the specific technical and operational requirements of the PACS have to be described. These should include the desired systems characteristics and components (subsystems), standards, interfaces, data protection and security, and type of project management. In addition, some information on cost expectation and the criteria used for evaluating the RFP may be given to the vendor. This information, however, is handled differently by different hospitals. A structural approach is particularly helpful in preparing the RFP, and subsequently the product and system evaluations. A suitable approach for creating a RFP can be derived from quality function deployment (QFD) techniques.

The QFD methodology is based on a strong involvement of the user in determining system requirements with clearly stated importance ratings. Suitable hardware and software attributes are selected to meet the user requirements (UR). Constructed as a HOQ template, it can be applied to the PACS environment. Contribution of QFD in a recent European project is shown next.

CASE EXAMPLE: SaxTeleMed PROJECT

Problem Description

PACS in Europe is moving toward a more strategic, rather than situational solution-seeking approach. According to Professor Lemke of Berlin University, this is best exemplified by a reference project in Saxony, Germany, called SaxTeleMed (Leuke, 2001). The project was initiated by the Ministry of Social Welfare, Health, Youth and Family of the Free State of Saxony. It covers seven regional projects distributed throughout Saxony. Each regional project is organized around so-called lead hospitals, which network with other cooperating hospitals and medical practices. The regional reference projects are designed to be largely independent, although in some instances, a network connection between them is also considered. Altogether, thirty-nine hospitals and medical centers are involved.

The aim of the program is to test the technical, organizational, legal, and economic problems in digitization and networking within Saxony. The knowledge gained from this project is expected to improve future PACS investment decisions in healthcare and, above all, to implement secure systems. An innovative aspect of the project is the development of a quality function deployment (QFD) method for PACS specification and selection.

Public healthcare in the Free State of Saxony is represented by 90 hospitals and two university clinics. When the state government came into office in the autumn of 1990, fundamental deficiencies in the hospitals of Saxony had to be remedied and the in-patient medical care of the population needed substantial improvement.

The initial situation was characterized by a dismal state of repair in the hospitals, often unacceptable hygiene conditions, and the deficient quality of the medical equipment as well as the lack of modern medical-technical equipment. Hospital administration faced the task of adjusting the overcapacity of hospital beds from the German Democratic Republic period (which had arisen because of a shortage of nursing home places and a lack of outpatient care) to a level of capacity suited to regional demand. In this restructuring, not only were overcapacities eliminated, but necessary new services were created, in heart surgery and cancer therapy, in particular.

As SaxTeleMed covers its seven telemedicine projects, the focus is on radiology. The seven hospitals in Saxony designated as lead hospitals correspond to the number of projects: Zwickau Heinrich Braun Hospital, Chemnitz General Hospital, Erlabrunn Hospital, Dresden-Neustadt City Hospital, Zittau District Hospital, Dresden-Friedrichstadt General Hospital, and Riesa District Hospital. In these lead hospitals, a restructuring into an almost filmless hospital is meant to take place by means of digitization and image communication that spreads out from radiology to other departments. Some of the aspects observed and investigated in this process include the following:

- Digital x-ray image evaluation and communication for faster delivery of therapy in the hospital and transmission to external medical institutions, from which patients are admitted;
- Carrying out of consultations by digital exchange of patient information;
- Digital transmission of image and report information from or to the medical institutions from which patients are admitted;
- Assessment and comparison of the use of telemedicine in emergency situations and in general medical processes; and
- Setting-up and testing of different forms of short- and long-term archiving of x-ray images and reports.

Supervision being carried out by a scientific advisory board is intended to ensure transparent and efficient project specification, selection, implementation and evaluation. Fifteen recognized experts from the fields of medicine, economics, and informatics have been appointed to this board from different regions of Germany. Appropriate standards and structural guidelines have been given by this board to the lead hospitals.

Call for Tenders and Implementation

Clearly defined digital modalities and KIS/RIS/PACS structures as well as agreed communication relations between the co-operation partners form the basis for a successful implementation of the projects (Saxony Ministry of Social Affairs, 2001). In 1999 tenders were invited for a regional development project concerning the networking of the hospitals and practices in order to mandate a general contractor for each of the seven projects who has to assume the overall responsibility for the hardware and software equipment as well as for the successful implementation of the digital picture communication. The call for tenders was based on a comprehensive specification including (applicable to all model projects in the same way) the general requirements to the standards, data protection, maintenance and repair, migration, business conditions etc. as well as the project-specific requirements. 49 firms applied as tenderers for the EU-wide awarding announcement. After a pre-selection of the applicants the project managers requested twelve firms to submit their offers. These offers were assessed on the basis of target criteria in assessment procedures developed for this (e.g. on the basis of the quality function deployment / QFD). The decision made on this basis as to the awarding was defended before the scientific board by each project.

RFP Through QFD

A working approach for creating a RFP was derived from QFD technique. The basic approach was to prepare an n-level hierarchical tree structure of the user requirements, referred to as the UR-tree. For a typical PACS, this may contain up to five levels of detail, with 0 as the highest and 4 as the lowest level. For one hospital of SaxTeleMed, almost 400 different requirements have been structured in this way. The selection of the requirements and their structure reflect the basic content of the RFP.

Some or all levels of the UR are assigned importance ratings (IR) and impact factors (IF). This facilitates the evaluation of the PACS technology and viability of the potential vendor solution. The IR parameter is given in percentages and describes the weight with which a specific requirement contributes to the UR of the next higher level in the hierarchy. It was determined by experts in the PACS project team independently of any expected solution offered in the tenders by the vendors.

Engineering attributes (EA) are features in the offering or tender of the vendor that are examined in relation to the fulfillment of the URs. For the Dresden-Friedrichstadt project, eight top level (level 0) UR's have been chosen. They are:

1. System Characteristics
2. Standards and Interfaces
3. Data Protection and Data Security
4. System Components
5. Project Management
6. Service
7. Integration into the Reference Project
8. Prices

The degree of fulfillment of these URs is parameterized by means of the widely accepted evaluation scale with the following parameter setting:

0: no fulfillment
1: low degree fulfillment
3: satisfactory fulfillment
9: complete fulfillment

This scale allows for a strong differentiation between no and complete fulfillment of the URs. After the successful implementation of the SaxTeleMed project, this RFP methodology has been used for PACS planning in other hospitals, such as the Zurich University Hospital in Switzerland. After evaluating the UR-tree, a suitable method of graphical representation of the result is a circle circumscribing a polygon whose corners represent the degree of fulfillment of the top level UR's.

Project Evaluation

Under the overall control of the scientific board a so-called three-level evaluation was developed for the assessment of the process and the results of the model programme. The evaluation levels 1 and 2 are established in a uniform, comparable and transferable way for and to all seven model projects. The evaluation of the use of the international communication standards (DICOM and HL7) required in the specification is the purpose of evaluation level 1.

At the second evaluation level a service process evaluation of the overall internal and external picture and findings communication as well as a cost analysis on the basis of an 'Activity Based Costing' (ABC) is made. The influence of the digital picture and findings communication is recorded as to the waiting period of transmission, on the one hand, and, on the other hand, the cost development of the service rendering considering the organizational concepts and the structural development (cooperation and division of labour) is evaluated.

At a third evaluation level specific questions of technical, medical and organizational nature are investigated which are related to the respective textual focal points of the individual projects.

Observations

A structural approach was carried out for the preparation of a RFP and evaluation of corresponding tenders. According to Lemke and his associates (2001), many questions, however, remain to be solved for a particular institution when actually applying the method. In particular, there are no recommendations on (i) the members responsible for assigning the values for the IR's and after tender examination, the values for the EA's, (ii) the method of reaching consensus on the parameter assignments, (iii) whether the detailed UR-tree structure with explicitly stated IR's and IF's could be communicated to the potential vendors, and (iv) what other criteria, for example trust between staff, social accountability, future trends of radio imaging, etc. in addition to the top UR levels should be considered for the final selection of the PACS vendor. As a general conclusion, it can be stated that the proposed QFD approach provides a valuable tool for a transparent discussion of UR's in a PACS environment.

A Modified QFD for PACS

To facilitate solving the remaining problems, it is recommended that scientific tools such as analytic hierarchy process (AHP) and theory of inventive problem solving (TRIZ) be used in combination with the QFD method. A brief description of these two tools is given below.

Analytic Hierarchy Process (AHP)

Rather than prescribing a "correct" decision, the AHP helps people to determine one. Based on mathematics and human psychology, it was developed by Thomas L. Saaty in the 1970s (Saaty, 1977; Saaty, 1996) and has been extensively studied and refined since then. The AHP provides a comprehensive and rational framework for structuring a problem, for representing and quantifying its elements, for relating those elements to overall goals, and for evaluating alternative solutions. It is used throughout the world in a wide variety of decision situations, and has been successfully applied in fields such as regulatory bodies, business, industry, healthcare, and education.

An important advantage of the AHP is that it allows for inconsistency in judgment. However, the AHP also measures the degree to which the judgments are inconsistent and establishes an acceptable tolerance level for the degree of inconsistency. Other advantages and the disadvantages of the AHP have been extensively described and debated elsewhere. For example, a series of articles in Management Science (Dyer, 1990; Harker and Vargas, 1990; Winkler, 1990) address the comparisons of the AHP and multi-attribute utility theory.

Eckman (1989) offers a critique of the AHP and argues that the pairwise comparisons are arbitrary, differences in factors such as costs and infection rates are subjectively interpreted, and the modeling approach does not adequately represent the decision making problem and produces a unitless, and therefore meaningless, score. Dolan (1990) and Dolan and Bordley (1993) have argued convincingly against these claims. A tutorial on the use of the AHP in medical decision making has been offered by Dolan et al. (1989). These authors also describe the theory of the AHP and demonstrate how it can be applied to a typical medical decision. Feeg (1999) reports that the AHP compares favorably with magnitude estimation scaling for developing the weights for a set of elements such as subjects' intensity of perceptions in nursing studies.

Several authors have discussed the use of the AHP across a broad range of applications in health and medical decision making. Hatcher (1994) describes how the AHP can be included within a group decision support process and how the resulting system can be applied in a variety of health care decision making settings. Sloane et al. (2002) discusses the applicability of the AHP for medical and hospital decision support and briefly describes three completed studies and three on-going studies.

The above review, together with other AHP applications to health care and medical decision making problems, suggest continued interest in the use of this method. It appears to be well suited to group decision making environments in health care. Although interest in diagnosis seems to have faded, patient participation and therapy/treatment are two application areas of continuing interest. For example, the AHP appears to be a promising support tool for shared decision making between patient and doctor. One major obstacle to implementation is physician acceptance. Physicians are not accustomed to using formalized methods to assist in decision making. It is expected that this barrier becomes less relevant as more and more successful applications are documented.

The AHP has seen extensive and on-going use in the evaluation and selection of medical technology, and capital and information systems projects (Liberatore & Nydick, 2008). Recently, there has been increased interest in its application for evaluating health care facilities. For instance, one could first decompose the RFP problem into a hierarchy of more easily comprehended sub-problems, each of which can be analyzed independently. The elements of the hierarchy can relate to any aspect of the decision problem—tangible or intangible, carefully measured or roughly estimated, well- or poorly-understood—anything at all that applies to the decision at hand. Once the hierarchy is built, decision makers can systematically evaluate its various elements, comparing them to one another in pairs. In making the comparisons, the decision makers can use objective data about the elements, or they can use their judgments about the elements' relative meaning and importance. It is the essence of the AHP that human judgments, and not just the underlying information, can be used in performing the evaluations. The AHP converts these evaluations to numerical data that can be processed and compared over the entire range of the problem. A numerical weighting factor or priority is derived for each element of the hierarchy, allowing diverse and often incommensurable elements to be compared to one another in a rational and consistent way. This capability distinguishes the AHP from other decision making techniques. In the final step of the process, numerical priorities are derived for each of the decision alternatives. Since these numbers represent the alternatives' relative ability to achieve targets.

Theory of Inventive Problem Solving (TRIZ)

Theory of inventive problem solving (TRIZ) was developed by Genrich Altshuller and his colleagues in the former USSR starting in 1946, and is now being developed and practiced throughout the world. TRIZ research began with the hypothesis that there are universal principles of invention that are the basis for creative innovations that advance technology, and that if these principles could be identified and codified, they could be taught to people to make the process of invention more predictable. The research has proceeded in several stages over the last 50 years. Over 2 million patents have been examined, classified by level of inventiveness, and analyzed to look for principles of innovation. The three primary findings of this research are as follows:

1.   Problems and solutions were repeated across industries and sciences.
2.   Patterns of technical evolution were repeated across industries and sciences.
3.   Innovations used scientific effects outside the field where they were developed.

In the application of TRIZ all three of these findings are applied to create and to improve products, services, and systems. It was noted that large and small companies are using TRIZ on many levels to solve real, practical everyday problems and to develop strategies for the future of technology. TRIZ is in use at Ford, Motorola, Procter & Gamble, Eli Lilly, Jet Propulsion Laboratories, 3M, Siemens, Phillips, LG, and hundreds more.

Altshuller believed that inventive problems stem from contradictions (one of the basic TRIZ concepts) between two or more elements, such as, "If we want to view high resolution images, we need a larger number of advanced display stations but that will increase the cost of the system," that is, more of something desirable also brings more of something less desirable, or less of something else also desirable (Altshuller et al, 2005). These are called Technical Contradictions by Altshuller. He also defined so-called physical or inherent contradictions: More of one thing and less of another may be needed. For instance, a higher temperature may be needed to melt a compound more rapidly, but a lower temperature may be needed to achieve a homogeneous mixture. An inventive situation might involve several such contradictions. In the case of PACS, the display station supplier typically trades one contradictory parameter for another; no special inventiveness is needed for that. Rather, he would develop some creative approaches for resolving the contradiction, such as inventing display stations that facilitates the generation of high resolution images without increasing the cost of the PACS.

Altshuller screened patents in order to find out what kind of contradictions were resolved or dissolved by the invention and the way this had been achieved. From this he developed a set of 40 inventive principles and later a Matrix of Contradictions. Rows of the matrix indicate the 39 system features that one typically wants to improve, such as speed, weight, accuracy of measurement and so on. Columns refer to typical undesired results. Each matrix cell points to principles that have been most frequently used in patents in order to resolve the contradiction. For readers interested in TRIZ method of creativity and innovation, they may refer to the online TRIZ journal, which contains the Contradiction Matrix and 40 principles, case studies and best practices (CTQ Media, 2008).

Hence one could combine TRIZ and AHP with QFD to generate more inventive solutions for PACS projects such as RFP.

CONCLUDING REMARK

The fundamental principle of a QFD is to gather all relevant information about the user requirements and use this information to drive the design of PACS services. Several tools can be integrated into the QFD process to facilitate the deployment of this information throughout the design and manufacturing processes, and to all relevant organizational functions. In the present context AHP and TRIZ have been suggested to combine with the traditional QFD to form the PACS-QFD.

In PACS design one could first use AHP to identify the user segments and to prioritize the users. Gathering the voice of the users and the context of use is an important second step. Again AHP can be used to prioritize the verbatim information. However, the context of use defines the location in which the PACS must function or the service be performed. These constraints often create design bottlenecks for which QFD provides no means for resolution. For this reason TRIZ could be employed as the innovation tool to overcome the psychological inertia or mental block commonly encountered. It is highly likely that through TRIZ the PACS team would be able to spawn new and perhaps unorthodox ideas in PACS design.

REFERENCES

Akao, Y. (1990) *Quality function deployment.* Cambridge: Productivity Press.

Altshuller, G., Clarke, D. W., Shulyak, L., & Lerner, L. (2005). *40 Principles: TRIZ Keys to Innovation* [Extended Edition] (Paperback), Technical Innovation Centre, Worcester, MA.

CTQ Media. (July 2008). *The TRIZ Journal* [Electronic Version]. Available from the CTQ Online Web Site, http://www.triz-journal.com/

DICOM WG24 November 29, 2005 Minutes. (2005). Retrieved on 31 January 2008 from http://medical.nema.org/DICOM/minutes/WG-24/2005/2005-11-29/Minutes_2005-11-29_Chicago_DICOM_WG-24.pdf.

Dolan, J. G. (1989). Medical decision making using the analytic hierarchy process: Choice of initial antimicrobial therapy for acute pyelonephritis. *Medical Decision Making, 9*(1), 51–56.

Dolan, J. G. (1990). Can decision analysis adequately represent clinical problems. *Journal of Clinical Epidemiology, 43*(3), 277–284.

Dolan J. G., & Bordley, D. R. (1993). Involving patients in complex decisions about their care: An approach using the analytic hierarchy process, *Journal of General Internal Medicine, 8*(4), 204–209.

Dyer, J. S. (1990). Remarks on the analytic hierarchy process. *Management Science, 36*(3), 249–258.

Eckman, M. H. (1989). A counterpoint to the analytic hierarchy process. *Medical Decision Making, 9*(1), 57–58

Feeg, V. D. (1999). Using the analytic hierarchy process as an alternative weighting technique to magnitude estimation scaling. *Nursing Research, 48*(6), 333–339.

Hallberg, N., Johansson, M., & Timpka, T. (1999). A prototype computer network service for occupational therapists.*Computer Methods and Programs in Biomedicine, 59*(1), 45-54.

Harker P. T., & Vargas, L. G. (1990). Reply to 'Remarks on the analytic hierarchy process' by J.S. Dyer. *Management Science, 36*(3), 269–273.

Hatcher, M. (1994). Voting and priorities in health care decision making, portrayed through a group decision support system, using analytic hierarchy process. *Journal of Medical Systems, 18* (5), 267–288.

Huang, H. K. (1999). *PACS basic principles and applications*. New York: Wiley-Liss.

Korb, W., Bohn, S., Burgert, O., Dietz, A., Jacobs, S., Falk, V., Meixensberger, J., Straus. G., Trantakis, C., & Lemke, H. U. (2005). H.U. Surgical PACS for the Digital Operating Room Systems Engineering and Specification of User Requirements. *Studies in Health and Informatics, 119*, 267-272.

Lemke, H. U. (2001). *Regional PACS projects take shape in Europe*. Retrieved 16 January, 2008 from http://www.dimag.com/pacsweb/printer_friendly/?articleID=47901454.

Lemke, H. U., Niederlag, W., Heuser, H., & Pollack, T. (2001). *PACS Planning and Evaluation using Quality Function Deployment*. Retrieved 16 January 2008 from http://www.uniklinikum-giessen.de/kis-ris-pacs/archiv/2001/di1015.pdf

Liberatore, L. J., & Nydick, R. L. (2008). The analytic hierarchy process in medical and health care decision making: A literature review. *European Journal of Operational Research, 189*(1), 194-207.

Maddux ,G. at al. (1991). Organizations can apply quality function deployment as strategic planning tool. *Industrial Engineering*, 33-37.

Marshall, M. (1999). An imaging department for the new millennium? *Developing a PACS system for King's College Hospital, Accessing the Futur*e, *4*, 9-118.

Mizuno, S., & Akao, Y. (1994). *QFD: The Customer Driven Approach to Quality Planning and Deployment.* Asian Productivity Organization.

Moores, B. M. (2006). Radiation safety management in healthcare – The application of Quality Function Deployment. *Radiography, 12*(4), 291-304.

Radharamanan, R., & Godoy, L. P. (1996). Quality function deployment as applied to a healthcare system. *Computers & Industrial Engineering, 31*(1-2), 443-446.

Saaty, T. L. (1977). A scaling method for priorities in hierarchical structures. *Journal of Mathematical Psychology, 15*, 234–281.

Saaty, T. L. (1996). *The Analytic Hierarchy Process.* Pittsburgh: RWS Publications.

Saxony Ministry of Social Affairs (2001) *SaxTeleMed - Thesis paper to the Model Program.* Retrieved 4 July 2008 from http://www.gesunde.sachsen.de/download/saxtelemed_eng.pdf

Sloane, E. B., Liberatore, M. J., & Nydick, R. L. (2002). Medical decision support using the Analytic Hierarchy Process, *Journal of Healthcare Information Management, 16*(4), 38–43.

Winkler, R. L. (1990). Decision Modeling and rational choice, AHP and utility theory. *Management Science, 36*(3), 247–248.

Chapter XI
Design for PACS Reliability

INTRODUCTION

Nowadays it is hard to think of any applications in modern society in which electronic systems do not play a significant role. In aerospace and aviation, defence, telecommunication and healthcare, to name a few, computers have already assumed the most life-critical tasks. Unlike most human beings, computers seem to do their job pretty well, at most times and under all environmental conditions. Sometimes, however, for some reason, the fresh water supply in a city stops, the mainframe computer of an international security exchange centre malfunctions, or the satellite television goes out abruptly. Possible sources for such dissatisfactory performances are physical deterioration or design faults in hardware components. Fortunately in the 1950s and 1960s quite a number of reliability models were developed for hardware. Another major source for malfunctioning of computer systems is the presence of bugs in the software that controls the system. The modelling of software reliability was only begun in the early 1970s.

This chapter presents a comprehensive approach to the development of a reliable PACS, which are capable of meeting the high-quality level required of mission-critical medical devices. To develop a preliminary design, the PACS team would begin with a system description and reliability evaluation of a baseline system, including implementation of hardware redundancy, software provisions, and acceptance test. Through detailed system analyses and electrical, electronic and mechanical reliability studies, a final preliminary design can be derived. In this chapter the essential mathematical and statistical aspects of hardware and software reliability predictions are first presented, followed by a spreadsheet-based approach to model hardware and software reliabilities. A method of designing higher system reliability through parallel and cross-linked configurations is then given. Finally a brief case on the acceptance test of a PACS software is illustrated.

BASIC CONCEPTS

Since the use of PACS raises both medical and social concerns, it cannot be instituted without addressing concerns related to the reliability and security issues. Reliability encompassed hardware and software reliability, including the retrieval of the previously obtained images. Reliability may be defined as the ability of a system to operate correctly according to its specification for a given time interval (Musa et al., 1987), under the precondition that the system operates correctly at the beginning of this time interval. Traditionally, system reliability is measured in terms of mean time between failures or the failure probability of a system function. To predict the reliability of component-based systems many methods have been proposed (Goseva-Popstojanova & Trivedi, 2001). The basic concept of these methods is to identify failure probabilities for each service of a component and determine the reliability of system functions based on the call sequences and dependencies between the low-level services and the specific system function.

PACS technologists are in many ways like soothsayers - they are expected to predict many things for the PACS: how many failures from this and that lot will occur within x number of years, how much of this and that lot will survive after x number of years, what will happen if a device is operated under these conditions, etc. Fortunately, they do not need any paranormal abilities to give intelligent responses to questions involving failures that have not yet happened. All they need is a good understanding of statistics and reliability mathematics to be up to the task.

In the present context, reliability is defined as the probability that software, component, device, or the entire PACS will perform its prescribed duty without failure for a given time when operated correctly in a specified environment. Reliability assessment, or the process of determining to a certain degree of confidence the reliability of a PACS, applies various statistical analysis techniques to analyze reliability data. If properly done, a reliability prediction using such techniques will match the survival behavior of the system, many years after the prediction was made.

By looking at the time to failure data or life distribution of a set of samples taken from a given population of PACS devices after they are operated in the field for some period, the PACS team can assess how the rest of the population will fail in future. Three important descriptors of PACS component life distributions should be understood by every PACS technologist. These are the cumulative failure distribution function F(t), the failure probability density function f(t), and the curve of failure rate λ(t).

The cumulative failure distribution function F(t), or simply cumulative distribution function, gives the probability of a failure occurring before or at any time, t. This function is also known as the unreliability function. If a population of PACS (or its devices) is operated from its initial use up to a certain time t, then the ratio of failures, c(t), to the total number of devices tested, n, is F(t). Thus, F(t) = c(t)/n. The unreliability function F(t) has an equivalent opposite function - the reliability function R(t). R(t) = 1 - F(t), so it simply gives the ratio of units that are still good to the total number of devices after these devices have operated from initial use up to a time t.

The failure probability density function f(t) gives the relative frequency of failures at any given time, t. It is related to F(t) and R(t) by the equation:

$$f(t) = dF(t)/dt = - dR(t)/dt$$

The curve of failure rate λ(t), also known as the failure rate function or the hazard function, gives the instantaneous failure rate at any given time t. It is related to f(t) and R(t) by this equation:

$$\lambda(t) = f(t)/R(t)$$

Thus, $\lambda(t) = f(t)/[1-F(t)]$

OVERVIEW OF FAILURE DISTRIBUTIONS

There are currently four failure distributions commonly used in electronic engineering and software reliability today, namely, the normal distribution, the exponential distribution, the lognormal distribution, and the Weibull distribution. Different failure mechanisms will result in time-to-failure data that fit different life distributions, so it is up to the PACS team to select which life distribution would best model the failure mechanism of interest. A review of recent literature would indicate the versatility of the Weibull distribution. Its application in mining, meteorology, manufacturing, non-destructive evaluation, electronic device reliability, materials science and engineering, environmental management, toxicology, etc. are shown below.

The performance of mining machines depends on the reliability of the equipment used, the operating environment, the maintenance efficiency, the operation process, the technical expertise of the miners, etc. As the size and complexity of mining equipments continue to increase, the implications of equipment failure become ever more critical. Therefore, reliability analysis is required to identify the bottlenecks in the system and to find the components or subsystems with low reliability for a given designed performance. It is important to select a suitable method for data collection as well as for reliability analysis. A case study describing reliability and availability analysis of the crushing plant number 3 at Jajarm Bauxite Mine in Iran was reported recently (Barabady & Kumar, 2008). In this study, the crushing plant number 3 is divided into six subsystems. The parameters of some probability distributions, such as Weibull, Exponential, and Lognormal distributions have been estimated by using a commercial software. The results of the analysis show that the conveyer subsystem and secondary screen subsystem are critical from a reliability point of view, and the secondary crusher subsystem and conveyer subsystem are critical from an availability point of view. The study also shows that the reliability analysis is very useful for deciding maintenance intervals.

An attempt was made to construct a database for the users of the wind power in Tunisia (Elamouri & Amar, 2008). It analyses 17 synoptic sites distributed over all the territory of Tunisia. From the meteorological data provided by the Meteorology National Institute, meteorological and Weibull methods are used to evaluate the wind speed characteristics and the wind power potential at a height of 10 m above ground level and in an open area. An extrapolation of these characteristics with the height is also carried out. The results obtained give a global vision of the distribution of the wind potential in Tunisia and define the windiest zones.

A comparative study of exponential distribution vs. Weibull distribution in machine reliability analysis within a cellular manufacturing system (CMS) design was carried out by Das (2008). The paper addresses machine reliability consideration by Weibull and exponential distribution approach in designing a CMS. A multi-objective mixed integer programming model that considers machine system reliability and system cost simultaneously is presented to implement the approach. When a part has the option to be processed in alternative routes, the route with the highest system reliability can be selected by considering individual machine reliabilities along each route. It is noted that a CMS design approach which selects processing routes for the part types with maximum system reliability, considering the machines along routes while optimizing system cost, will improve the overall performance of the system. The rerouting provision of the part types, integrated with the approach, will also help the user/designer to solve machine breakdown problems during processing of a part. This study offers the capability to model different failure characteristics, such as, an increasing, decreasing or constant machine failure rate.

A non-destructive evaluation method for predicting the residual tensile strength of erosion damaged fiber-reinforced composites was developed based on monitoring the acoustic emission (AE) activity of the composite specimens during uniaxial tensile loading (Yang et al, 2008). The developed method was used for estimating the residual strength of E-glass/epoxy composite. A mixture of air and SiC particles with diameter of 400–500 μm was blasted to the composite specimens at various impact angles and durations to induce the local damage. Subsequently, uniaxial tensile tests were carried out on the specimens subjected to solid particle erosion as well as undamaged specimens while monitoring the acoustic emission activity. The extent and mechanisms of damage due to tensile loading of composite specimens were explored by examining the failure surface upon completion of tensile tests under a scanning electron microscope (SEM) and by measuring the distribution of AE events by event duration, ring down counts and energy distribution during tensile tests. Weibull distribution and AE stress delay parameter models were developed to relate the AE activity to the erosion damage and residual strength. The results show that the developed non-destructive method is capable of predicting the residual strength of composites subjected to solid particle damage.

The dielectric breakdown field is one of the important concerns for device reliability. The breakdown of dielectric is originated at a fatal flaw that grows to cause failure and can be explained by the weakest-link theory. In a study on metal-insulator-metal (MIM) capacitors with plasma enhanced chemical vapor deposited (PECVD) SiN_x, ammonia (NH_3) plasmas were applied after the deposition of the dielectric SiN_x. The Weibull distribution function, which is based on the weakest-link theory, is employed to analyze the effect of the electrode area as well as the plasma treatment on the breakdown of the MIM capacitors (Ho & Chiou, 2008). The time dependent dielectric breakdown testing indicates a decrease in both the leakage current and the lifetime of the MIM capacitors treated with plasma. Possible dielectric degradation mechanisms are also explored.

It is claimed in almost every experimental work on ceramics that the strength is Weibull distributed. The literature demonstrates that this is not valid in any case, but it is up to now the backbone in the design of brittle components. An overview on situations that deviate from Weibull statistics is shown, such as multi-modal flaw distribution, R-curves, etc. (Danzer et al. 2007). It is also shown that testing specimens with different volumes may help to understand the real strength distribution. Inaccuracies that arise from using the Weibull's theory are noted. Monte Carlo simulations on the basis of the standardized testing procedure (30 specimens) clearly reveal that these deviations can hardly be detected on the basis of small samples.

A research was conducted to create a baseline model of soil compaction response to trampling and a methodology to model the effects of trampling on soil (McDonald & Glen, 2007). Although trampling studies have been conducted in the past, the analysis of military training in part provides a different perspective and approach. The data showed bulk densities remained relatively constant for a time and then began to increase at an increasing rate for several hundred passes and finally levelled and remained at or below 1.30 g/cm^3 through the remainder of the experiment. Mathematical models were created based on empirical data from a trampling experiment using a more standard logistical growth curve as well as curves based on Weibull and gamma cumulative distribution functions. The experiment and the resulting models give quantifiable continuous inference on the effects of trampling, as opposed to the existing qualitative assessments. These baseline models would serve as the foundation for future studies of land management when trampling occurs.

A study comparing two statistical methods of estimating tumor latency using the Weibull distribution model and the Kaplan-Meier method was conducted (McKee et al., 1990). Parallelism of dose-response curves of different materials and quantitative reproducibility of dermal carcinogenesis data were also examined. The Weibull method has the advantage of producing parameter estimates, even when tumor yield is low. The Kaplan-Meier method, on the other hand, is free of distribution assumptions. It was noted that since the comparisons of potency are made on the basis of parameters from the same assumed distribution on the same strain of animal, the Weibull estimates were favored. A comparison of dose-response data for benzo[a]pyrene and catalytically cracked clarified oil indicated that the slopes of the two dose-response curves were significantly different. Thus the relative carcinogenic potencies of different materials vary with dose, and potency comparisons must necessarily be dose-specific. The dose-response curves from the three studies of one material had significantly different slopes. Thus the results suggested that there were sources of biological variability which could contribute to experimental error.

It can be proved that the Weibull distribution can be used to describe the failure characteristics of the other three commonly used distributions, i.e. normal, exponential and lognormal distributions. In general, its parameters may be determined by the maximum likelihood method or the special graph paper. However, the former method involves intensive mathematical treatment and the latter method produces subjective results. In this regard, a practical approach which does not require advanced mathematical background and capable of producing objective parameters is suggested. A description of this practical approach is shown below, followed by a PACS case illustration.

Methods of Estimating Weibull Parameters

Most of the work on estimation of the Weibull parameters may be grouped into one of three categories. One approach is to use methods based on the maximum likelihood estimates. These methods tend to have good properties and often satisfy certain optimality properties as the sample size of failure data increases. A disadvantage is that the maximum likelihood estimates cannot be solved in closed form, hence considerable mathematical treatment is involved. For instance, iterative procedures such as the Newton-Raphson technique are required to find the maximum likelihood estimators. A second approach is to consider methods based on best linear estimators. This approach also suffers from difficulties similar to those associated with the first approach.

Many engineers therefore prefer to use the third approach - graphical methods. Frequently a frequency diagram can represent the available failure data and the required statistical model may be determined by visually comparing a density function with the frequency diagram constructed. Alternatively, the data may be plotted on probability papers specially prepared for the Weibull distribution. These are graph papers for plotting observed data and their corresponding cumulative frequencies or probabilities. The linearity, or lack of linearity, of sample data plotted on such papers would indicate the appropriateness of a given distribution for modeling the population. However, the graphical approach is rather subjective in that the determination of whether or not the data contradict the assumed model is based on a visual inspection of the freehand fit to a sample data, which differs from person to person.

Having estimated the Weibull parameters, traditionally the next step is to verify the assumed distribution in the light of available data using certain statistical tests, known as goodness-of-fit tests. Indeed, when two or more distributions appear to be plausible distribution models, such tests can be used to delineate the relative degree of validity of the different distributions. There is a variety of statistical tests for determining the goodness of fit of data to the Weibull distribution. A commonly used procedure for evaluating the Weibull assumption is the chi-square (χ^2) goodness-of-fit test. To use this test, the observed data are grouped into frequency cells and compared to the expected number of observations based on the proposed distribution. From this comparison, a test statistic that approximately follows a chi-square distribution only if the assumed model is correct is calculated. The test statistic will tend to exceed a chi-square variate if the assumed model is not correct. The major advantage of the chi-square test is its versatility. It can be applied simply to test any distributional assumption, without any knowledge of the values of the distribution parameters. Its major shortcomings are its lack of sensitivity in detecting inappropriate models when few observations are available, the frequent need to arrange the data into arbitrary intervals, which can affect the outcome of the test, and there is arbitrariness in the choice of the significance level. Although this procedure allows us to reject a model as inadequate, the main problem is that it does not allow us to prove that the model is correct. In fact, the outcome of a statistical test depends highly upon the amount of available data - the more data there are, the better are the chances of rejecting an inadequate model.

To provide an objective and non-complicated method of estimating the Weibull distribution, a moment-based approach is suggested below. Such a technique allows us to verify the Weibull assumption, without using complex mathematics and at the same time to estimate the distribution parameters objectively. Contrary to the conventional approach, the proposed moment-based approach verifies the applicability of the Weibull distribution to the PACS operational data first and then estimates the model parameters.

Verification of Weibull Assumption

In order to verify the applicability of the Weibull distribution, the mean value (μ) of the available data, the second, third and fourth central moments are required. If we have no knowledge of the form or parameters of the probability density function concerned, the required central moments may be calculated as follows:

$$m_2 = [1/(n-1)]\sum_{i=1}^{n}(t_i - \mu)^2 \tag{1}$$

$$m_3 = (1/n)\sum_{i=1}^{n}(t_i - \mu)^3 \tag{2}$$

$$m_4 = (1/n)\sum_{i=1}^{n}(ti - \mu)^4 \tag{3}$$

Where t_i, $i = 1,2, \ldots n$, are the values of n given observations; m_2, m_3 and m_4 are the second, third and fourth central moments of the observed data respectively. It can be seen that m_2 is slightly modified as an unbiased estimate of the variance, i.e. $m_2 = \sigma^2$. From these three central moments, we can determine the moment coefficient of skewness (S) and the moment coefficient of kurtosis (K) as follows:

$$S = m_3/(m_2)^{1.5} \tag{4}$$

$$K = m_4/m_2^2 \tag{5}$$

Figure 1. A kurtosis-skewness squared (K-S²) diagram showing the Weibull Region

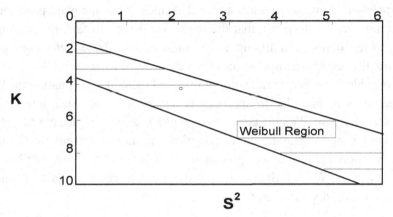

The moment coefficient of skewness (S) measures the skewness of a distribution. Skewness characterizes the degree of asymmetry of a distribution around its mean. Positive skewness indicates a distribution with an asymmetric tail extending towards values that are more positive and a negative skewness indicates a distribution with an asymmetric tail extending towards values that are more negative.

The moment coefficient of kurtosis (K) measures the kurtosis of a data set. Kurtosis characterizes the relative peakedness or flatness of a distribution compared to the normal distribution. For the normal distribution, K is found to be equal to 3. Hence the kurtosis is sometimes defined by $(K - 3)$, in which case a positive kurtosis indicates a relatively peaked distribution and a negative kurtosis indicates a relatively flat distribution.

Once the sample estimates of S and K are determined, one can plot the point (K, S²) on a K-S² diagram (Wong, 1985). A K–S² diagram showing the Weibull region is shown in Fig. 2. If the plotted point falls within the Weibull region, then the Weibull distribution is a logical candidate to model the observed data. We might then proceed to obtain estimates for the distribution parameters.

Proposed Weibull Estimation

This is the process of obtaining estimates for the parameters υ, β and θ. Assume that there are *n* statistically independent observed values of a random variable T that we believe has a Weibull distribution. Since υ is the smallest possible value of T, it is reasonable to estimate υ by the smallest observed value t_{min} of T. That is,

υ =minimum of t_1, t_2, ... t_n.
$= t_{min}$

The mean (μ) and variance (σ^2) of the Weibull distribution may be shown to be

$$\mu = \upsilon + \theta\Gamma[1 + (1/\beta)] \tag{6}$$

And

$$\sigma^2 = \theta^2 \{\Gamma(1 + (2/\beta)] - \{\Gamma[1 + (1/\beta)]\}^2\} \tag{7}$$

Where the complete gamma function $\Gamma(\alpha)$ is given by

$$\Gamma(\alpha) = \int_0^\infty \rho^{\alpha-1} \times \exp(-\rho) \, d\rho$$

For $\alpha > 1$, $\Gamma(\alpha)$ can be obtained from the identity:

$$\Gamma(\alpha) = (\alpha-1) \, \Gamma(\alpha-1) \tag{8}$$

From Eqn. (6),

$$\mu - \upsilon = \theta\Gamma[1 + (1/\beta)] \tag{9}$$

And from Eqn. (7)

$$\sigma^2 + (\mu - \upsilon)^2 = \theta^2 \{\Gamma(1 + (2/\beta)]\} \tag{10}$$

Divide the square of Eqn. (9) by Eqn. (10), we have

$$(\mu - \upsilon)^2 / [\sigma^2 + (\mu - \upsilon)^2] = \{\Gamma[1 + (1/\beta)]\}^2 / \{\Gamma(1 + (2/\beta)]\} \tag{11}$$

Subsituting sample values of υ, μ and σ into the L.H.S. of Eqn. (11), we can solve for β by using a table tabulating values of $\{\Gamma[1+(1/\beta)]\}^2 / \Gamma[1+(2/\beta)]$. Once an estimate of β has been determined, we can obtain an estimate of θ through the expression:

$$\theta = (\mu - \upsilon)/\Gamma[1 + (1/\beta)] \tag{12}$$

Spreadsheet Procedure

Based on the principles mentioned above, one can achieve Weibull estimation through the following procedure:

- **Step 1:** Use any spreadsheet software to compute the mean (μ), second (m_2), third (m_3) and fourth (m_4) central moments of the observed data. While the mean value can be obtained through the built-in statistical function, the second to fourth central moments are to be obtained by means of Eqn. (1) to (3).
- **Step 2:** Compute the squared moment coefficient of skewness S^2 and moment coefficient of kurtosis K by substituting values of m_2, m_3 and m_4 into Eqn. (4) and (5).
- **Step 3:** Plot the point (S^2, K) on Figure 2. If this plotted point falls within or reasonably close to the Weibull region, then the Weibull distribution is a logical candidate to model the observed data.
- **Step 4:** Estimate the location parameter υ by choosing the smallest value t_{min} of given data.
- **Step 5:** Estimate the L.H. S. term of Eqn. (10) by substituting the sample values of σ^2, μ and υ. Then use Appendix 2A to find the corresponding value of β.
- **Step 6:** With the value of β obtained, get the respective gamma function $\Gamma[1 + (1/\beta)]$ by means of Appendix 2B.
- **Step 7:** Substitute estimated values of μ, υ, and $\Gamma[1 + (1/\beta)]$ into the R.H.S. of Eqn.(12) in order to estimate the scale parameter θ.

CASE ILLUSTRATION: PACS IMAGE REJECTS

Digital radiography systems are in common use for medical imaging, yet few studies have examined computed radiography quality performance in terms of reject rates. This lack is due primarily to difficulty in modeling the image reject rates. A recent reject analysis shows that this problem has been further compounded by the lack of software infrastructure necessary to centrally compile data for radiology departments that have multiple digital capture devices. In this study each database record contains image information such as body part and view position, exposure level, technologist identifier, and reason for rejection. Reject analysis was performed on 288,000 computed radiography (CR) image records collected from two local hospitals. Each record contains image information, such as body part and view position, exposure level, technologist identifier, and, if the image was rejected, the reason for rejection. Extensive database filtering was required to ensure the integrity of the reject-rate calculations.

Accurate reject analysis provides a platform from which to develop targeted training programs designed to mitigate the largest sources of patient repeat exposures. It was suggested that comprehensive digital radiography QA requires that a mechanism be put into place to force technologists to enter reject data information into a database, preferably before another image can be scanned. Also, standardized terminology and definitions for QA deficiencies must be established, along with the associated training, to eliminate inconsistent and inappropriate labelling of rejected images. To illustrate the user-friendliness of the proposed Weibull estimation method, a spreadsheet-based reject rate modeling is given below.

The Problem

The main server or the network attached server (NAS) of the PACS can handle most of the data storage capacity for a large hospital; however, there are medical legal requirements for long-term storage of medical information that must also be considered. In the United States of America, some states require medical information to be stored for up to 5-7 years and for pediatric patients until after their 22nd birthday. These regulations include medical images and radiology reports. Almost all of us can imagine purging hundreds of outdated x-ray files to make room on shelves for current year files. Moving these files and reorganizing file room space takes time and a lot of muscle. The PACS system must carry out similar functions of data storage that include long-term storage of records. These records can easily be retrieved from PACS just as a film jacket can be retrieved from a remote location if needed or purged if outdated.

A storage function not easily accomplished with analog films is the recording of back-up files in case of a disaster that destroys the main systems. A back-up disaster image file for analogue film is primarily accomplished using a microfilm scanner or a minifier system. These may require some darkroom processing and a lot of time to produce and store duplicate images. PACS is able to provide disaster file using optical disk technology and/or digital linear tape technology.

Imaging data can be stored indefinitely on the NAS server if enough memory is provided. Most institutions save data on network servers, optical disk within an optical disk jukebox (ODJ), and on digital linear tape (DLT), or in a DLT jukebox, or combinations of all of the methods mentioned. An optical disk jukebox is a long-term storage hardware device which encompasses optical disk drives, optical disk storage slots, and associated robotic arms and software for fetching data disk (s).

In a large hospital with many imaging modalities transferring data over the network, there may be delays in images reaching the radiologist for viewing depending on the cable system's capacity to move data. To avoid delays most PACS networks use Ethernet, twisted pair cables, coaxial cables and fiber optic cables. The

Figure 2. Frequency of PACS image rejects

TBR(Days)	No. of Rejections
1 - 25	24
26 - 50	16
51 - 75	8
76 - 100	8
101 - 125	5
126 - 150	1
151 - 175	7
176 - 200	2
201 - 225	1
226 - 250	3
251 - 275	1
276 - 300	2
301 - 325	1
326 - 350	0
351 - 375	2
376 - 400	2
401 - 425	1
Total	84

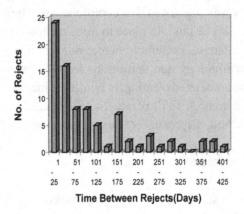

PACS administration team is able to track the flow of images and data through the network, and can spot and correct cable malfunctions, and numerous errors such as duplicate files that tax server memory as they occur.

In this illustration, it is assumed that the PACS administrator is interested in estimating the average number of rejecting a certain type of radiology images in two district hospitals in a local hospital network. Figure 2 shows the frequency diagram of the number of image rejects for a period of eight years.

Weibull Estimation

A Weibull analysis of the observed data would proceed as follows:

- **Step 1:** By means of any commercially available spreadsheet software, the mean (μ), second (m_2), third (m_3) and fourth (m_4) central moments of the observed data can be found as follows:
  $\mu = 96.435$
  $m_2 = 11109.61$
  $m_3 = 1,683,730$
  $m_4 = 518,285,854$
- **Step 2:** By substituting values of m_2, m_3 and m_4 into Eqn. (4) and (5), the squared moment coefficient of skewness (S^2) and moment coefficient of kurtosis (K) were found to be 2.068 and 4.199 respectively.

- **Step 3:** Plot the point (S^2, K) on Figure 1. As shown in Figure 1, the plotted point (indicated as a tiny circle) falls within the Weibull region. Hence the Weibull distribution is a logical candidate to model the observed data.
- **Step 4:** A review of the collected data would show that the minimum time between callbacks is 3 days, hence the location parameter υ is taken as 3 days.
- **Step 5:** By substituting the estimated values of m_2, μ and υ into the L.H.S. of Eqn.(11), the L.H.S. can be calculated to be 0.440. By looking up the value of 0.440 in Appendix C1, it is found that the nearest value is 0.441 and the corresponding value of β can be found to be 0.89 approximately.
- **Step 6:** By means of Appendix C2, the gamma function $\Gamma[1 + (1/0.89)]$, i.e. $\Gamma(2.12)$, can be found to be 0.886.
- **Step 7:** Substituting values of μ, υ and $\Gamma[1 + (1/\beta)]$ into the R.H.S. of Eqn(12), the scale parameter θ can be calculated to be 105.46.

Hence, the Weibull model based on the given data would be of the form:

$$(0.0084)[(t - 3)/105.46]^{-0.11} \exp[-(t - 3/105.46)^{0.89}]$$

It can be seen that the mean time between rejects is approximately 106 days and the failure rate is decreasing (since magnitude of β is less than unity), although most components in the system are having constant failure rates.

IMPROVING PACS HARDWARE RELIABILITY

Since PACS is made up of a number of components, the reliability of the system will depend crucially on the reliability of the components present. The concept of fault tolerance (Avrin et al. 2000; Liu et al. 2001; Tellis & Andriole, 2001; Liu et al., 2003; Huang, 2005; Mukai, 2007) has been introduced to PACS design not long ago. Basically it is the implementation of redundant systems, such that in the event of a system failure, maximum availability and reliability – without the loss of transactional data – can be achieved. PACS redundancy can be defined as the provision of multiple interchangeable components to perform a single function in order to cope with failures and errors. Redundancy normally applies primarily to hardware. For example, one might install two or even three computers to do the same job. There are several ways these could be used. They could all be active all the time thus giving extra performance through (parallel processing) as well as extra availability; one could be active and the others simply monitoring its activity so as to be ready to take over if it failed (this is called "warm standby"); the "spares" could be kept turned off and only switched on when needed (this is "cold standby").

Another common form of hardware redundancy is "disk mirroring". Redundancy can also be used to detect and recover from errors, in either hardware or software. A well-known example of this is the cyclic redundancy check, which adds redundant data to a block in order to detect corruption during storage or transmission. If the cost of errors is high enough, e.g. in a safety-critical system, redundancy may be used in both hardware and software with three separate computers programmed by three separate teams and some system to check that they all produce the same answer, or some kind of majority voting system.

While archival systems require good compression, their administrators must also ensure that data is reserved over long periods. As shown in previous chapters, compression techniques, while they save storage space, also have the potential to reduce reliability. We can improve system reliability by introducing redundancies into a large storage system in different ways such as erasure correcting codes used in RAID levels 5 and 6, and by introducing different data placement, failure detection and recovery disciplines. We do not consider these here mainly because they offer intricate trade-offs between speed of recovery, ease of recovery, and computational and storage overhead. In the PACS context, it is clear that different types of redundancy configurations can be arranged to achieve a high degree of reliability and the PACS reliabilities (Rs) can be determined in the following manner:

Series Components

$$Rs = \prod_1^n R_i$$

Where R_i = individual reliability of components

Parallel Components

$$Rs = 1 - \prod_i^n (1 - R_i)$$

Where R_i = individual reliability of components

Cross-Linked Components

To analyze the system reliability of the cross-linked configuration, two situations have to be considered:

Figure 3. A cross-linked system

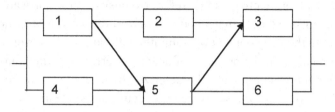

- when the crucial component is failed; and
- when the crucial component is operating.

Assume that:

- R^- as the system reliability, given the failure of the crucial component, and
- R^+ as the system reliability, given the successful operation of the crucial component.

When the crucial component 5 is failed, the reduced system comprises a series of 3 components, 1, 2 and 3; components 4 and 6 no longer contribute to the value of R^-.

When component 5 is operating, we have a series combination of 2 parallel configurations, 1 and 4 in the first and 3 and 6 in the second; since component 2 is always bypassed, it has no effect on R^+.

The system reliability is therefore the sum of two mutually exclusive states, component failed and component operational. Since $(1 - R_5)$ is the probability that the crucial component 5 will fail and R_5 the probability that it will not,

$$R = R^-(1 - R_5) + R^+R_5$$

SOFTWARE RELIABILITY MODELS

Despite all attempts to ensure that the PACS accompany software is free from errors, some residual errors (bugs) often persist. This is mainly due to fact that software testing can mount up to more than a third of the total development time and the test time seems not productive and therefore expensive to the software developer. Besides, there exists the risk, that a competitor will release the same product a bit earlier. Efforts in the development of computer software models over the past two decades have resulted in the proposal of dozens of error-counting and debugging models. Each model is completely characterized by a set of assumptions. Often it is assumed that failures in the software will occur independently and that when a failure is detected, the fault is fixed immediately with no new faults introduced. This is the case for some well-known models: the Jelinski-Moranda model and the Goel-Okumoto model (Pham, 2006).

In practice, assumptions underlying these models like independence of the occurring faults, negligible repair time and perfect repair are of course, not quite realistic. It is unknown how large the impact on the outcome is of such an assumption as the independence. Without this assumption, however, the mathematical problem becomes a lot more complicated. A new and interesting idea seems to be the modeling of imperfect repair and software growth simultaneously. With software growth the PACS software is no longer a static object, but on the contrary changes in time. Not only does each repair cause a change in the software, but also in practice at certain moments in the testing/operating new modules will be added to the software as well. In the Poisson Growth and Imperfect Repair Model (Van Pul, 1991), it is assumed that the expected number of new faults introduced at a certain point in time, is proportional to the size of the change in the software at that moment. This assumption makes it possible to model imperfect repair and software growth simultaneously. Readers might like to refer to the literature (e.g. Pham, 2006) for a more advanced treatment of the software reliability models.

A major statistical problem confronting the PACS teams is the comparison of different models. This is usually done by goodness of fit testing. In the PACS operating environment, the test statistics involved are rather complicated, and the derivation of their distributions can cause considerable difficulties. Not only does the choice of the best model confront us with many questions, but also the estimation of the parameters in the chosen model is a difficult task. We usually use the maximum likelihood estimation procedure for this purpose. Broadly speaking, the likelihood of a set of data is the probability of obtaining that particular set of data, given the chosen probability distribution model. This expression contains the unknown model parameters. The values of these parameters that maximize the sample likelihood are known as the Maximum Likelihood Estimator. We derive the chance (likelihood) function and maximize this likelihood as a function of the parameters. The derivation of the likelihood function is not always possible analytically and the numerical computation of its maxima can be unstable. Often tedious iterative techniques like the Newton-Raphson procedure or the down-hill simplex method are used to approximate the roots of a system of equations. In view of the mathematical complexity involved, the moment-based approach suggested above for the PACS hardware can be applied to the software as well, though distributions other than Weibull might be used.

A PACS SOFTWARE CASE STUDY

In this case study the failure characteristic of an application software for PACS, during an early phase of the testing process in a Hong Kong hospital is analyzed. The main objective is to evaluate the duration adequacy of each test phase.

Software Development and Testing

The hospital started the development of PACS software packages in the late nineties. Of these products about every year an updated version is released. Each release supports new hardware, introduces new functionality, and also includes internal structural improvements. From annual project plan one can approximately distinguish the following development and test phases:

- development phase 1 (several months)
- installation-test (several weeks): Installation test. This test aims to get a basic part of the system operational and ready for a clinical tryout on some sites.
- development phase 2 (several months)
- alpha-test (several weeks): This is a software test conducted by the software developers. Hardware was not tested, but only used to test the software.
- system integration test (several weeks): Software was run on specified hardware with the aim of evaluating the complete system.
- Beta-test (several weeks): During this test the entire system is tested by the software management group and it serves mostly as acceptance test.

In practice there is some limited overlap between development and testing phases. In this case study the failure characteristic of the application software during the installation and alpha-test; these are the phases where most of the software failures are detected and corrected. The application software is grouped into 6 segments. Before alpha testing started, the test-leader had made a complete alpha test plan. It stated exactly which segment would be tested by whom and when. Time was also provided for problem solving. Test specifications for each test session were prepared by the software developers. Software errors (bugs) were collected in a problem report (PR) database. Testers had to fill in a log-form detailing information such as times of start and end of test, description of test items, which of them were successful and which not, and other comments concerning hardware malfunctioning.

Both the installation and alpha tests under consideration lasted about 6 weeks. For each software error the following data were collected:

- The problem report number that identifies the error.
- Occurrence date and time.
- Segment to which the PR is assigned.
- The priority of the error ranges from routine (RO), urgent (UR) to very urgent (VU). Minor display problems were typically considered routine, and memory stack dumps were very urgent. The priority of errors might be changed as deadlines came closer.
- The total test effort per day in testing hours.

Figure 4 shows the distribution of errors associated with each software segment.

In Figure 5, the failure characteristics of individual segments during alpha test is compared. The two most critical segments, 3 and 6, have similar failure behavior. The same can be said for the two smallest segments, 2 and 5. The two remaining segments, 1 and 4, show, however, different failure histories. The failure intensity of segment 4 is decreasing gently, whereas the failure intensity of segment 1 is still growing. This suggests, that at least for this segment, the alpha test duration was inadequate. Indeed, in sequel tests (system integration and beta tests) relatively large numbers of segment 1 errors were recorded.

Figure 4. Error distribution of software segments

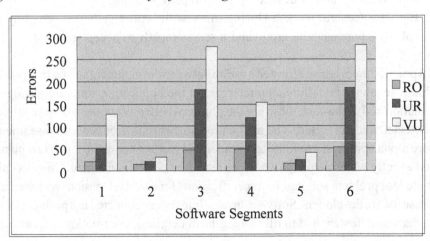

Figure 5. Software error trend during alpha test

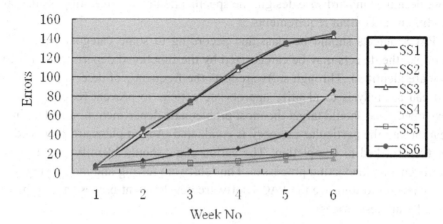

Figure 6. Trend of software errors during alpha test

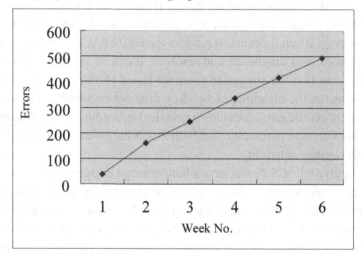

Figure 6 shows the trend of the total software errors during throughout the six weeks of alpha test. It can be seen that the error rate is gradually decreasing.

IMPROVING PACS SOFTWARE RELIABILITY

Many of the errors recorded during software testing originate in the specification. The PACS software specification must describe fully and accurately the requirements of the modality programs. As there are no safety factor provisions in software design as in hardware design, the specification must cover all possible input conditions and output requirements.

PACS defects should be classified according to some category scheme, for example, the defects may be categorized by the functional departments in which they are identified. Through software tests the frequency of defects per category and causal analysis to identify appropriate actions to prevent reoccurrence are developed. One should target the most problematic department first and an investigation into the particular category is conducted. Action plans are produced and are then tracked to completion. The action plans should identify and carry out improvements to existing processes. Thus software testing and monitoring offers a mechanism to improve the PACS software development process and to mature the software test process.

CONCLUDING REMARK

Hardware and software failures frequently occur in PACS. For instance, a significant point of hardware failure in PACS is at the PACS controller, or the main archive server. When it occurs, it renders the entire PACS inoperable and crippled until the problem is diagnosed and resolved. It can be seen from the above PACS modeling case that the suggested moment-based method, an objective approach that emphasizes the matching of two key distribution coefficients, viz. skewness and kurtosis coefficients, provides a practical procedure to the estimation of the Weibull distribution parameters for both PACS hardware and software, as well as the overall system reliability.

Many current PACS do not have a fault-tolerant design or adequate backup system for the main archive server due to several issues including cost. This chapter shows that higher system reliability can be achieved through simple redundancy arrangements of the key components. Since modality additions are foreseeable developments in PACS, one would need to spend more time on associated software tests. As indicated through the software case study, besides the need to evaluate failure characteristics of individual software segments, the adequacy of test duration during software acceptance testing also needs to be addressed.

REFERENCES

Avrin, D. E., Andriole, K. P., Yin, L., Gould, R., & Arenson, R. L. (2000). Simulation of disaster recovery of a picture archiving and communications system using off-site hierarchal storage management. *J. Digit Imaging,* 13(2 Suppl 1), 168-70.

Barabady, J., & Kumar, U. (2008). Reliability analysis of mining equipment: A case study of a crushing plant at Jajarm Bauxite Mine in Iran. *Reliability Engineering & System Safety, 93*(4), 647-653.

Danzer, R., Supancic, P., Pascual, J., & Lube, T. (2007). Fracture statistics of ceramics – Weibull statistics and deviations from Weibull statistics. *Engineering Fracture Mechanics, 74*(18), 2919-2932.

Das, K. (2008). A comparative study of exponential distribution vs Weibull distribution in machine reliability analysis in a CMS design. *Computers & Industrial Engineering, 54*(1), 12-33.

Elamouri, M., & Amar, F. B. (2008). Wind energy potential in Tunisia. *Renewable Energy, 33*(4), 758-768.

Foos, D. H., Sehnert, W. J., Reiner, B, Siegel, E. L., Segal, A., & Waldman, D. L. (2008). Digital Radiography Reject Analysis: Data Collection Methodology, Results, and Recommendations from an In-depth Investigation at Two Hospitals. *J. Digital Imaging.* [Epub ahead of print]. Retrieved on 30 June 2008 from http://www. springerlink.com/content/92m24u782p586611/

Goseva-Popstojanova, K., & Trivedi, K. S. (2001). Architecture-based approach to reliability assessment of software systems. *Performance Evaluation, 45*(2–3), 179–204.

Ho, C. C., & Chiou, B. S. (2008). Effect of size and plasma treatment and the application of Weibull distribution on the breakdown of PECVD SiNx MIM capacitors. *Microelectronic Engineering, 85*(1), 110-114.

Huang, H. K. (2005). *PACS and Imaging Informatics.* New York: John Wiley & Sons.

Liu, B. J., Cao, F., Zhang, J. Q., Huang, H. K., Zhou, M. Z., & Mogel, G. (2001). Fault-tolerant PACS server design and evaluation. *International Congress Series, 1230*, 760-766.

Liu, B. J., Cao, F., Zhou, M. Z., Mogel, G., & Documet, L. (2003). Trends in PACS image storage and archive. *Computerized Medical Imaging and Graphics, 27*(2-3), 165-174.

McDonald, K. W., & Glen, A. (2007). Modeling military trampling effects on glacial soils in the humid continental climate of southern New York. *Journal of Environmental Management, 84*(4), 377-383.

McKee, R. H., Nicolich, M. J., Scala, R. A., & Lewis, S. C. (1990). Estimation of epidermal carcinogenic potency. *Fundamental and Applied Toxicology, 15*(2), 320-328.

Mukai, M., Tanikawa, T., Uemura, K., & Ando, Y. (2007). Development and Evaluation of PACS, a Parallel Operation System with Improved Fault-tolerance. *Medinfo 2007: Proceedings of the 12th World Congress on Health (Medical) Informatics; Building Sustainable Health Systems*, Amsterdam, 2035-2036.

Musa, J. D., Iannino, A., & Okumoto, K. (1987). *Software Reliability: Measurement, Prediction, Application*. New York: McGraw-Hill.

Pham, H. (2006) *System Software Reliability*. London: Springer-Verlag.

ReliaSoft Corp. (2001) Limitations of the Exponential Distribution for Reliability Analysis. *ReliaSoft's Reliability Edge Newsletter*. Retrieved on 16 January, 2008 from http://www.reliasoft.com/newsletter/4q2001/exponential.htm.

Tellis, W. M., & Andriole, K. P. (2001). Finding the optimal picture archving and communciation system (PACS) architecture: A comparison of three PACS designs. *J. Digital Imaging, 14*(2), 72-76.

Wong, T. T. (1985). Reliability Modeling of Lifts. *Proc. of 2nd International Conf. on Planned Maintenance, Reliability and Quality*, University of Oxford, 2-3 April, 1998, 239-244.

Wong, T. T. (2000). Weibull Estimation: A Moment-Based Approach in *Industrial Engineering Applications and Practice: Users' Encyclopedia* [CD ROM].

Yang, N. H., Nayeb-Hashemi, H., & Vaziri, A. (2008). Non-destructive evaluation of erosion damage on E-glass/epoxy composites. *Composites Part A: Applied Science and Manufacturing, 39*(1), 56-66.

Chapter XII
PACS Failure Mode and Effects

BACKGROUND

There are some medical errors for which preventability is rarely questioned. These include medical errors such as wrong site surgery, wrong procedure, wrong patient operations (Seiden & Barach, 2006; Michaels et al., 2007; Lee et al., 2007), wrong drug/dose/duration (Pugh et al., 2005) or incompatible organ transplantation (Cook et al., 2007). Less preventable medical errors include judgment type errors such as case studies reported in journals, where one or more experts review the treatment decisions of a clinician and conclude that the clinician's judgment was incorrect (Lukela et al., 2005).

Many healthcare managers first heard about Failure Mode and Effects Analysis FMEA when Joint Commission on Accreditation of Healthcare Organizations (JCAHO) released its Leadership Standards and Elements of Performance Guidelines in July 2002 (JCAHO, 2002). The purpose of performing an FMEA for JCAHO was to identify where and when possible system failures could occur and to prevent those problems before they happen. If a particular, failure could not be prevented, then the goal would be to prevent the issue from affecting healthcare organizations in the accreditation process.

FMEA is a tool that when performed adequately, can reduce the risk of preventable medical errors. Hospitals in the United States that are accredited by JCAHO are required to perform at least one FMEA each year. The main output of FMEA is a series of mitigations, each of which is some process change implemented to reduce the risk of error. Because resources are limited, implementing all mitigations is not possible so the challenge is to find the set of mitigations that provides the highest reduction in risk for the least cost. Hence, preventability may be viewed in terms of the cost and effectiveness of mitigation. A low-cost and effective mitigation is associated with a highly preventable medical error, whereas a high-cost and or less effective mitigation is associated with a less preventable medical error.

Currently AAPM TG 100 (2007) is reviewing reports from previous task groups and from several professional organizations. This group is also reviewing ISO guidelines in an effort develop a suitable general QA approach that "balances patient safety and quality versus resources commonly available and strikes a good balance between prescriptiveness and flexibility." The TG 100 initiative identifies three industrial engineering–based tools as potential components of a QA management system in radiation therapy and FMEA is one of them.

There are a few potential problems with these recommendations, however. The first is that the general radiation therapy community is concerned that the use of these tools to reduce the risks or hazards associated with radiation therapy will require a considerable amount of additional resources. Although this should be a concern, process mapping, flowcharting tools, and FMEA (Stamatis, 1995; Fletcher, 1997; Thomadsen et al, 2003; Latino, 2004; JACHO, 2005; Hansen, 2007; Huq, 2007) have been used for decades by the medical device and pharmaceutical industries, among others, to reduce the level or risks or hazards in products and processes with many positive results. Also if the organizations are trained in the use of these tools and if these tools are applied with the assistance of experienced facilitators, there are few if any additional resources required, and the resulting process improvements will increase the effectiveness and productivity of the organization. A second potential problem is TG 100's recommendation that these tools be used for risk and hazard analysis versus overall process improvement. This might prevent the realization of significant improvements in processes and the resulting increase in quality and productivity.

Although FMEA has been applied in the medical community, its use appears to have the highest potential for assisting the radiation therapy community in improving overall process quality and in reducing and controlling the risk of injury without overtaxing resources. In the modern environment the number and sophistication of possible tests and measurements have increased dramatically. There is a need to prioritize quality management activities in a way that will strike a balance between being reasonably achievable and optimally beneficial to patients. A systematic understanding of possible errors over the course of a radiation therapy treatment and the potential clinical impact of each is needed to direct limited resources in such a way to produce maximal benefit to the quality of patient care. In a recent report's guidelines on risk assessment approaches with emphasis on failure mode and effect analysis (FMEA) are provided. Examples of FMEA applied to intensity-modulated radiation therapy and high-dose-rate brachytherapy are presented (Hug et al. 2008).

BASIC CONCEPT

To consider the effects of PACS hardware/software integration, one needs to predict the field performance. This is usually done through a FMEA. FMEA is a methodology designed to identify potential failure modes for a product or process, to assess the risk associated with those failure modes, to rank the issues in terms of importance and to identify and carry out corrective actions to address the most serious concerns (Wong, 2005).

In general, FMEA requires the identification of the following basic information:

- Items
- Functions
- Failures
- Effects of Failure
- Causes of Failure
- Current Controls
- Recommended Actions
- Plus other relevant details

Most analyses of this type also include some method to assess the risk associated with the issues identified during the analysis and to prioritize corrective actions. A popular method is the risk priority numbers (RPNs).

There are a number of published guidelines and standards for the requirements and recommended reporting format of FMEAs. Some of the main published standards for this type of analysis include SAE J1739, AIAG FMEA-3 and MIL-STD-1629A. In addition, many industries and companies have developed their own procedures to meet the specific requirements of their products/processes.

FMEA PROCEDURE

The process for conducting an FMEA is straightforward. The basic steps are outlined below.

1. Assemble the PACS team.
2. Establish the ground rules and procedures.
3. Gather and review relevant information.
4. Describe the PACS process and its intended function. An understanding of the radiological process is important to have clearly articulated. This understanding simplifies the process of analysis by helping the PACS engineer identify those product/process uses that fall within the intended function and which ones fall outside. It is important to consider both intentional and unintentional uses since product failure often ends in litigation, which can be costly and time consuming.
5. Create a functional block biagram (FBD) of the product or process. A block diagram of the PACS process should be developed. This diagram shows major components or process steps as blocks connected together by lines that indicate how the components or steps are related. The diagram shows the logical relationships of components and establishes a structure around which the FMEA can be developed. Establish a coding system to identify system elements. The block diagram should always be included with the FMEA form. A Sample FBD are shown in Appendix B.
6. Complete the entries on a FMEA Form worksheet: Product/System, Subsystem/Assembly, Component, Design Lead, Prepared By, Date, Revision (letter or number), and Revision Date. Modify these headings as needed.
7. Use the FBDs prepared above to begin listing items and their functions.
8. Identify failure modes. A failure mode is defined as the manner in which a component, subsystem, system, process, etc. could potentially fail to meet the design intent. Examples of potential failure modes include disc failure in the RAID, electrical short circuits, etc.
9. A failure mode in one component can serve as the cause of a failure mode in another component. Each failure should be listed in technical terms. Failure modes should be listed for functions of each component or process step. At this point, the failure mode should be identified whether or not the failure is likely to occur. Looking at similar products or processes and the failures that have been documented for them is a good starting point.
10. Describe the effects of those failure modes. For each failure mode identified, the engineer should determine what the ultimate effect would be. A failure effect is defined as the result of a failure mode on the function of the product/

process as perceived by the hospital management. Keep in mind the internal as well as the external customer. Examples of failure effects include injury to the user, inoperability of the hardware or software, patient complaints, etc.

11. Establish a numerical ranking for the severity of the effect. A common industry standard scale uses 1 to represent no effect and 10 to indicate very severe with failure affecting system operation and safety without warning. The intent of the ranking is to help the analyst determine whether a failure would be a minor nuisance or a catastrophic occurrence to the customer. This enables the engineer to prioritize the failures and address the real big issues first.

12. Identify the causes for each failure mode. A failure cause is defined as a design weakness that may result in a failure. The potential causes for each failure mode should be identified and documented. The causes should be listed in technical terms and not in terms of symptoms. Examples of potential causes include improper torque applied in assembly of PACS components, unsteady current, excessive voltage, erroneous algorithms, improper operating conditions, etc.

13. Estimate the probability factor. When there is inadequate operational data, a numerical weight would be assigned to each cause that indicates how likely that cause is (probability of the cause occurring). A common industry standard scale uses 1 to represent not likely and 10 to indicate inevitable. After operating the PACS for a while and when some failure models can be developed, then the Probability factor should be estimated from the failure model rather than subjective judgment of certain PACS team members.

14. Identify current controls. Current controls are the mechanisms that prevent the cause of the failure mode from occurring. The engineer should now identify testing, analysis, monitoring, and other techniques that can or have been used on the same or similar products/processes to detect failures. Each of these controls should be assessed to determine how well it is expected to identify or detect failure modes. After a new product or process has been in use previously undetected or unidentified failure modes may appear. The FMEA should then be updated and plans made to address those failures to eliminate them from the product/process.

15. Determine the likelihood of detection. Detection is an assessment of the likelihood that the current controls will detect the cause of the failure mode or the failure mode itself. If the HSSH model is followed, the occurrence of escaped user defects associated with certain software offers an indication of the detection likelihood.

16. Review risk priority numbers (RPN). The risk priority number is a mathematical product of the numerical Severity, Probability, and Detection ratings:

$$RPN = (Severity) \times (Probability) \times (Detection)$$

The RPN can then be used to compare issues within the analysis and to prioritize problems for corrective action to be carried out on the PACS, as shown in the following case illustration.

17. Determine recommended actions to address potential failures that have a high RPN. These actions could include specific inspection, testing or quality procedures; selection of different components or materials; de-rating; limiting environmental stresses or operating range; redesign of the item to avoid the failure mode; monitoring mechanisms; performing preventative and/or condition-based maintenance; and inclusion of back-up systems or redundancy.

18. Assign responsibility and a target completion date for these actions. This makes responsibility clear-cut and facilitates tracking.

19. Indicate actions taken. After these actions have been taken, re-assess the severity, probability and detection and review the revised RPN's for any further actions.

20. Update the FMEA as the design or process changes, the assessment changes or new information becomes known.

CASE ILLLUSTRATION: PACS FMEA

The following case is based on the work carried out by a hospital in Hong Kong.

Problem Description

The PACS system consists of four subsystems: hardware, software, network, environment, and these are shown in Figure 1. The following report describes the failure mode and effect analysis (FMEA) study carried out since early 2003 (Tong & Wong, 2005). The FMEA study aims at identifying the potential failure modes for the PACS system and assessing the risk associated with each failure mode. Each potential failure mode is ranked according to priority and corrective actions have been carried out to address high-risk failure modes.

Then the Functional Block Diagram (FBD) for each of the four major subsystems is prepared and these are shown in Figures 2 through 5 respectively.

Based on the function of each equipment, an output list is prepared and shown in Table 1.

In order to determine the RPN and the effectiveness of recommended actions in respect of each selected component, the Automotive Industry Action Group

Figure 1. PACS block diagram

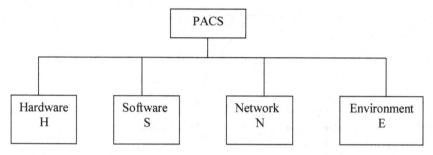

Figure 2. Hardware functional block diagram

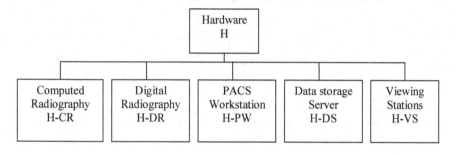

Figure 3. Software functional block diagram

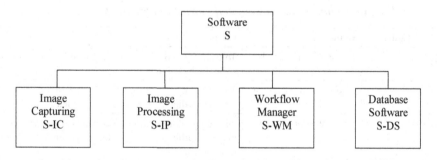

(AIAG) FMEA-3 format was adopted. Details of the analysis of each fault code are shown in Appendix B.

Potential failure modes for the PACS system were identified and a risk priority number was assigned to each potential failure mode. Recommendations and target completion dates were assigned for each potential failure mode and new risk priority number was calculated once the PACS leader's acceptance of recommended actions had been obtained. It was found that there were generally reductions in risk priority

Figure 4. Functional block diagram of network

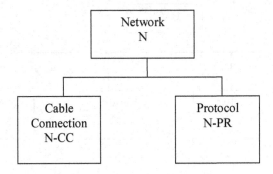

Figure 5. Functional block diagram of environment

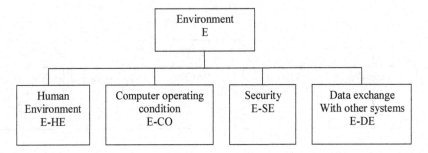

Table 1. Function output list for selected subsystem elements

Fault Code.	Function	Output
H-CR	Computed radiography	To capture radiographic images to the PACS system via radiography equipment.
H-DR	Digital radiography	To capture digital radiographic images to the PACS system via digital radiography equipment.
H-PW	PACS Workstation	Direct digital images and associated information about clients to different viewing stations according to hospital procedure and rules.
H-DS	Data storage Server	Store database: including radiographic images, client personal data, diagnostic data, medical reports, treatment procedures and billing information in hard disks, magnetic tapes or other computerized means.
H-VS	Radiographic images display	To allow diagnostic review of radiographic images electronically for authorized personnel such as physicians within the hospital network or medical experts overseas.
S-IC	Image capturing	To operate the DR and CR machine to capture digital images into the PACS system

continued on following page

Table 1. continued

Fault Code.	Function	Output
S-IP	To edit digital images	To edit captured images such as contrast, color and sizing.
S-WM	Workflow Manager	To oversee the operation of the whole system, central control of equipment within the system.
S-DS	Database input and management	To store, retrieve and amend relevant client records within the system. To generate reports and to import/ export data from other database system within or outside hospital network.
N-CC	Cable Connection	All necessary hardware such as servers, routers, hardware links, communication lines to construct a local area network, wide area network or internet to connect all relevant users.
N-PR	To set up standards, procedure and rules of communication	To allow communication be established and maintained within the network by observing the preset rules and procedures.
E- HE	To produce a good working environment for the operator	To enhance the efficiency of operator.
E-CO	To produce a good physical environment for computer	To maintain a proper condition for efficient computer operation.
E-SE	To protect client information	To allow authorized personnel to access the client information, use of firewalls to prevent hacking of computer system and loss of data.
ET-DE	Data exchange with other systems	To share database with all other computer systems within institution to maintain records properly and reduce costs of data storage.

numbers if the recommendations were taken. Encouraging results could be found by referring to Figures 6 through 9.

A comparison of the RPNs for each subsystem is shown in Figures 6 through 9, it can be seen that the FMEA is a useful tool for prioritization of PACS defects and corrective action planning

CONCLUDING REMARK

FMEA was developed outside of health care and is now being used in health care to assess risk of failure and harm in processes and to identify the most important

Figure 6. Hardware RPNs before and after corrective actions

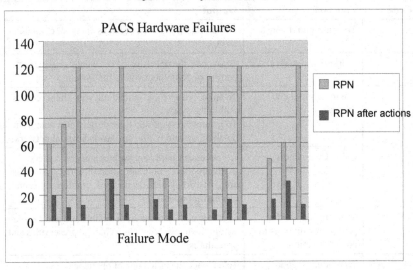

Figure 7. Software RPNs before and after corrective actions

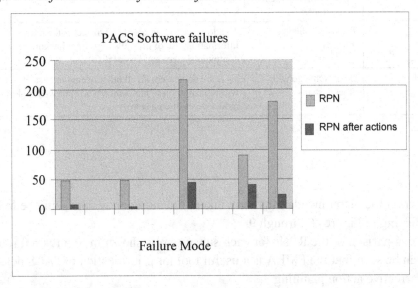

Figure 8. Network RPNs before and after corrective actions

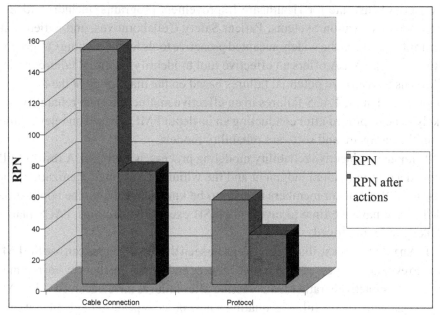

Figure 9. Environment RPNs before and after corrective actions

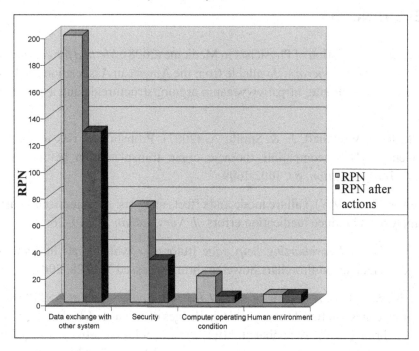

areas for process improvements. FMEA has been used by hundreds of hospitals in a variety of Institute for Healthcare Improvement programs, including Idealized Design of Medication Systems, Patient Safety Collaboratives, and Patient Safety Summits. Based on the widely accepted proactive tools for developing QA programs (Rath, 2008), FMEA offers an effective tool to identify potential failure modes. It allows us to prioritize potential failures based on the magnitude of the RPNs, such that we can handle PACS failures in an effective manner. System reliability would likely to be improved after conducting an in-depth FMEA based on relevant inputs from the hardware and software reliability models.

Without an objective reliability modeling process, actual FMEA results will be dependent on individual judgment and the whims of varying organization priorities. If all PACS team members happen to be knowledgeable in the application of FMEA and have the time to invest in HSSH execution meetings, PACS planning is likely to be improved.

From the above case illustration it can be seen that PACS teams can use the FMEA Tool to evaluate processes for possible failures and to prevent them by correcting the processes proactively rather than reacting after failures have occurred. The FMEA Tool is particularly useful in evaluating a new process prior to implementation and in assessing the impact of a proposed change to an existing process.

REFERENCES

American Association of Physicists in Medicine (2008). *Method for evaluating QA needs in radiation therapy.* Available from the American Association of Physicists in Medicine Web site, http://www/aapm.org/org/structure/default.asp?committee code=100.

Cook, R. I., Wreathall, J., & Smith, A. (2007). Probabilistic risk assessment of accidental ABO-incompatible thoracic organ transplantation before and after 2003. *Transplantation, 84,* 1602-1609.

Fletcher, C. E. (1997). Failure mode and effects analysis: An interdisciplinary way to analyze and reduce medication errors. *J. Nurs. Admin.,* 27, 19–26.

Hansen, D. A. *Flowcharting help page* [tutorial]. Available at: http://home.att. net/_dexter.a.hansen/flowchart/flowchart.htm. Accessed May 28, 2007.

Huq, M. S. (2007). *A Review of AAPM TG 100.* Presentation at ASTRO Quality Assurance of Radiation Therapy and Challenges of Advanced Technology Symposium, February 2007. Available at: http://www.oncologymeetings.org/quality_assurance/scientific_program.htm#sched. Accessed June 5, 2007.

Huq, M. S., Fraass, B. A., Dunscombe, P. B., Gibbons Jr., J. P., Ibbott, G. S., Medin, P. M., Mundt, A., Mutic, S., Palta, J. R., Thomadsen, B. R., Williamson, J. F., & Yorke, E. D. (2008). A Method for Evaluating Quality Assurance Needs in Radiation Therapy. *International Journal of Radiation Oncology, 71*(1), Supplement 1, S170-S173

Joint Commission on Accreditation of Healthcare Organizations (JCAHO) (2002). *Hospital Accreditation Standard*, LD 5.2, 200-201.

Joint Commission on the Accreditation of Healthcare Organizations (JCAHO) (2005). *Failure mode and effects analysis in healthcare: Proactive risk reduction*, 2nd ed. Oakbrook Terrace, IL: JCAHO.

Latino, R. J. (2004). Optimizing FMEA and RCA efforts in health care. *ASHRM Journal, 24*(3), 21-27.

Lee, J. S., Curley, A. W., & Smith, R. A. (2007). Prevention of wrong-site tooth extraction: clinical guidelines. *J. Oral Maxillofac Surg., 65*, 1793-1799.

Lukela, M., DeGuzman, D., Weinberger, S., & Saint, S. (2005). Unfashionably Late. *New Eng J Med, 352*, 64-69

Michaels, R. K., Makary, M. A., & Dahab, Y. (2007). Achieving the National Quality Forum's "Never Events": prevention of wrong site, wrong procedure, and wrong patient operations. *Ann. Surg., 245*, 526-532.

Pugh, M. J., Fincke, B. G., & Bierman, A. S. (2005). Potentially inappropriate prescribing in elderly veterans: are we using the wrong drug, wrong dose, or wrong duration? *J. Am. Geriatr. Soc., 53*, 1282-1289.

Rath, F. (2008). Tools for developing a quality management program: proactive tools (process mapping, value stream mapping, fault tree analysis, and failure mode and effects analysis. *Int. J. Radiation Oncology Biol. Phys., 1*(71), Supplement, S187–S190.

Seiden, S. C., & Barach, P. (2006). Wrong-side/wrong-site, wrong-procedure, and wrong-patient adverse events: are they preventable? *Arch. Surg., 141*, 931-939.

Stamatis, D. H. (1995). *Failure mode and effect analysis: FMEA from theory to execution*. Milwaukee, WI: American Society for Quality Control.

Thomadsen, B., Lin, S. W., & Laemmrich, M. S. (2003). Analysis of treatment delivery errors in brachytherapy using formal risk analysis techniques. *Int J Radiat Oncol, 57*, 1492–1508.

Tong, C. K. S., & Wong, E. T. T. (2005). Picture Achiving and Communication System in Healthcare. In M. Pagani (Ed.) *Encyclopedia of Multimedia Technology and Networking,* Idea Group Reference, 821-828.

Wong, E. T. T. (2005). Risk Modeling for Airport Hazard Management, *Proceedings of the Airport Council International-Pacific Best Practice Seminar & CEO Forum,* [CD-ROM], April 18-21, 2005, Beijing.

Chapter XIII
PACS Network Traffic Control

NETWORK STANDARDS

Economically speaking, it is interesting to see that over the years, the question as to whether PACS is cost-justifiable has not been easier to answer. The early work at the hospital of the University of Pennsylvania, as well as at Washington University in Seattle, provided some early numbers and a framework to use, however, a clear "savings-model" is still difficult to formulate. The challenge is that one cannot just look at how much is saved by eliminating film, but that the true savings lie more in the increases in efficiency. Productivity studies by the VA in Baltimore in the early 1990's have helped in this regard. However, one has to realize that, as Dr. Eliot Siegel from the VA in Baltimore strongly advocates, one has to re-engineer a department and its workflow to make use of the advantages of this new technology to really realize the benefits.

As one can imagine, the early PACS only replaced their film-based operation with a softcopy environment without emphasizing re-engineering. That brings us to one of the big "drivers" in this technology: network standardization. In the early 1980's, there was no one single standard. Transmission Control Protocol and the Internet Protocol (TCP/IP) was just one of the several options available. The United States government was pushing for the Open Systems Interconnection (OSI) standard.

The OSI was an effort to standardize networking that was started in 1982 by the International Organization for Standardization (ISO), along with the International Telecommunication Union (ITU). The OSI reference model was a major advance in the teaching of network concepts. It promoted the idea of a common model of protocol layers, defining interoperability between network devices and software.

However, the actual OSI protocol suite that was specified as part of the project was considered by many to be too complicated and to a large extent unimplementable. Taking the "forklift upgrade" approach to networking, it specified eliminating all existing protocols and replacing them with new ones at all layers of the stack. This made implementation difficult, and was resisted by many vendors and users with significant investments in other network technologies. In addition, the OSI protocols were specified by committees filled with differing and sometimes conflicting feature requests, leading to numerous optional features; because so much was optional, many vendors' implementations simply could not interoperate, negating the whole effort. Even demands by the USA for OSI support on all government purchased hardware did not save the effort.

Major manufacturers, notably General Motors, were also trying to enforce broadband instead of Ethernet standards. As a matter of fact, the first PACS by Philips used broadband technology. There were also "ad-hoc" developments using inventive solutions in the 1980's, such as the one at Michigan State University, whereby images from three CT scanners were sent to the University diagnostic center for reading leasing bandwidth from the commercial CATV cable system; a predecessor to cable modems! The early versions of DICOM, called ACRNEMA, only specified a dedicated point-to-point connection, leaving it up to the manufacturer to exchange the data via their network of choice. It took about ten years for the network standard to emerge, something we take for granted now. Today, everyone uses the TCP/IP as the basis for network communication, making it easy for new developments at the physical level such as gigabit/sec Ethernet to be deployed.

As with all other communications protocol, TCP/IP is composed of layers (Yale, 1995):

- **IP** - is responsible for moving packet of data from node to node. The Internet authorities assign ranges of numbers to different organizations. The hospital authority assign groups of their numbers to PACS departments.
- **TCP** - is responsible for verifying the correct delivery of data from client to server.
- **Sockets** - is a name given to the package of subroutines that provide access to TCP/IP on most systems.

TCP and IP were developed by a US Department of Defense (DOD) research project to connect a number different networks designed by different vendors into the Internet". It was initially successful because it delivered a few basic services that PACS staff needs, e.g. imaging file transfer, across a very large number of client and server systems. A small number of computers in a PACS department can use TCP/IP on a single local area network (LAN). The IP component provides routing from the department to the Medical Authority network, then to regional networks, and finally to the global Internet. Owing to the growing Internet traffic, a quality problem frequently occurs and it is relating to the congestion control in TCP.

TCP CONGESTION CONTROL

Liu (2008) has given a clear explanation on congestion control. According to his online information, each user wishes to transmit as many packets as possible. However, the Internet is a resource by billions of users, and the links which connect the computers and routers, have only limited capacity, which means that the links can only transmit data at no more than certain maximum rates. When many users simultaneously transmit at very high data rates, their total transmission rate may exceed the capacity of some link on their paths, in which case the arriving packets to that link wait in a queue before they are processed. However, due to memory limitations, each link can only store a certain number of packets in its queue and when the number of packets exceeds the maximum allowed queue limit, newly arriving packets are dropped. If the transmission rate of senders is not regulated, a lot of packets are dropped, and the packets which are not packet also experience a very large latency, and the network may completely fail to work. Since a sender does not know how much bandwidth is available, TCP chooses a trial and error method: TCP increases its packet transmission rate very slowly and linearly, till the network starts to drop packets. Upon detecting packet loss, TCP judges that the network is congested, and it drastically reduces its transmission rate (reduces its transmission rate to half of its original size). After the congestion, TCP slowly increases the transmission rate again, till the next occurrence of packet loss. This linear increase and reduction by half mechanism is called AIMD: additive increase and multiplicative decrease.

Consider the case of a hospital gateway, a router connecting the hospital network to the rest of the Internet (Figure 1). All traffic leaving the hospital network must pass through a single router outgoing port. The gateway router can become congested because the hospital network provides larger bandwidth than the link connecting the hospital with the rest of the Internet.

Figure 1. A simplified diagram of a hospital network

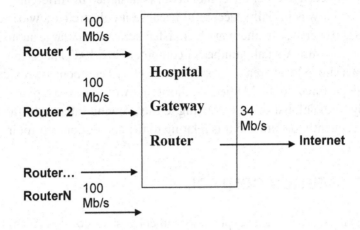

Any protocol that runs on top of IP (Internet Protocol), such as TCP (Transmission Control Protocol), can detect packet drops and interpret them as indications of congestion in the network. In particular, a TCP sender will react to these packet drops by reducing its sending rate. This slower sending rate translates into a decrease in the incoming packet rate at the router, which effectively allows the router to clear up its queue.

Queues are used to smooth spikes in incoming packet rates and to allow the router sufficient time for packet transmission. When the incoming packet rate is higher than the router's outgoing packet rate, the queue size will increase, eventually exceeding available buffer space. When the buffer is full, some packets will have to be dropped -- but which ones? A straightforward solution is to drop the packets that are just arriving at the input port; that is, if a packet arrives and finds the queue full it will be dropped. This policy is known as drop tail or tail-drop (DT). Other solutions include dropping the first packet in the queue ("drop front on full") (Lakshman et al. 1996) or dropping a random packet already stored in the queue. Each of these solutions has certain advantages and disadvantages (which we will not elaborate on due to space limitations), but DT is the most widespread dropping policy.

While every PACS team is still searching for an ideal TCP congestion control method which can achieve reasonably small queue length and stable window size, a cost-effective solution, based on a free and open software "Scilab", is proposed.

Scilab is a numerical computational package developed by INRIA and École natio-
nale des ponts et chaussées (ENPC). It is a high level programming language in that
most of its functionality is based around the ability to specify many computations
with few lines of code. It is similar in functionality to MATLAB, but is available
for download at no cost (Scilab, 2008). Readers are welcome to contact the authors
for any download difficulties.

QUEUE MANAGEMENT

With the evolvement of the Internet, the number of users and applications using
Internet increases very quickly. Congestion has become an important issue. To keep
the stability of the whole network, congestion control algorithms have been extensively studied. Queue management employed by the routers is one of the important
components in congestion control study. Numerous Active Queue Management
(AQM) algorithms have been proposed in the literature to address the problem of
congestion in the Internet. Their performance is highly dependent on parameters'
setting and tuning. Besides that, most of the AQM algorithms focus on throughput
optimization and fail to provide bounded transmission delay while providing high
link utilization to popular TCP-based radio/video streaming applications.

Tackling the aforementioned concerns, Aoul et al. (2007) proposed and evaluated a novel self-configuring AQM algorithm based on fuzzy logic. The proposed
approach simplifies significantly the deployment and management of such complex
control mechanisms in the Internet providing at the same time a good tradeoff between link utilization and queuing latency. The introduced algorithm is compared
with the most efficient adaptive AQM algorithms proposed to date such as ARED,
REM, PID and LRED. The performance analysis demonstrates that the proposed
"Fast and Autonomic Fuzzy Controller" (FAFC): (1) minimizes queue fluctuation,
(2) optimizes the throughput regardless of the traffic load variation and the presence
of unresponsive UDP/RTP based voice and video communications, and (3) suggests
the best compromise between link utilization and queuing delay.

A two-dimensional discrete-time Markov chain was introduced to model the
random early detection (RED) mechanism for two traffic classes where each dimension corresponds to a traffic class with its own parameters (Guan et al, 2007). This
mechanism takes into account the reduction of incoming traffic arrival rate due
to packets dropped probabilistically with the drop probability increasing linearly
with system contents. The stochastic analysis of the queue considered could be of
interest for the performance evaluation of the RED mechanism for the multi-class
traffic with short-range dependent (SRD) traffic characteristics. The performance
metrics including mean system occupancy, mean packet delay, packet loss prob-

ability and system throughput are computed from the analytical model for a dropping policy that is a function of the thresholds and maximum drop probability. Typical numerical results are included to illustrate the credibility of the proposed mechanism in the context of external burst and correlated traffic. These results clearly demonstrate how different threshold settings can provide different trade-offs between loss probability and delay to suit different service requirements. The effects on various performance measures of changes in the input parameters and of burstiness and correlations exhibited by the arrival process are also presented. It was claimed that the model would be applicable to high-speed networks, which use slotted protocols.

In TCP/IP networks, the packet-dropping probability function is considered as a control input. Therefore, a TCP AQM controller was modeled as a time-delayed system with a saturated input (Chen et al. 2007). The objective of the work was to design robust controllers capable of achieving the desired queue size and guaranteeing asymptotic stability of the operating point. To achieve this aim, two control strategies, namely a static state feedback controller and an observer-based controller, were proposed. By applying the Lyapunov–Krasovskii functional approach and the linear matrix inequality technique, control laws and delay-independent stability criteria for the AQM controllers were derived. The performance of the two control schemes was evaluated in various network scenarios via a series of numerical simulations. The simulation results confirm that the proposed schemes outperform other AQM schemes.

Another work focuses on deriving the necessary and sufficient stability condition of transmission control protocol (TCP) network with a proportional-integral (PI) active queue management (AQM) scheme via a parameter space approach was done (Wang, 2007). First, a fluid-flow TCP nonlinear model was converted into a linear time-delay system of neutral type. Second, the stability of the closed-loop system was characterized in terms of the networks and the controllers parameters. By simulation studies the boundary relations of these two kinds of parameters in the parameter space were studied and it was shown how PI controller's parameters affect the stability. Finally, different stability conditions are compared to show the less conservatism of the necessary- and sufficient-condition-based method, and simulation experiments by both Matlab and NS-2 were conducted to prove the author's claim.

It has been observed that TCP connections that go through multiple congested links (MCL) have a smaller transmission rate than the other connections. Such TCP behavior is a result of two components (i) the cumulative packet losses that a flow experiences at each router along its path; (ii) the longer round trip times (RTTs) suffered by such flows due to non-negligible queuing delays at congested routers. This double "bias" against connections with MCLs has been shown to approximate the so-called minimum potential delay fairness principle in the current Internet. Despite the recent proliferation of new congestion control proposals for TCP in high-speed networks, it is still unclear what kind of fairness principle could be achieved with such newly proposed congestion control protocols in high-speed networks with large-delays. Studies already show that some high-speed TCP variants may cause surprisingly severe RTT unfairness in high-speed networks with DropTail (DT) routers.

Chen & Bensaou (2007) studied the problem of unfairness in high-speed networks with some well-known high-speed TCP variants in presence of multiple congested links and highlights the severity of such unfairness when DropTail queue management is adopted. Through a simple synchronized loss model analysis, we show how synchronized losses with DropTail in high-speed networks could lead to severe RTT unfairness and drop probability (DP) unfairness; while random marking AQM schemes, which break the packet loss synchrony mitigate such unfairness dramatically by ensuring that the packet loss probability of a flow is the sum of the loss probabilities on the congested routers it crosses. Extensive simulations were carried out and the results support their findings.

Queue Management

From the above, it may be seen that two popular queue management methods are: Drop tail and RED (Random Early Detection) and they are explained below.

Drop Tail (DT)

Drop Tail, is a simple queue management algorithm used by Internet routers to decide when to drop packets. In contrast to the more complex algorithms like RED and WRED, in TD all the traffic is not differentiated. Each packet is treated identically. With TD, when the queue is filled to its maximum capacity, the newly arriving packets are dropped until the queue has enough room to accept incoming traffic. The name arises from the effect of the policy on incoming datagrams. Once a queue has been filled, the router begins discarding all additional datagrams, thus dropping the tail of the sequence of datagrams. The loss of datagrams causes the TCP sender to enter slow-start, which reduces throughput in that TCP session until the the sender begins to receive ACKs again and increases its congestion window. A more severe problem occurs when datagrams from multiple TCP connections are dropped, causing global synchronization, i.e., all of the involved TCP senders enter slow-start. This happens because, instead of discarding many segments from one connection, the router would tend to discard one segment from each connection (Corner, 2006).

Random Early Detection (RED)

RED is an AQM mechanism, which is not designed to operate with any specific protocol, but performs better with protocols that perceive drops as indications of congestion (e.g. TCP). RED gateways require the user to specify five parameters: the maximum buffer size or queue limit (QL), the minimum (min_{th}) and maximum (max_{th}) thresholds of the "RED region", the maximum dropping probability (max_p), and the weight factor used to calculate the average queue size (w_q). QL can be defined in terms of packets or bytes. Note that when DT is implemented at a router, QL is the only parameter that needs to be set. A RED router uses early packet dropping in an attempt to control the congestion level, limit queuing delays, and avoid buffer overflows. Early packet dropping starts when the average queue size exceeds min_{th}. RED was specifically designed to use the average queue size (*avg*), instead of the current queue size, as a measure of incipient congestion, because the latter proves to be rather intolerant of packet bursts, as we will see shortly. If the average queue size does not exceed min_{th} a RED router will not drop any packets. *avg* is calculated as an exponentially weighted moving average using the following formula (Pentikousis 2001):

$$avg_i = (1 - w_q) \times avg_{i-1} + w_q \times q$$

where the weight w_q is commonly set to 0.002, and q is the instantaneous queue size. This weighted moving average captures the notion of long-lived congestion better than the instantaneous queue size. Had the instantaneous queue size been used as the metric to determine whether the router is congested, short-lived traffic spikes would lead to early packet drops. So a rather underutilized router that receives a burst of packets can be deemed "congested" if one uses the instantaneous queue size. The average queue size, on the other hand, acts as a low pass filter that allows spikes to go through the router without forcing any packet drops (unless, of course, the burst is larger than the queue limit). The user can configure w_q and min_{th} so that a RED router does not allow short-lived congestion to continue uninterrupted for more than a predetermined amount of time. This functionality allows RED to maintain high throughput and keep per-packet delays low.

Figure 4 shows a more complex data flow diagram, which describes the functions of the "Multi-sender simulation" mode. Under this mode, more interfaces are designed as more than one sender and router are configured and each sender or router may have different configuration. Similar to the previous mode, all the input data are gathered and sent to the calculation model, and the results are returned and charts are plotted.

As the most widely used reliable transport in today's Internet, TCP has been extensively studied in the past decade. However, previous research usually only considers a small or medium number of concurrent TCP connections. The TCP behavior under many competing TCP flows has not been sufficiently explored. There are three commonly used approaches to study the TCP protocol: developing analytical models, conducting Internet measurements, and running simulations. In the present context, results of various simulations to systematically investigate the performance of many TCP flows were analyzed. In their paper, Qiu et al (2001) used extensive simulations to systematically investigate the performance of a large number of concurrent TCP flows. They started with a simple scenario, in which all the connections had the same roundtrip time (RTT), and the gateways used drop-tail policy. The way the aggregate throughput, goodput, and loss rate varied with different underlying topologies were examined. They also looked at the behavior of each individual connection when competing with other connections. They broke the synchronization by either adding random processing time or using random early detection (RED) gateways, and examine their effects on the TCP performance. Finally TCP performance with different RTTs was observed and the roundtrip bias was quantified using both analysis and simulations. Notable findings include:

- When all the connections have the same propagation delay, without adding random processing time, global synchronization occurs in the large pipe case.
- Adding random processing time or using RED gateways makes both synchronization and consistent discrimination less pronounced.
- For both drop-tail and RED gateways, the aggregate throughput of TCP flows is close to link bandwidth, except when there are too few connections to fill up the pipe. There is a small variation in the throughput as the number of connections increases, but most variation is within 2%.
- For both drop-tail and RED gateways, the aggregate goodput of TCP flow decreases slightly with the number of connections due to the increase in the unnecessary retransmissions. The only exception occurs when there are too few connections to fill up the pipe.

Based on these results, several observations were made. First, since adding random processing time makes both synchronization and consistent discrimination less pronounced, these dramatic behaviors are not severe problems in the Internet. Second, for bulk transfers, the aggregate throughput, goodput, and loss rate under drop-tail gateways are comparable to those under RED gateways. Third, for bulk transfers, RED tends to reduce the bias against long-RTT connections, making the bandwidth sharing more fair than with drop-tail.

TCP/AQM NETWORK MODEL

Since their inception in the late 1980s, the congestion control mechanisms in TCP have been extremely successful in keeping the Internet under control while it underwent a dramatic growth. One of the problems is that TCP is not able to provide operational information (e.g. router queue length) of networks. To enable such a function within TCP, Active Queue Management (AQM) techniques have recently been proposed to alleviate some of the congestion control problems for IP networks as well as enhancing quality of service (Misra et al. 2000). Modeling and analysis of such networks is important to understand their dynamics.

Recently, Campbell and his colleagues have proposed a nonlinear time-delay system which was developed by using Scilab to represent a fluid model for a TCP/AQM network (Campbell, 2006). The Scicos diagram was used to realize this system. In most of the cases, single sender and single/multi-level routers were considered. However, it did not consider the complexity of the real life network involving multiple senders and multi-level routers. In the proposed approach, the simplified model developed by Campbell et al. (2006) has been modified by the authors and research associates. AQM/RED and DT algorithms have been added to the router, and implementation of multi-routers and multiple TCP flows have also been considered.

In Campbell's work, the fluid model for a TCP/AQM network showed a good agreement between predictions from this model and measurements in some of the real cases (Misra et al., 2000). The model takes the following functions:

$$W(t) = \frac{1}{R} - \frac{W(t)W(t-R)}{2R}KQ(t-R) \tag{1}$$

$$Q(t) = \begin{pmatrix} N\dfrac{W(t)}{R}-C, & Q>0 \\ \max(N\dfrac{W(t)}{R}-C,0) & Q=0 \end{pmatrix} \tag{2}$$

Where W refers to the TCP window size, Q refers to queue length in the router, and R refers to round-trip time.

A shortcoming of this model is that when the queue gets excessively large, the packet loss process, which is made to be proportional to the queue length with coefficient K, would be inappropriate. Additionally, in this model the round-trip time is assumed time-invariable, which does not represent the real-life situation.

Proportional AQM Scheme

Active queue management (AQM) is a process wherein packets are marked as function of queue length (Hollot and Chait, 2001). The purposes of marking packets in this way are to reduce TCP source rates as queue length grows, to maintain a relatively stable queue length in the router and avoid the buffer gets full. RED is one of the recent AQM schemes. In RED, the loss is made roughly to be proportional to the average queue length. For a single congested router with a transmission capacity C, the packet discard function p(x) takes an estimate of the average queue length at the router as its argument. In RED, p(x) takes the following function:

$$
\left(
\begin{array}{ll}
0, & 0 < x < q^{min} \\
\dfrac{x - q_{min}}{q^{max} - q^{min}} p^{max}, & q^{min} < x < q^{max} \\
1, & q^{max} < x
\end{array}
\right)
\tag{3}
$$

Where q^{min}, q^{max} and p^{max} are configurable parameters and refer to the minimum queue length, the maximum queue length, and the maximum drop probability respectively.

A TCP FLUID-FLOW MODEL

Hollot and Chait (2001) considered a system with single congested router. A dynamic model of TCP behavior was developed by using fluid-flow and stochastic differential equation analysis. The model is described by the following coupled nonlinear differential equations:

$$
\dot{W}(t) = \frac{1}{R(t)} - \frac{W(t)W(t - R(t))}{2R(t - R(t))} p(t - R(t))
\tag{4}
$$

$$
\dot{q}(t) = N(t)\frac{W(t)}{R(t)} - C
\tag{5}
$$

Where the queue length q and window-size W are positive and bounded quantities; i.e. $q \in [0, q_{max}]$ and $w \in [0, w_{max}]$, the value of the marking probability p is only in the range $\{0, 1\}$, and R (t) is the time-variant round-trip time delay, which takes the following function:

$$R(t) = \frac{q(t)}{C} + T_p \tag{6}$$

Where Tp is the propagation delay. It shows that the round-trip time delay depends on both router's queue length and capacity.

MULTI-ROUTER AND MULTIPLE TCP FLOW SIMULATION

The extension to the more complex network situation is straightforward. Let V be a collection of routers. Each router $v \in V$ has a transmission capacity of C_v. Router v has an AQM policy. The queue length for router v is $q_v(t)$. For TCP flows with a workload of N, the flows are labeled with i=1...N, and the average round trip time of flow I is approximated equal to:

$$R_i(q,t) = a_i + \sum_{v \in V} q_v(t) / C_v \tag{7}$$

For each TCP flow, the combined loss seen by a particular flow is

$$1 - \prod (1 - AP(x)_v) \tag{8}$$

Where $P(x)_v$ is the pack loss probability in router v.
Thus, (4) is modified to

$$W(t) = \frac{1}{R(t)} - \frac{W(t)W(t-R(t))}{2R(t-R(t))} (1 - (\prod (1 - AP(x)_v))) \tag{9}$$

For each router, (5) is modified to:

$$q(t) = \sum \frac{W(t)_i}{R(t)} - C \tag{10}$$

Data Flow Diagrams (DFD)

In this section, data flow diagrams are developed to illustrate the relationships among blocks in the model and how the fluid flow TCP/AQM model works during the simulation.

As shown in Figure 2, the primary interfaces in the model and the relationships among them are presented. Any two of the four interfaces are related by a link.

Figure 2. Links between main interfaces

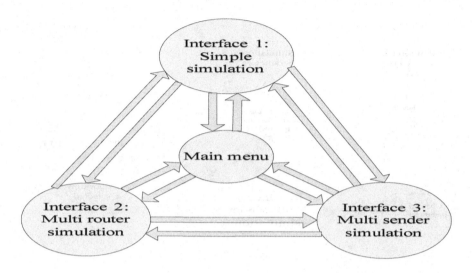

Figure 3. DFD in "simple simulation" mode

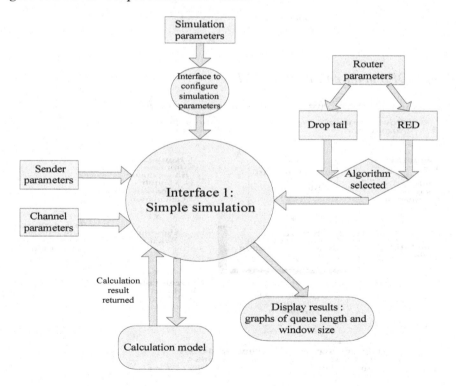

Figure 4. DFD in "multi sender" mode

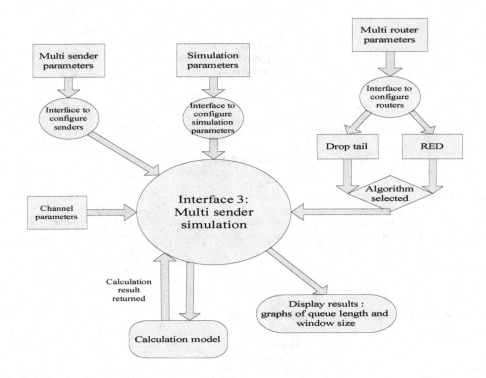

Figure 5. DFD in the calculation model

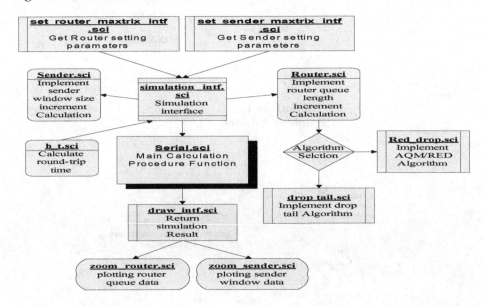

In Figure 3, the data flow diagram in the "Simple simulation" mode is presented. Under this mode, there is only one sender and only one router. The circle represents interfaces which are showed to user, and the rectangle represents input data. The arrow shows the direction of data flow in the model. What should be mentioned here is that the calculation model returns the results to the main interface, and then the display units plot charts.

Data flows among Scilab files are shown in Figure 5.

Simulation Results

In the model, users in the interfaces before the simulation process can set all necessary parameters of senders and routers. After simulating, the display units can plot the charts of the simulation results: queue length for the router and window size for the sender such as Figure 6.

Figure 6. Simulation results displays

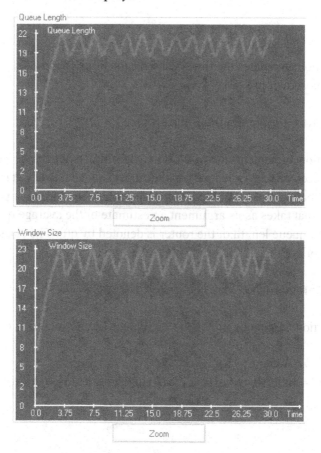

Core Function Descriptions

Function draw_intf (router_index,sender_index)

This function is called by the interface model to transfer the required router queue and sender window for displaying. As in the GUI, when simulating the situation for multi-router and multi-sender, only the window of one sender and the queue of one router could be displayed at one time. This function receives the parameters: router_index sender_index, and send back the queue and window data for the required router and sender for displaying.

Function p = drop_tail(buffer,q)

This function implements the droptail algorithm in the router. When the buffer of the router is full, the router would drop all its received packets (returned p=1); otherwise the router accepts all the packets and stores them in the buffer (returned p=0).

Function delay = h_t(Qv,C,Tp,N_R)

This function calculates the time-delay for the fluid TCP model. It implements the calculation shown in Eqn. (7).

Function p = Red_drop(q,q_min,q_max,p_max)

This function implements the AQM/RED algorithm in the router. The drop probability of its received packet depends on the current queue linearly. It implements an active queue management (AQM) policy that is characterized by a packet discard function p(x) that takes as its argument an estimate of the average queue length at the router. The queue length of the router is denoted by q(t). The classical example of an AQM policy is RED for which p(x) takes the form in (3)

Function d_q=router(t,Wv_Matrix,C,t_step,delay,N_S)

This function calculates the queue increment of one router. It takes the form in (9)

Function d_W=sender(Pi_Matrix,Wi_Matrix,t,delay,t_step,h_Matrix)

This function calculates the window size increment of one sender. It takes the form in (8).

CONCLUDING REMARK

In recent years, one of the major objectives in the networking research area is to find an ideal TCP congestion control method, which can achieve reasonably small queue length and stable window size. The simulation results of the authors' work, which are realized by using inside tcl/tk script executed from Scilab, show that at certain level of traffic flow, one can achieve the objective by combining TCP with the AQM algorithms. The algorithms work even in complex environments involving multiple senders, multi-level routers and multiple TCP flows. Based on the preliminary success in fluid-flow simulations, the objective of achieving optimum resource allocation between TCP flows can be pursued.

REFERENCES

Aoul, Y. H., Mehaoua, A., & Skianis, C. (2007). A fuzzy logic-based AQM for real-time traffic over internet. *Computer Networks*, *51*(16),4617-4633.

Campbell, S., Chancelier, J. P., & Nikoukhah, R. (2006). Modeling and simulation in Scilab/Scicos. 2nd Edn., Springer.Chen, S. & Bensaou, B. (2007) Can high-speed networks survive with DropTail queues management? *Computer Networks*, *51*(7), *763-1776.*

Chen, C. K., Hung, Y. C., Liao, T. L., & Yan, J. J. (2007). Design of robust active queue management controllers for a class of TCP communication networks. *Information Sciences*, *177*(19), 4059-4071.

Comer, D. E. (2006). *Internetworking with TCP/IP, 5.* Upper Saddle River, NJ: Prentice Hall.

Guan, L., Awan, I. U., Woodward, M. E., & Wang, X. G. (2007). Discrete-time performance analysis of a congestion control mechanism based on RED under multi-class bursty and correlated traffic. *Journal of Systems and Software, 80*(10), 1716-1725.

Hollot, C. V., & Chait, Y. (2001). Nonlinear Stability Analysis for a Class of TCP/AQM Network. *Proc. IEEE Conference on Decision and Control.* Orlando. Lakshman. (pp. 2309-2314).

Liu, S. (2008). *What is Congestion Control?* Retrieved on 16 January 2008 from http://www.ews.uiuc.edu/~shaoliu/tcpillinois/background1.html#congestioncontrol.

Misra, V., Wei-Bo, G., & Towsley, D. (2000). Fluid-based analysis of a network of AQM routers supporting TCP flows with an application to RED. *Proc. ACM/SIG-COMM.* Stockholm, Sweden, pp.151--160.

Neidhardt, T. V., & Ott, T. (1996). The Drop From Front Strategy in TCP Over ATM and its Interworking with Other Control Features. *Proceedings of IEEE INFOCOM 1996*. San Francisco, California, April 1996.

Pentikousis, K. (2001) *Active Queue Management*. Retrieved on 16 January 2008 from http://www.acm.org/crossroads/columns/connector/july2001.html

Qiu, L., Zhang, Y., & Keshav, S. (2001). Understanding the performance of many TCP flows. *Computer Networks, 37*(3-4), 277-306.

Scilab (2008). *Scilab Software*. Available from Scilab Online Web site. www.scilab.org

Wang, D. J. (2007). Stability Analysis of PI TCP/AQM Networks: A Parameter Space Approach. *Acta Automatica Sinica, 33*(7),756-760.

Yale University (1995). *Introduction to TCP/IP*. Retrieved on 16 January 2008 from http://www.yale.edu/pclt/COMM/TCPIP.HTM

Chapter XIV
Human Factors and Culture

BACKGROUND

Human factors engineering (HFE) is the science of designing systems to fit human capabilities and limitations. These include limitations in perception, cognition, and physical performance. HFE involves the application of specific methods and tools in the design of systems.

Human information processing is influenced by multiple factors:

- **Attention:** May be limited in duration or focus, especially if attention to several things is necessary.
- **Memory constraints:** Working memory is limited, especially when active processing of information is required.
- **Automaticity:** Consistent, over learned responses may become automatic, and completed without conscious thought.
- **Situation awareness:** A person's perception of elements in the environment may affect their processing of information.

Humans have certain tendencies and biases that can predispose them to error. These heuristics are usually very useful and successful, but at times can get us into trouble. The objectives of this chapter are to provide practical Human Factors guidance to professionals concerned with PACS operation and management and to introduce the non-specialist to Human Factors issues in PACS operation and management. It is intended to show how human capabilities and limitations can influence field performance and quality within the PACS environment.

This chapter also discusses the quality improvement likely to result from the provision of a proper work environment. First the importance of communications and information exchange among PACS users, maintenance staff, manufacturers, suppliers, and so forth, is discussed. The need to introduce self-paced computer-based PACS training for hospital staff is stressed. Then a comparison of the western and eastern cultural dimensions is illustrated through a case study. Finally a feasible PACS HF model is suggested. Obviously, a PACS environment that works for one hospital does not necessarily work for another; hence it is imperative that the organizational culture must be considered when a PACS project is being planned.

COMMUNICATION AND INFORMATION EXCHANGE

Communication is probably the most important Human Factor issue in PACS operation and management. Without communication among referring clinicians, radiologists, technologists, nursing staff, maintenance engineers and suppliers, high PACS quality standards would be difficult to maintain. In the PACS environment, there is an enormous volume of information that must be created, conveyed, assimilated, used and recorded in delivering quality medical imaging service. A frequently quoted example in the aviation sector is the paper stack, supposedly exceeding the height of Mt. Everest, that the Boeing Aircraft Company produces annually in order to support its aircraft operators. Airlines literally have warehouses full of paper that contain the historical records of maintenance of their aircraft.

As part of a national program in the Department of Veterans Affairs to improve communication within the healthcare environment, a Medical Team Training questionnaire was developed to assess organizational culture, communication, teamwork, and awareness of human factors engineering principles (Mills et al. 2008). First, the Medical Team Training questionnaire was pilot tested with 300 healthcare clinicians. The final version of the Medical Team Training questionnaire was administered to an interdisciplinary group of 384 surgical staff members in 6 facilities as part of the Medical Team Training pilot project in the Department of Veterans Affairs. The results revealed a pattern of discrepancies among physicians and nurses in which surgeons perceive a stronger organizational culture of safety, better communication, and better teamwork than either nurses or anesthesiologists do. It was concluded that the Medical Team Training questionnaire was helpful in identifying hidden problems with communication before formal team training learning sessions, and it would be useful in focusing efforts to improve communication and teamwork in the operating room.

It is most important that operation and management information be understandable to the target audience. For PACS operation, the primary members of this audience are the technologists and radiologists, who choose patient from modality worklist, obtain images, check images for quality, and review images and reports, as well as dictate examination with voice recognition systems. New manuals, operation and maintenance service bulletins, job cards and other information to be used by this audience should be tested before distribution to make sure that they will not be misunderstood or misinterpreted. Sometimes operation information is conveyed through a less-than-optimum selection of words. Anecdotal evidence suggests a case where a certain procedure was "proscribed" (i.e. prohibited) in an operation manual. The technologist reading this concluded that the procedure was "prescribed" (i.e. defined, laid down) and proceeded to perform the forbidden action. These types of problems are becoming more prevalent now that PACS are being employed all over the world. Sometimes the technical language of the manufacturer does not translate easily into the technical language of the customer and the result can be operation documentation that is difficult to understand.

Communication with the PACS manufacturers, as well as between hospitals, can be crucial. If one PACS user discovers a problem in operating its PACS that could degrade quality, then that problem should be communicated to the manufacturer and to other PACS users of the same type. This is not always easy to do. Industry cost control measures and competitive pressures may not place a premium on communication among hospitals. However, medical regulatory bodies can play an important role by encouraging PACS operators under their jurisdiction to interact frequently with one another and the manufacturer of the PACS they operate. An operation-related incident in one hospital, if made known to other operators, could easily prevent an accident from happening. The accident record has no shortage of accidents that could have been prevented if incident information from hospitals had been made known to the healthcare industry.

Lack of communication within a hospital's medical imaging department can also have a very serious negative impact on the hospital's operation. Indeed many occurrences indicated that lack of proper communication of action taken or action that needed to be taken was rampant, adding to the series of errors and, thus, the accident occurrences.

Patients do not like treatment delays due to PACS defects and if they happen too often in a certain hospital, business may be lost to a competitor. PACS maintenance staff are keenly aware of this pressure and strive to accomplish their work in a timely manner. Clearly this can sometimes lead to compromised maintenance especially when, as so often happens, things do not go according to plan. Hospital administrators' role is to ensure that their PACS maintenance departments are provided with adequate personnel and resources to prevent the type of work that results in degraded imaging service. This problem, while not — strictly speaking — a communication issue, highlights the importance of an open, two-way exchange within relevant departments. Hospital management needs to develop procedures and ensure their application to prevent dispatch of poor quality images. One of the best ways of facilitating this activity is to maintain an ongoing dialogue with PACS users and maintenance team, encouraging them to report hazardous situations or practices.

PACS TRAINING

The growing complexity of newer generations of PACS makes it necessary to provide more formal classroom-type training. With, for example, sophisticated DICOM networks, it is important to provide extensive classroom-based training on underlying system principles. This is difficult to do with on-the-job training. Here, as well, it is very important that PACS instructors be extensively prepared for their task. It is not enough to simply dub a senior engineer an instructor. In addition to being a subject matter expert, the instructor must also know how to teach, i.e. how to present information clearly, how to seek feedback from the participants to ascertain that they are learning, how to determine problem areas and be able to provide remedial instruction.

Today's healthcare trainees have greater expectations from interactive computer systems including training systems. In many countries including a number of developing countries, secondary or high school students have already had some exposure to personal computers and to computer games available for home televisions. These devices do provide considerable feedback and performance rating features found in new technology training systems. Similarly, newer computer-based instruction (CBI) systems offer training that adapts to the students' knowledge and skill. However, advanced technology CBI must have a reasonable degree of intelligence comparable to that of a human instructor. More than the instructions and feedback on what needs to be done or on how one is performing; new technology should be able to provide systemic tutoring. Systems capable of such endeavours are now available in some high-technology training establishments. These new systems are called Intelligent Tutoring Systems (ITS). The features that set ITS apart from the less proficient CBI systems are software modules that emulate students, subject matter experts and instructors. In view of the growing integration of the PACS and imaging modalities with the hospital and Radiological Information System (RIS), such ITS systems would need to be implemented for PACS.

ITS have been found to be very effective for training in the diagnosis and maintenance of complex high-technology equipment and software. They have a number of advantages over traditional training methods including the capacity to provide "just-in-time" training or refresher training immediately before maintenance work is started. Also with ITS, training is under the students' control and can be scheduled, paced or repeated at the students' discretion. There is a feeling, in some circles, that these systems may prove to be too complex for widespread use. It is possible that these feelings spring from lack of experience with this technology rather than from an evaluation of technical and training staff capabilities. Hospital administrators are required to keep an open mind about the use of these new education and training technologies lest they deprive their hospitals of important capabilities that could have very significant safety and quality implications.

EFFECTS OF ORGANIZATION CULTURE

The importance of organizational culture is not new. In 1967 Peter Drucker noted that "developing executive effectiveness challenges directions, goals, and purposes of the organization. It raises the eyes of its people from preoccupation with problems to a vision of opportunity." Dr. Deming (1986) developed 14 Points that were an interrelated system of paradigms, processes and procedures to achieve maximum effectiveness and quality of product and service from people. Organization culture is the personality of the organization. Culture is consisted of the assumptions, values, norms and tangible signs (artifacts) of organization members and their behaviors. Members of an organization soon come to sense the particular culture of an organization. Culture is one of those terms that are difficult to express distinctly, but everyone knows it when they sense it. For instance, the culture of a large, for-profit corporation is quite different from that of a hospital.

A survey of the quality literature would reveal that people are a vital but missing link in most continuous improvement initiatives. Sustainable PACS operation requires the combination of individual staff and organizational skills. The success of any quality initiative, whether it is a Kaizen, Lean Manufacturing or Six Sigma effort, depends on the effective integration of relationship management skills with process improvement tools. Organizations that have implemented quality programs have invested substantially in learning all of the tools, processes and systems. Despite this commitment, results are remained to be seen.

The globalization of business has placed new demands on management thinking and process improvement techniques, making a basic understanding of cultural differences and their management implications a prerequisite for the quality expert. With this in mind, the impact of cultural differences on PACS quality is examined. Within the context of Six Sigma implementation, the impact of four major cultural dimensions have been examined, viz. power distance, individualism, uncertainty avoidance, and company long-term orientation (Hofstede, 1983).

The TQM method is a project-driven management approach to improve the organization's products, services, and processes by continually reducing defects in the organization. It is a business strategy that focuses on improving customer requirements understanding, business systems, productivity, and financial performance. Dating back to the mid 1980s, applications of the TQM methods allowed many organizations to sustain their competitive advantage by integrating their knowledge of the process with statistics, engineering, and project management (Anbari, 2002).

Researchers and practitioners are trying to integrate Six Sigma with other existing management practices that have been around to make TQM method more attractive to organizations that might have not started or fully implemented the Six Sigma method. Integrating and comparing principles and characteristics of Six Sigma with Total Quality Management (Revere and Black, 2003; Hammer and Goding, 2001), Human Resource Functions (Wyper and Harrrison, 2000), Lean Manufacturing (Anthony et al., 2003; He, 2005), ISO 9000 (Cathewood, 2002), ISO 9001 (Dalgleish, 2003), and the capability maturity model (Murugappan and Keeni, 2003) are all part of the quality community's effort to maximize the positive effect of TQM. Key factors for the successful deployment of TQM and Six Sigma have been widely documented in the literature, e.g. Fok and Wong (2005). Some are obvious, such as the extensive use of statistical techniques by practitioners known as Blackbelts. However, other more subtle, but very important, features of TQM are concealed within the hospital culture. It is clear to those who have participated in this success, which any organization embarking on TQM will not succeed if it focuses on statistical tools whilst failing to develop a supporting culture. The objective of this chapter is to illustrate the effect of human factors on the adoption of modern TQM methods in Hong Kong.

According to Hofstede (1983), culture is "the collective programming of the human mind, obtained in the course of life, which is common to members of one group and opposed to another". Culture is acquired knowledge that people use to interpret social behaviour. Many problems facing businesses on the international stage may be caused by a lack of understanding or familiarity with cultural differences.

From the initial results and later additions, Hofstede developed a model that identifies four primary Dimensions to assist in differentiating cultures: Power Distance Index (PDI), Individualism (IDV), Masculinity (MAS), and Uncertainty Avoidance Index (UAI). Geert Hofstede added a fifth Dimension after conducting an additional international study with a survey instrument developed with Chinese employees and managers. That Dimension, based on Confucian dynamism, is Long-Term Orientation (LTO) and was applied to 23 countries. In the following comparison of company culture, four communication and team-conducive cultural dimensions are used, viz. PDI, IDV, UAI and LTO.

- **Power Distance Index (PDI):** Power distance measures how much a culture has respect for authority. This dimension focuses on the degree of equality, or inequality, between staff in various business organizations. A high Power Distance ranking indicates that inequalities of power have been allowed to grow within the organization. These organizations are more likely to follow a superior-subordinate system that does not allow significant modifications of existing strategies or polices.

- **Individualism (IDV):** This dimension focuses on the degree the organization reinforces individual or collective achievement and interpersonal relationships. A high Individualism ranking indicates that individual opinions are respected within an organization. Individualism these organizations may tend to form a larger number of looser relationships.

- **Uncertainty Avoidance Index (UAI):** This dimension focuses on the level of tolerance for uncertainty and ambiguity within the organization—i.e. unstructured situations. A high Uncertainty Avoidance ranking indicates the organization has a low tolerance for uncertainty and ambiguity. This creates a rule-oriented organization that institutes rules, regulations, and controls in order to reduce the amount of uncertainty.

- **Long-Term Orientation (LTO):** This dimension focuses on the degree the organization embraces long-term devotion to traditional, forward thinking values. High Long-Term Orientation ranking indicates the organization prescribes to the values of long-term commitments and respect for tradition. This is thought to support a strong work ethic where long-term rewards are expected because of today's hard work. However, business initiatives may take longer to develop in this organization, particularly for new quality management initiatives such as Six Sigma method.

CASE ILLUSTRATION: CULTURAL COMPARISON

Background

A comparison of the cultural dimensions in Hong Kong, USA and the world is shown in Figure 1.

Power Distance Index (PDI)

The PDI for the United States is 40, compared to the world Average of 55 and Hong Kong's score of 68.

To understand this dimension, think about some experience you have had in your work life where the director you worked for was inspiring, and you really enjoyed working for this person. As you do this, perhaps you will see that this experience was probably a situation where you felt more like a colleague to this individual (and to your fellow employees) than a subordinate. You also probably felt free to try new things without fear of reprisal. This individual, in his or her management role, probably looked out for you and was someone you felt you could rely on, just as you were a person he or she could rely on as well. The employees probably felt they could be most productive and satisfied on the job under these circumstances.

Now reflect on the times when you have had a director who tried to assert his or her authority over you. Maybe this was in enforcing seemingly mindless policies without much thought as to their value or purpose for getting things done. In either of these situations, you no doubt felt frustrated and limited in your ability

Figure 1. A comparison of cultural dimensions

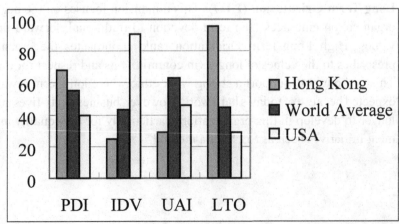

to contribute. The relatively high PDI associated with Hong Kong reveals that this latter scenario is a common operating procedure in many local companies.

Effects of High PDI on Corporate Communication

A major consequence of a high PDI on TQM implementation is that as long as the mentality behind superior-subordinate relationships exists in the organizational culture, staff would not express freely what is on their minds. In other words, active communication forums between employees and management would rarely occur and there will not be any truly two-way communication allowing the flow of negative information without fear for disseminating it. This would affect the degree of truth reflected through the voice of the customers in PACS design.

Another effect of a high PDI is that organizations would retain their hierarchies and chains of command. Consequently, it takes more energy to keep information flowing via these chains than the effort may be worth. Who needs a middle manager to dispense information when employees can punch a few buttons and find out what they need to know? There it is either from on-line files or directly from the person who knows the information.

Members of an organization decide what to do base on information and what that information implies about the situations in which they find themselves. Limited information means that decisions will be more speculative and thus more likely to introduce additional uncertainty into the company and its processes. Just think about when you or one of your colleagues made a poor decision. It probably happened because you did not have enough information. It is also likely that the information you needed was available but maybe you did not have access to it.

Despite the fact that open communication and access to information about, for example, the hospital's available modalities, patient records, finances, delivery of medical images, image retakes, what different people and teams are doing, and how the progress of your team is affecting other teams and vice versa, have already been documented for successful implementation of quality management systems, limited access to information is still a common practice in high PDI organizations.

Individualism-Collectivism

There are only seven (7) countries in Hofstede's research that have Individualism (IDV) as their highest Dimension: USA (91), Australia (90), United Kingdom (89), Netherlands and Canada (80), and Italy (76). The high Individualism (IDV) ranking for the United States indicates a society with a more individualistic attitude and relatively loose bonds with others. The populace is more self-reliant and looks out for themselves and their close family members.

Hong Kong has an Individualism (IDV) ranking of 25, second highest for Far East Asian countries, behind Japan's 46 ranking, and compared to an average of 24. Hong Kong's Individualism ranking indicates a high level of emphasis on a Collectivist society as compared to one of Individualism. This explains the slow adoption of TQM initiatives such as Six Sigma in the Hong Kong healthcare community.

Effect of Low IDV on Teamwork

US companies at home and elsewhere practice teamwork widely, especially in the form of self-directed teams, in which employees themselves are responsible for managing their groups and their work, and for making production-related decisions. By the mid-1990s, around 70 percent of Fortune 1,000 companies were relying on teams and planning to expand such usage, according to a study by the American Productivity and Quality Center in Houston, Texas. Companies organized around work teams have reported a number of benefits, including better productivity, higher-quality output, less absenteeism, less employee turnover, leaner plant structures, and substantial improvements in production-cycle time.

A study of the factors that determine the success of a team-based structure in the People's Republic of China is useful to the study of cultural influences on teamwork in general (Chen and Barshes, 2000). Chinese culture – the dominant culture in Hong Kong, on one hand, encompasses a collectivist orientation that emphasizes the importance of group structure and values. This orientation may support crucial aspects of teamwork such as a common purpose and cooperative effort. The importance of relationships in a collectivist society such as Hong Kong may also prompt individuals to place group (e.g., work team) interests ahead of their own. Thus traditional Chinese values may be expected to facilitate teamwork, especially when teams are assigned by the hospital managment and have strong appointed leaders.

On the other hand, the very elements of Chinese culture that create and sustain group attachment and conformity also support a rigid social hierarchy. Top-down control (as indicated by a high PDI) contravenes the principle and practice of true teamwork. Such a system of workplace control reinforced other Confucian cultural and social traditions, such as highly centralized decision-making, poor horizontal communication, suppressed individual initiatives, and mistrust of and lack of co-operation among coworkers. To the extent that these Confucian influences linger today in Hong Kong, they could undermine the factors necessary for successful TQM implementation in local hospitals.

Uncertainty Avoidance Index (UAI)

The UAI for the US is 46, compared to the world average of 64. A low ranking in the Uncertainty Avoidance Dimension is indicative of a society that has fewer rules and does not attempt to control all outcomes and results. It also has a greater level of tolerance for a variety of ideas, thoughts, and beliefs.

However, Hong Kong's is having an even lower UAI , only 29, compared to an average of 63 for the Far East Asian countries. This very low level of Uncertainty Avoidance is the fourth lowest in the World, with only Denmark (23), Jamaica (13), and Singapore (8) having lower scores for this Dimension.

Effect of Low UAI on TQM Implementation

The low Uncertainty Avoidance ranking indicates an organization that not only tolerates uncertainty and a freedom of opinions, but also uses this strength, in the case of Hong Kong, to be a place where many varying cultures and ideas such as quality improvement initiatives can come together. An additional reflection of a culture with low Uncertainty Avoidance is a population with less emotion, which may appear as apathy, and a more introspective nature. This explains the skeptical attitude in the implementation of advanced TQM technique among healthcare organizations in Hong Kong.

Long-Term Orientation

The LTO is the lowest Dimension for the US at 29, compared to the world average of 45. This low LTO ranking is indicative of the societies' belief in meeting its obligations and tends to reflect an appreciation for cultural traditions.

Hong Kong's has the highest-ranking (96) LTO, which is true for all Far East Asian cultures. This Dimension indicates a society's and its business community's time perspective and an attitude of persevering; that is, overcoming obstacles with time, if not with will and strength.

Effect of High LTO on TQM Initiatives

For public and private organizations in a high LTO society, new quality improvement initiatives may take longer to develop, particularly for modern technology transferring from foreign countries. A high LTO ranking indicates the organization and its management reinforces the concept of long-term, traditional orientation. In this culture, change would occur very slowly as long-term traditions and commitments might become impediments to change.

IMPLICATIONS FOR LOCAL PACS COMMUNITY

The findings of this case study carry significant implications and lessons for the healthcare community in Hong Kong, especially for their expatriate managers. A key lesson is that long-term growth and success in Hong Kong depends on how companies initiate and manage—an important shift from a business-based to a human-oriented approach. The team-based structures that have proven successful in many US companies may also be effective mechanisms in Hong Kong.

However, with a large number of local hospital departments still in the early stages of corporate governance development, it may be too soon to transfer western-style, self-directed teamwork with peer-based control and decision-making by individual team members to Hong Kong. To evaluate the individual user acceptance of PACS by the radiology department staff of a hospital, one may refer to the real-life application of the unified theory of acceptance and use of technology at the Ghent University Hospital (Duyck et al. 2008). Effective strategies should be developed to create, nurture, and synthesize the four communication and team-conducive cultural dimensions identified in this study. This will ensure that a unique PACS-TQM system that fits Hong Kong will evolve over time and produce benefits for both employees and companies.

It was found that a high power distance in local organizations would suppress open, honest communication and would create obtacles for effective TQM implementation. Although the dominant culture in Hong Kong encompasses a collectivist orientation that emphasizes the importance of group structure and values, the presence of Confucian influences could undermine the factors necessary for successful TQM implementation. A low Uncertainty Avoidance among staff explains the indifferent attitude in the implementation of TQM initiatives such as Six Sigma within the local healthcare community. Finally, in a high long-term orientation society, implementation of changes in organizations would occur rather slowly as long-term traditions and commitments might become impediments to change.

To ensure the success of any quality initiative in a mixed-culture city like Hong Kong it is clear that, additional to the individual effects, the combined effect of the above-mentioned human factors would merit further research.

PROPOSED HUMAN FACTOR APPROACH

A Sociotechnical System Approach

Based on the above observations, it is obvious that the ideal quality practice is one in which all PACS staff will cease to be silent loners, and will openly communicate with one another. This communication would, ideally, be with PACS management, and with other clinicians, technologists, radiologists, medical clerks, nurses, and maintenance technicians, about their own human errors, about technological flaws and about how to prevent them. Despite the increasing number of human factor programs operated in the medical community, a quality culture of open communication and error reduction is still a long way to go. This is because three obstacles limit the cultural change efforts. First, these programs are limited by the focus on awareness of what is good, rather than on acting to do good; second, they are reactive and must wait for an incident or accident to occur before learning can take place, and third, they deal with the individual hardware/software maintenance team and ignore the fact that these staff working together are an essential part of a sociotechnical system (STS).

The sociotechnical systems (STS) approach is devoted to the effective blending of both the technical and social systems of an organization. These two aspects must be considered interdependently, because arrangements that are optimal for one may not be optimal for the other and trade-offs are often required. Thus, for effective organization design, there is need for both dual focus and joint optimization. The approach has more relevance today than ever before, as organizational personnel seek more fruitful means of empowerment and as their organizations strive for greater productivity and viability in increasingly turbulent environments.

Many unintended and undesired consequences of healthcare information technologies (HIT) flow from interactions between the HIT and the healthcare organization's sociotechnical system—its workflows, culture, social interactions, and technologies. Harrison et al. (2007) developed and illustrated a conceptual model of these processes called Interactive Sociotechnical Analysis (ISTA). ISTA captures common types of interaction with special emphasis on recursive processes, i.e., feedback loops that alter the newly introduced HIT and promote second-level changes in the social system. ISTA draws on prior studies of unintended consequences, along with research in sociotechnical systems, ergonomics, social informatics, technology-in-practice, and social construction of technology. Five types of sociotechnical interaction were presented and each type were illustrated with cases from published research. It was noted that familiarity with the model can foster medical practitioners' awareness of unanticipated consequences that only become evident during HIT implementation.

The design and implementation of a multimethod evaluation model to assess the impact of computerized order entry systems on both the technical and social systems within a healthcare organization was reported (Westbrook, 2007). Designing an effective evaluation model requires a deep understanding of the nature and complexity of the problems that information technology interventions in healthcare are trying to address. Adopting a sociotechnical perspective for model generation improves the healthcare professional's ability to develop evaluation models that are adaptive and sensitive to the characteristics of wicked problems and provides a strong theoretical basis from which to analyze and interpret findings.

In the aviation industry, STS has been applied successfully to overcome the about-mentioned obstacles by designing organizational structures and processes to develop a safety culture and the maintenance department social system has been treated as an essential ingredient – mechanics and managers are seen as system members collaborating for a shared purpose, rather than individuals laboring to external regulations. In view of STS success in aviation, suggestions are made below to (i) introduce a process of developing structured communication within the PACS environment and (ii) develop an organizational structure that would work toward the hospital mission.

A Structured Communication Process

To facilitate PACS team decision-making, it is proposed that a specific structure and a process are used. The PACS department's structure in the proposed approach is to mandate regular briefings among radiologists, among technicians, and between radiologists and technicians. This process, called the Concept Alignment Process (CAP), is a way of ensuring that all parties act on the same concept. Its main objective is to mitigate errors—minimize the effects of past errors, prevent current errors, and increase the body of safety information to ensure the PACS deliver a high quality imaging service.

According to this process, a concept is an idea or a piece of information presented by a party to, or observer of, a technical PACS decision. All members are expected to present their concepts. If the members present different concepts, validations from a third-party source are required. If only one concept can be validated, it is executed; if none of the concepts can be validated, the most conservative concept is executed. If multiple concepts can be validated, the senior ranking person has the authority to choose any one of the valid concepts. Additionally, when multiple concepts are stated, whether valid or not, the PACS members are required to study the reasons for the existence of multiple concepts. Such a study is aimed at providing systemic feedback to minimize the occurrence of multiple ideas, at least the non-validated ones. In addition, once one concept is selected as the course of action, the CAP enters a "Judgment Phase" wherein the strengths and weaknesses in that course of action are monitored by the team. Such action monitoring may necessitate a change in direction, encourages the team members to be assertive if any new information becomes available.

The CAP successfully addresses the following causes of human error accidents: incorrect tactical decisions, complacency or inattention, non-adherence to procedure, and failure to challenge another member's error (Lynch, 1996). Through its objective procedures, the use of the process is transparent to all. It provides team members with decision-making and conflict-resolution methodology. With collective effort from all members, it reduces chances of acting on incorrect concepts and there is a way of changing the course when variances from original concept are detected. It reduces interpersonal conflict and defensiveness through the understanding that what is challenged is the concept and not the individual. However, it is to be noted that acknowledging one's lack of knowledge or uncertainty in a new situation requires a level of trust in the process and in one's co-workers and managers.

A PACS Organizational Structure

The proposed structure consists of a Director of Quality Assurance (QA) and a multi-discipline PACS workforce. QA Inspectors are to be identified from the ranks of the most experienced and senior technicians. When inspection tasks are required, these staff immediately become responsible to the QA Department and act as Inspectors. At all other times they act as technicians and reported to the Hospital Maintenance Supervisor. They are technicians working beside and with other technicians most of the time, but perform inspection tasks on others' work when it is required. As the most experienced technicians, the inspectors usually have comprehensive and unique knowledge of the PACS hardware and software they are inspecting and are expected to provide some information and training for correcting defects to the people (e.g. radiological clerks, transport aides, etc.) whose work they are inspecting. These technicians/inspectors are fully aware of the disruption caused by this dual responsibility and will develop procedures for reducing its effects.

It is anticipated that the skill-level of the PACS-related departments would be raised through this focused application of on-the-job training. Likewise, the level of defects will diminish over time as the skill level increased. More efficient use of skilled labor would raise the productivity and quality of the PACS. Further, the inspectors/technicians would experience a higher level of satisfaction from the greater contribution they will make to PACS excellence, and because of collaborative and cooperative nature of the relationship between QA inspectors and technicians, PACS-related departments would display a better morale.

A Common Business Understanding

Researchers such as Wigand et al. (1997) and Fuehrer & Ashkanasy (2001) note that an important element in any business cooperation is the establishment of common business understanding. An earlier work suggests that there are three specifications necessary for the establishment of a common business understanding in the internet context. The first is a clear service specification: the design, quality, and functionality of the service. The second is specification of the level of cooperation, which requires agreement about deadlines, liability, prices, profit allocation, and staff and resource input. The third is formal specification of agreements between the PACS partners. In a PACS regional or global network, these specifications need to be communicated clearly between the partners to achieve a common business understanding. There is always varying uncertainty between members, however. Therefore, there is a need to guard against opportunistic behavior varies between the partners (Wicks et al., 1999). This depends on the risk that the member is prepared to sustain as a potential loss, and also the partner's fear of opportunistic exploitation and the uncertainty of their behavior.

The three specifications (production, cooperation, and agreements between partners) can be achieved by negotiating relational contracts that guide the formation, operation, and dissolution of the PACS network, thereby facilitating an increase in the level of collaboration-enabling trust. Other mechanisms to establish a common business understanding in a virtual service network (VSN) include development of an organization handbook, design of a mutual Internet site, chat room technology, or the use of team addresses for e-mail. A specific example is Livelink, a software selected by Siemens to enable creation of a common business understanding through a standard computer interface.

Scott and Lane (2000) emphasize that a common business understanding requires the creation of a shared vision, together with communication of mutual aims through clear definition of the roles and expectations within the team, especially in the early stages of the partnership. In this respect, the process is typically initiated by agreement on a symbolic logo and/or design for the PACS service. This is because understanding each member's role, together with group identification, determines critical behaviors such as willingness to cooperate with others, and willingness to engage in mutual goal setting. The PACS partners thus need rapidly to establish group identity and an awareness of mutual needs and expectations, along with the clarification of tasks and responsibilities. In traditional partnerships, awareness and identity are in part shaped by the legal framework that regulates organizational relationships, as well as by networks, artifacts, and the organization chart.

These examples illustrate how the creation of a sense of shared meaning, member identification, and mission identity, especially in an early stage of the partnership, facilitates collaboration at an individual level and the operation and productivity of the PACS network as a whole. As such, a common business understanding provides an essential condition for the development of trust within the organization. In effect, a common business understanding provides the PACS network members with an opportunity to share their perceptions of the organization's defined features, and creates a feeling of ownership and trust.

Mutual Forbearance Amongst PACS Partners

Some researchers approach the issue of trust by defining cooperation as co-ordination effected through mutual forbearance. Forbearance is refraining from cheating. Cheating may take a weak form — failing to perform a beneficial act for the other party, or a strong form — committing a damaging act. The incentives for forbearance arise from the possibility of reciprocity, leading to mutual forbearance. Parties that are observed to forbear may gain a reputation for this behavior, which makes them potentially attractive partners for others. The parties to a successful agreement may develop a commitment to mutual forbearance, which cements the partnership, and, in this way, mutual trust is created, which alters the preferences of the parties towards a mutually cooperative mode. Thus, short-term, self-interested behavior becomes converted to cooperative trusting behavior.

Ability of PACS Partners

In a PACS network participating institutions will be more willing to share knowledge when they trust in others' ability. It is only natural that they would want to converse with others who have the knowledge and skills regarding the PACS topic at hand.

CONCLUDING REMARK

Effective and quality PACS occur when the people responsible for achieving the work understand the common ground between their goals and the mission of the hospital and where those people also know how they specifically contribute to achieve those common goals, and with whom they must collaborate to reach them. A joint optimization between the technical and the social entities is only possible when the purpose and values of the enterprise are both shared among its people and served directly by its technology. Purpose and value comprise the working culture, and working culture can effectively drive the simultaneous design of both the technology and the social system.

STS, in operation, would be successful when they equip their members to have the motives and the ability to make decisions and to act rapidly and accurately in new situations. In order to do this, PACS members must be skilled in understanding the purpose and service of their system in order to have the confidence to make modifications or replacements for events that have never occurred before. To create a successful PACS network, long-term trust between PACS partners is a critical factor, which can be achieved through a common business understanding and mutual forbearance amongst partners.

REFERENCES

Anbari, F. T. (2002). Six Sigma Method and Its Applications in Project Management. *Proceedings of the Project Management Institute Annual Seminars and Symposium [CD]*, San Antonio, Texas. Oct 3–10, 2002. Newtown Square, PA: Project Management Institute.

Antony, J., Escamilla, J. L., & Caine, P. (2003). Lean Sigma. *Manufacturing Engineer, 82*(4), 40–42.

Antony, J., & Banuelas, R. (2002). Key ingredients for the effective implementation of six sigma program. *Measuring Business Excellence, 6*(4), 20–27.

Catherwood, P. (2002). What's different about Six Sigma. *Manufacturing Engineer, 81*(8), 186–189.

Chen, X., & Barshes, W. (2000). *To team or not to team?* China Business Review, March-April 2000. Retrieved July 6, 2005, from http://www.chinabusinessreview.com/public/0003/chen.html.

Dalgleish, S. (2003). My ideal quality system. *Quality, 42*(7), 1-6.

Deming, W. E. (1986). *Out of the Crisis*. MIT Press.

Duyck, P, Pynoo, B., Devolder, P., Voet, T., Adang, L., & Vercruysse, J. (2008). User acceptance of a picture archiving and communication system. Applying the unified theory of acceptance and use of technology in a radiological setting. *Methods Inf Med., 47*(2), 149-56.

Fok, T. S., & Wong, E. T. T. (2005). Deployment of Six Sigma in SMEs in Hong Kong. *Proceedings of the 1st International Conference on Quality Management and Six Sigma,* Hong Kong, pp.114-116.

Fox, W. M. (1995). Sociotechnical System Principles and Guidelines: Past and Present. *Journal of Applied Behavioral Science, 31*(1), 91-105.

Fuehrer, E. C., & Ashkanasy, N. M. (2001). Communicating trustworthiness and building trust in interorganizational virtual organizations. *Jr. of Management, 27*(3), 235-254.

Hammer, M., & Goding. J. (2001). Putting six sigma in prospective. *Quality, 40*(10), 58–62.

Harrison, M. I., Koppel, R., & Bar-Lev, S. (2007). Unintended Consequences of Information Technologies in Healthcare An Interactive Sociotechnical Analysis. *J. Am. Med. Inform. Assoc., 14*(5), 542 – 549

He, J., Zhang, Z. H., & Che, J. G. (2005). A Study of the Integration of Lean Production and Six Sigma. *Proceedings of the 11ᵗʰ Hong Kong Quality Management and 1ˢᵗ Six Sigma Convention,* Hong Kong, June 2005, pp.116-125.

Hofstede, G. (1983). The Cultural Relativity of Organizational Practices and Theories. *Journal of International Business Studies,* Fall, (pp. 75-89).

Hofsteda, G. (2005). *Geert Hofstede™Cultural Dimensions.* Retrieved July 6, 2005, from http://www.geert-hofstede.com/hofstede_united_states.shtml.

Lynch, K. (1996). Management systems: A positive, practical method of Cockpit Resource Management. *Proceedings of the 41ˢᵗ Corporate Aviation Safety Seminar.* Orlando, FL: The Flight Safety Foundation, pp.244-254.

Mills, P., Neily, J., & Dunn, E. (2008). Teamwork and Communication in Surgical Teams: Implications for Patient Safety. *Journal of the American College of Surgeons, 206(1),* 107-112

Murugappan, M., & Keeni, G. (2003). Blending CMM and six sigma to meet business goals. *IEEE Software,* March 2003.

Revere, L., & Black, K. (2003). Integrating six sigma with total quality management: A case example for measuring medication errors. *Journal of Healthcare Management, 48*(6), pp. 377–391.

Scott, S. C., & Lane, V. R. (2000). A stakeholder approach to Organizational Identity. *Academy of Management Review, 25,* 43–62.

Westbrook, J. I., Braithwaite, J., Georgiou, A., Ampt, A., Creswick, N., Coiera, E., & Iedema, R. (2007). Multimethod Evaluation of Information and Communication Technologies in Health in the Context of Wicked Problems and Sociotechnical Theory. *J. Am. Med. Inform. Assoc., 14*(6), 746 - 755.

Wicks, A. C., Berman, S. L., & Jones, T. M. (1999). The structure of optimal trust: moral and strategic implications. *Academy of Management Review, 29,* 99–116.

Wigand, R., Picot, A., & Reichwald, R. (1997). *Information, organization and management: expanding markets and corporate boundaries.* Chichester, UK: Wiley.

Wong, E. T. T., & Fok, T. S. (2005). A Six Sigma Implementation Plan for SMEs. In J. Chan, R. Kwan, & E. Wong (Eds), *Quality Management: A New Era.* (pp. 65-79). Singapore: World Scientific.

Wyper, B., & Harrison, A. (2000). Deployment of six sigma methodology in human resource function: a case study. *Total Quality Management and Business Excellence, 11*(4 and 5), S720–S727.

Chapter XV
PACS Monitoring

BACKGROUND

The present study advocates the application of statistical process control (SPC) as a performance monitoring tool for a PACS. The objective of statistical process control (SPC) differs significantly from the traditional QC/QA process. In the traditional process, the QC/QA tests are used to generate a datum point and this datum point is compared to a standard. If the point is out of specification, then action is taken on the product and action may be taken on the process. To move from the traditional QC/QA process to SPC, a process control plan should be developed, implemented, and followed. Implementing SPC in the PACS environment need not be a complex process. However, if the maximum effect is to be achieved and sustained, PACS-SPC must be implemented in a systematic manner with the active involvement of all employees from line associates to executive management. SPC involves the use of mathematics, graphics, and statistical techniques, such as control charts, to analyze the PACS process and its output, so as to take appropriate actions to achieve and maintain a state of statistical control. While SPC is extensively used in the healthcare industry, especially in patient monitoring, it is rarely applied in the PACS environment. One may refer to a recent SPC application that Mercy Hospital (Alegent Health System) initiated after it implemented a PACS in November 2003

(Stockman & Krishnan, 2006). The anticipated benefits characteristic to PACS through the use of SPC include:

- Reduced image retake and diagnostic expenditure associated with better process control.
- Reduced operating costs by optimizing the maintenance and replacement of PACS equipment components.
- Increased productivity by identification and elimination of variation and out-of-control conditions in the imaging and retrieval processes.
- Enhanced level of quality by controlled applications.

SPC involves using statistical techniques to measure and analyze the variation in processes. Most often used for manufacturing processes, the intent of SPC is to monitor product quality and maintain processes to fixed targets. Hence besides the HSSH techniques, the proposed TQM approach would include the use of SPC. Although SPC will not improve the reliability of a poorly designed PACS, it can be used to maintain the consistency of how the individual process is provided and, therefore, of the entire PACS process.

A primary tool used for SPC is the control chart, a graphical representation of certain descriptive statistics for specific quantitative measurements of the PACS process. These descriptive statistics are displayed in the control chart in comparison to their "in-control" sampling distributions. The comparison detects any unusual variation in the PACS delivery process, which could indicate a problem with the process. Several different descriptive statistics can be used in control charts and there are several different types of control charts that can test for different causes, such as how quickly major vs. minor shifts in process means are detected. These control charts are also used with service level measurements to analyze process capability and for continuous process improvement efforts.

RELEVANT WORK

During recent years there has been a growing interest and debate in the application of SPC for improving the quality of software products. Given the need for clarification about the role of SPC in the debate surrounding software quality, several published case studies in software development and maintenance were discussed. It was found there is a need for greater awareness and analysis of the statistical characteristics of software quality data prior to the use of SPC methods. In addition, a more widespread understanding of the inherent limitations of the basic SPC methods as well as knowledge of the usable alternatives needs to be fostered within the software engineering community. Where measurements are limited, the data intensive techniques of SPC may not be applicable (Lewis, 1999).

Although originally developed to evaluate quality in manufacturing, SPC techniques may be applicable to other frequently performed standardized processes. SPC analysis has rarely been used in medicine. SPC charts were employed to analyze the outcomes of one- and two-muscle horizontal strabismus surgery for esotropia and exotropia. During a 33-month period between October 1, 1998 and July 1, 2001, 95 patients undergoing strabismus surgery on either one or two previously unoperated eye muscles in one or both eyes were evaluated. SPC charts were used to evaluate the success and validity of the surgical guidelines for horizontal recession and resection procedures. Data were divided into 2 groups, patients with esotropia and patients with exotropia, for computerized statistical analysis using QI Analyst (SPSS, Chicago, IL). The results after horizontal strabismus surgery, both esotropia and exotropia repair, appeared to follow the laws of statistical fluctuation or normal random variation. The dose-response schedule produced a resultant ocular alignment or exit angle that appeared to be in statistical control, i.e., variation from orthotropia that can be expected simply from normal random chance error with only a limited number of outliers. It was found that the resultant ocular alignment or exit angle after one- or two-muscle strabismus surgery may be described by standard models of statistical fluctuation. SPC was suggested to be a valuable method to analyze the variability of the results of many ophthalmologic procedures or treatments over time with the ultimate goal of producing better patient outcomes by decreasing variability (Self & Enzenauer, 2004).

In his book, Stapenhurst (2005) illustrates the use of "p" charts in the healthcare industry. Purpose of the p chart is to evaluate process stability when counting the fraction defective. It is used when the sample size varies: the total number of PACS records, image orders delivered varies from one sampling period to the next. The principles of SPC were applied to manage calcineurin inhibitor (CNI) blood levels. It was hypothesized that the use of SPC would increase the proportion of CNI blood levels in the target range. The study population consisted of 217 patients more than 3 months after liver transplantation. After demonstration of proof of concept using the rapid cycle improvement process, SPC was applied to the entire population. The change package included definition of target ranges for CNI, implementation of a web-based tool that displayed CNI blood levels on a control chart, and implementation of a protocol and a checklist for management of CNI blood levels. The principal outcome measured was the proportion of CNI blood levels in the target range. In the pilot study, the proportion of CNI blood levels in the target range increased from 50% to 85%. When the protocol was spread to the entire population, the proportion of drug levels in the target range increased to 77% from 50% (P <.001), whereas the range of CNI levels decreased. The rate of allograft rejection did not change. It was concluded that utilization of SPC increased the proportion of CNI blood levels in target range. These observations may be applicable to the care of other chronic healthcare problems (Bucuvalas, 2005).

Rehabilitation psychology embraces the scientist-practitioner model as its professional philosophy. This model's original intent was that the diagnosis and treatment of each individual case was to be regarded as a single and well-controlled experiment. Executing this ideal in rehabilitation has been problematic owing to practical, ethical, and technical concerns. SPC is offered as a means to deploy single-subject designs on the front lines of rehabilitation. Case examples relevant to rehabilitation practice (ambulation, depression, cognitive rehabilitation, agitation were illustrated with SPC control charts and it was suggested that SPC charts are a time-tested, scientifically validated, and pragmatic tool to achieve and document patient outcomes (Callahan & Barisa, 2005).

SPC techniques were applied to simulate monitoring the process of outpatient service delivery at two mental health centers using data collected 23 years earlier (Green, 1999). Clients included in this study received between two and 21 psycho-therapy visits during the previously conducted evaluation study. Global outcomes for clients were derived from weekly ratings of functioning provided by the client and therapist. The self-report and therapist ratings were aggregated, then combined across visits to estimate the rate of linear change in functioning. Rates of change were plotted in a control chart format, using the moving average of two scores to estimate the range. Special causes of high variability and a downward trend were noted for all discharges at both centers. Control limits were re-estimated for the discharges following the downward trend in scores. Subsequently, the service processes supporting global client outcomes no longer varied uncontrollably. However, upon estimating specification limits for global client outcomes, it was noted that the mean level of client outcome fell below the mean specified as the target and that some discharges yielded unacceptable outcomes.

CONTROL CHARTS

The control chart was invented by Walter A. Shewhart while working for Bell Labs in the 1920s. The company's engineers had been seeking to improve the reliability of their telephony transmission systems. Because amplifiers and other equipment had to be buried underground, there was a business need to reduce the frequency of failures and repairs. By 1920 they had already realized the importance of reducing variation in a manufacturing process. Moreover, they had realized that continual process-adjustment in reaction to non-conformance actually increased variation and degraded quality. Shewhart framed the problem in terms of common- and special-causes of variation and, in May 1924, wrote an internal memo introducing the control chart as a tool for distinguishing between the two.

Dr. Shewhart's superior, George Edwards, recalled: "Dr. Shewhart prepared a little memorandum only about a page in length. About a third of that page was given over to a simple diagram which we would all recognize today as a schematic control chart. That diagram, and the short text which preceded and followed it, set forth all of the essential principles and considerations which are involved in what we know today as process quality control" (Western Electric, 2008). Shewhart stressed that bringing a production process into a state of statistical control, where there is only common-cause variation, and keeping it in control, is necessary to predict future output and to manage a process economically.

Dr. Shewhart created the basis for the control chart and the concept of a state of statistical control by carefully designed experiments. While Dr. Shewhart drew from pure mathematical statistical theories, he understood data from physical processes never produce a "normal distribution curve" (a Gaussian distribution, also commonly referred to as a "bell curve"). He discovered that observed variation in manufacturing data did not always behave the same way as data in nature (Brownian motion of particles). Dr. Shewhart concluded that while every process displays variation, some processes display controlled variation that is natural to the process, while others display uncontrolled variation that is not present in the process causal system at all times (British Deming Association, 1992).

In 1925, Shewhart's innovation came to the attention of W. Edwards Deming, then working at the Hawthorne facility. Deming later worked at the United States Department of Agriculture and then became the mathematical advisor to the United States Census Bureau. Over the next half a century, Deming became the foremost champion and exponent of Shewhart's work. After the defeat of Japan at the close of World War II, Deming served as statistical consultant to the Supreme Commander of the Allied Powers. His ensuing involvement in Japanese life, and long career as an industrial consultant there, spread Shewhart's thinking, and the use of the control chart, widely in Japanese manufacturing industry throughout the 1950s and 1960s.

More recent use and development of control charts in the Shewhart-Deming tradition has been championed by Donald J. Wheeler. A control chart is a statistical tool used to distinguish between variation in a process resulting from common causes and variation resulting from special causes. It presents a graphic display of process stability or instability over time. Every PACS process has variation. Some variations may be the result of causes which are not normally present in the process. This could be special cause variation. Some variation is simply the result of numerous, ever-present differences in the process. This is common cause variation. Control Charts differentiate between these two types of variation.

One aim of using a control chart is to achieve and maintain process stability. Process stability is defined as a state in which a process has displayed a certain degree of consistency in the past and is expected to continue to do so in the future. This consistency is characterized by a stream of data falling within control limits based on plus or minus 3 standard deviations (3 sigma) of the centerline (Montgomery, 2005).

Control Chart Limits

Control limits represent the limits of variation that should be expected from a process in a state of statistical control. When a process is in statistical control, any variation is the result of common causes that effect the entire production in a similar way. Control limits should not be confused with specification limits, which represent the desired process performance.

Shewhart sets 3-sigma limits on the following basis:

- The coarse result of Chebyshev's inequality that, for any probability distribution, the probability of an outcome greater than k standard deviations from the mean is at most $1/k^2$.
- The finer result of the Vysochanskii-Petunin inequality, that for any unimodal probability distribution, the probability of an outcome greater than k standard deviations from the mean is at most $4/(9k^2)$.
- The empirical investigation of sundry probability distributions reveals that at least 99% of observations occurred within three standard deviations of the mean.

PACS Application

A stable process is one that is consistent over time with respect to the center and the spread of the data. Control charts help the PACS administration monitor the behavior of each process to determine whether it is stable.

Run charts display process performance over time. Upward and downward trends, cycles, and large aberrations may be spotted and investigated further. In a run chart, events, shown on the y axis, are graphed against a time period on the x axis. Hence a PACS example might involve plotting the frequency of image retrieval delays against the day of the week. The results might show that there are more delays at noon than at 3 p.m. Investigating this phenomenon could unearth potential for improvement. Run charts can also be used to track improvements that have been put into place, checking to determine their success. Also, an average line can be added to a run chart to clarify movement of the data away from the average.

Like run charts, control charts display data in the time sequence in which they occurred. However, control charts are more efficient that run charts in assessing and achieving process stability.

The PACS team can benefit from using a control chart than the run chart when the following objectives are pursued:

- Monitor process variation over time.
- Differentiate between special cause and common cause variation.
- Assess the effectiveness of changes to improve a process.
- Communicate how a process performed during a specific period.

Types of Control Charts

There are two main categories of control charts, those that display attribute data, and those that display variables data.

- **Attribute Data:** This category of control chart displays data that result from counting the number of occurrences or items in a single category of similar items or occurrences. These "count" data may be expressed as pass/fail, yes/no, or presence/absence of a defect.
- **Variables Data:** This category of control chart displays values resulting from the measurement of a continuous variable. Examples of variables data are image transfer time, temperature, and radiation dose.

While these two categories encompass a number of different types of control charts, there are three types that will work for the majority of the data analysis cases the hospital administration will encounter, viz.

- X-Bar and R Chart
- Individual X and Moving Range Chart for Variables Data
- Individual X and Moving Range Chart for Attribute Data

As the construction procedure is quite similar for all these types, the construction of the X-Bar and R Chart, which is considered to be most useful in the PACS environment will be considered. The decision tree shown in Figure 1 would help the reader in determining when to use these three types of control charts.

X-Bar and R Control Chart for Variables Data

The X-Bar (arithmetic mean) and R (range) control chart can be used with variables data when subgroup or sample size is between 2 and 15. The steps for constructing this type of control chart are:

1. Determine the data to be collected. Decide what questions about the process you plan to answer.
2. Collect and enter the data by subgroup. A subgroup is made up of variables data that represent a characteristic of a product produced by a process. The sample size relates to how large the subgroups are.
3. Calculate and enter the average for each subgroup.
4. Calculate and enter the range (difference between the largest and the smallest value in each subgroup) for each subgroup.
5. Calculate the grand mean of the subgroup's average by Eqn. (1) The grand mean of the subgroup's average (X-Bar) becomes the centerline of he upper plot.

$$\mu_x = (\sum x_i)/k \tag{1}$$

Where: μ_x = The grand mean of all the individual subgroup averages
x_i = The average for each subgroup
k   = The number of subgroups

Figure 1. Decision tree for PACS control charts

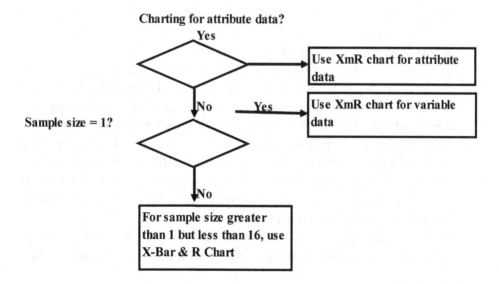

6. Calculate the average of the subgroup ranges by Eq. (2). The average of all subgroups becomes the centerline for the lower plotting area.

$$R = (\sum R_i)/k \tag{2}$$

Where
R = The average of the ranges for all subgroups
R_i = The individual range for each subgroup
k = The number of subgroups

7. Calculate the upper control limit (UCL) and lower control limit (LCL) for the averages of the subgroups. At this point, the chart will look like a run chart. However, the uniqueness of the control chart becomes evident as you calculate the control limits. Control limits define the parameters for determining whether a process is in statistical control. To find the X-Bar control limits, use the following formula:

$$UCL_X = \mu_x + A_2 R$$
$$LCL_X = \mu_x - A_2 R \tag{3}$$

Where the constant A_2, based on the subgroup size, is used in determining control limits for variables charts. Details of the constants can be found in Gitlow's book (1999).

8. Calculate the upper control limit for the ranges. When the subgroup or sample size is less than 7, there is no lower control limit. To find the upper control limit for the ranges, use the formula:

$$UCL_R = D_4 R \tag{4}$$

Where D_4 depends again on the subgroup size.

9. Select the scales and plot the data points and centerline in each plotting area. Before the data points and centerline can be plotted, the scales must first be determined. Once the upper and lower control limits have been computed, the easiest way to select the scales is to have the current spread of the control limits take up approximately two-thirds of the vertical (Y) axis. The scales for both the upper and lower plotting areas should allow for future high or low out-of-control data points. Plot each subgroup average as an individual data point in the upper plotting area. Plot individual subgroup range data points in the lower plotting area (see Figure 2).

10. Provide the appropriate documentation. Each Control Chart should be labeled with who, what, when, where, why, and how information to describe where

Figure 2. A sample X-Bar and R chart

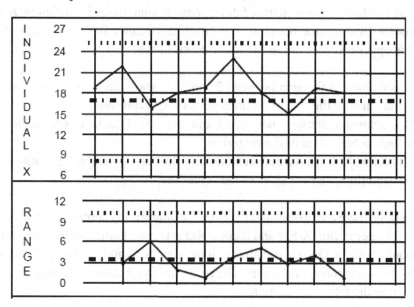

the data originated, when it was collected, who collected it, any identifiable equipment or work groups, sample size, and all the other necessary information.

Interpretation of PACS Control Charts

Process stability is reflected in the relatively constant variation exhibited in control charts. Basically, the data fall within a band bounded by the control limits. If a process is stable, the likelihood of a point falling outside this band is so small that such an occurrence is taken as a signal of a special cause of variation. In other words, something abnormal is occurring within the PACS process. However, even though all the points fall inside the control limits, special cause variation may be at work. The presence of unusual patterns can be evidence that the process is not in statistical control. Such patterns are more likely to occur when one or more special causes are present. Control charts are based on control limits which are 3 standard deviations (3 sigma) away from the centerline.

One should resist the urge to narrow these limits in the hope of identifying special causes earlier. Experience has shown that limits based on less than plus and minus 3 sigma may lead to false assumptions about special causes operating in a process (Montgomery, 2005). In other words, using control limits which are less than 3 sigma from the centerline may trigger a hunt for special causes when the process is already stable. The three standard deviations are sometimes identified by zones. Each zone's dividing line is exactly one-third the distance from the centerline to either the upper control limit or the lower control limit.

Zone A is defined as the area between 2 and 3 standard deviations from the centerline on both the plus and minus sides of the centerline.

Zone B is defined as the area between 1 and 2 standard deviations from the centerline on both sides of the centerline.

Zone C is defined as the area between the centerline and 1 standard deviation from the centerline, on both sides of the centerline.

Generally, there are two basic set of rules for interpreting control charts. One set of rules for interpreting X-Bar and R control charts and another set for interpreting XmR control charts. One must realize that these rules should not be confused with the rules for interpreting run charts. The rules for interpreting X-Bar and R charts are shown in the following section.

Rules for Interpreting X-Bar and R Charts

When one is interpreting X-Bar and R Control Charts, he or she should observe the following set of rules:

- **Rule 1:** Whenever a single point falls outside the 3 sigma control limits, a lack of control is indicated. Since the probability of this happening is rather small, it is very likely not due to chance.
- **Rule 2:** Whenever at least 2 out of 3 successive values fall on the same side of the centerline and more than 2 sigma units away from the centerline, a lack of control is indicated. Note that the third point can be on either side of the centerline.
- **Rule 3:** Whenever at least 4 out of 5 successive values fall on the same side of the centerline and more than one sigma unit away from the centerline, a lack of control is indicated. Note that the fifth point can be on either side of the centerline.
- **Rule 4:** Whenever at least 8 successive values fall on the same side of the centerline, a lack of control is indicated.

Having considered the construction of the X-Bar and R chart, one would want to know when would be more appropriate to use the Individual X and Moving Range (XmR) control chart and what are the conditions governing the use of this chart.

Timing For Individual X and Moving Range (XmR) Control Charts

One can use Individual X and Moving Range (XmR) Control Charts to assess both variables and attribute data. XmR charts reflect data that do not lend themselves to forming subgroups with more than one measurement. One might want to use this type of control chart if, for example, a PACS process repeats itself infrequently, or it appears to operate differently at different times. If that is the case, grouping the data might mask the effects of such differences. One can avoid this problem by using an XmR chart whenever there is no rational basis for grouping the data. However there is an essential condition which must be satisfied before using an XmR control chart for attribute data - the average count per sample must be greater than one. There is no variation within a subgroup since each subgroup has a sample size of 1, and the difference between successive subgroups is used as a measure of process variation. This difference is called a moving range. There is a corresponding moving range value for each of the individual X values except the very first value.

Similar to the X-Bar and R chart, the construction procedure for the XmR chart is:

1. Determine the data to be collected.
    Decide what questions about the process you plan to answer.
2. Collect and enter the individual measured data (X_i). These measurements will be plotted as individual data points in the upper plotting area.
3. Calculate and enter the moving ranges. Use the following formula to calculate the moving ranges between successive data entries. The moving range data will be plotted as individual data points in the lower plotting area

$$mRi = \left| X_i - X_{i1} \right| \qquad (5)$$

Where: X_i = an individual value
X_{i1} = the next sequential value following X_i
Note: The brackets ($|\ \ |$)refer to the absolute value of the numbers contained inside the bracket. Hence the difference is always a positive number.

4. Calculate the overall average of the individual data points. The average of the individual X data becomes the centerline for the upper plot.

$$\mu_x = (\sum x_i)/k \qquad (6)$$

Where

μ_x = The average of the individual measurements
xi = An individual measurement
k = The number of subgroups of one

5. Calculate the average of the moving ranges. The average of all moving ranges becomes the centerline for the lower plotting area.

$$mR = (\textstyle\sum mr_i)/(k\text{-}1) \tag{7}$$

Where
mR = The average of all the Individual Moving Ranges
mr_i = The Individual Moving Range measurements
k = The number of subgroups of one

6. Calculate the upper and lower control limits for the individual X values. The calculation will compute the upper and lower control limits for the upper plotting area. To find these control limits, use the formula:

$$UCL_X = X + 2.66*mR$$
$$LCL_X = X - 2.66*mR \tag{8}$$

The constants used for formulae in Steps 6 and 7 are based on a two-point moving range.

7. Calculate the upper control limit for the moving ranges. This calculation will compute the upper control limit for the lower plotting area. There is no lower control limit. To find the upper control limit for the moving ranges, use the formula:

$$UCLm_R = 3.268*mR$$
$$LCLm_R = \text{none} \tag{9}$$

8. Select the scales and plot the data points and centerline in each plotting area. Plot each Individual X value as an individual data point in the upper plotting area. Plot moving range values in the lower plotting area.

9. Provide the appropriate documentation.

10. Check for *inflated* control limits. One should analyze the XmR control chart for inflated control limits. When either of the following conditions exists, the control limits are said to be *inflated*, and one must recalculate them:

    •   If any point is outside of the upper control limit for the moving range (UCLmR)
    •   If two-thirds or more of the moving range values are below the average of the moving ranges computed in Step 5.

11. If the control limits are inflated, calculate 3.144 times the median moving range. For example, if the median moving range is equal to 8, then

$$3.144*8 = 25.152$$

The centerline for the lower plotting area is now the median of all the values when they are listed from smallest to largest.

12. Depending on the magnitude of the product of 3.144 times the median of moving range, take one of the following actions:

- Do not compute new limits if the product of 3.144 times the median of moving range value is greater than the product of 2.66 times the average of the moving ranges.

- Re-compute all of the control limits and centerlines for both the upper and lower plotting areas if the product of 3.144 times the median moving range value is less than the product of 2.66 times the average of the moving range. The new limits will be based on the following formulae:

Upper Plot –
$UCL_X = X + 3.144*\text{median of mR}$
$LCL_X = X - 3.144*\text{median of mR}$
Centreline = μ_x (10)

Lower Plot –
$UCL_{mR} = 3.865*\text{median of mR}$
$LCL_{mR} = \text{None}$
$Centreline_{mR} = \text{median of mR}$ (11)

These new limits must be redrawn on the corresponding charts before one wants to identify signals of special causes. The old control limits and centerlines should be ignored in any further assessment of the collected data.

PACS CAPABILITY INDICES

Once a process is in control, we can determine the PACS capability through an eclectic use of capability indices. Again, the approach to answering this question is based on statistical reasoning.

Potential Capability (C$_p$)

This is the simplest and most straightforward indicator of process capability. It is defined as the ratio of the specification range to the process range; using ± 3 sigma limits one can express this index as:

C$_p$ = (USL-LSL)/(6*Sigma)

Put into words, this ratio expresses the proportion of the range of the normal curve that falls within the engineering specification limits (provided that the mean is on target, that is, that the process is centered, see below).

Bhote (1988) reports that prior to the widespread use of statistical quality control techniques (prior to 1980), the normal quality of US manufacturing processes was approximately C$_p$ = .67. This means that the two 33/2 percent tail areas of the normal curve fall outside specification limits. As of 1988, only about 30% of US processes are at or below this level of quality (see Bhote, 1988, p. 51). Ideally, of course, we would like this index to be greater than 1, that is, we would like to achieve a process capability so that no (or almost no) items fall outside specification limits. Interestingly, in the early 1980's the Japanese manufacturing industry adopted as their standard C$_p$ = 1.33! The process capability required to manufacture high-tech products is usually even higher than this; Minolta has established a C$_p$ index of 2.0 as their minimum standard (Bhote, 1988, p. 53), and as the standard for its suppliers. Note that high process capability usually implies lower, not higher costs, taking into account the costs due to poor quality.

Capability Ratio (C$_r$)

This index is equivalent to C$_p$; specifically, it is computed as 1/C$_p$ (the inverse of C$_p$).

Lower/Upper Potential Capability: C$_{pl}$, C$_{pu}$

A major shortcoming of the C$_p$ (and C$_r$) index is that it may yield erroneous information if the process is not on target, that is, if it is not *centered*. We can express non-centering via the following quantities. First, upper and lower potential capability indices can be computed to reflect the deviation of the observed process mean from the LSL and USL. Assuming ± 3 sigma limits as the process range, we compute:

C$_{pl}$ = (Mean - LSL)/3*Sigma

And

$C_{pu} = (USL - Mean)/3*Sigma$

Obviously, if these values are not identical to each other, then the process is not centered.

Non-Centering Correction (K)

We can correct C_p for the effects of non-centering. Specifically, we can compute:

$K=abs(D - Mean)/(1/2*(USL - LSL))$

where

$D = (USL+LSL)/2$

This correction factor expresses the non-centering (target specification minus mean) relative to the specification range.

Demonstrated Excellence (C_{pk})

Finally, we can adjust C_p for the effect of non-centering by computing:

$C_{pk} = (1-k)*C_p$

If the process is perfectly centered, then k is equal to zero, and C_{pk} is equal to C_p. However, as the process drifts from the target specification, k increases and C_{pk} becomes smaller than C_p.

Potential Capability II: C_{pm}

A recent modification (Chan, Cheng, & Spiring, 1988) to C_p is directed at adjusting the estimate of *sigma* for the effect of (random) non-centering. Specifically, we may compute the alternative *sigma (Sigma$_2$)* as:

$Sigma_2 = \{\sum (x_i - TS)^2/(n-1)\}^{1/2}$

where:
$Sigma_2$ is the alternative estimate of *sigma*

x_i is the value of the i'th observation in the sample

TS   is the target or nominal specification

n   is the number of observations in the sample

We may then use this alternative estimate of sigma to compute C_p as before; however, we will refer to the resultant index as C_{pm}.

Experiments to Improve Process Capability

As mentioned before, the higher the C_p index, the better the process -- and there is virtually no upper limit to this relationship. The issue of quality costs, that is, the losses due to poor quality, is discussed in detail in the context of Taguchi robust design methods (Montgomery, 2005). In general, higher quality usually results in lower costs overall; even though the costs of production may increase, the losses due to poor quality, for example, due to customer complaints, loss of market share, etc. are usually much greater. In practice, two or three well-designed experiments carried out over a few weeks can often achieve a C_p of 5 or higher. If you are not familiar with the use of designed experiments, but are concerned with the quality of a PACS process, we strongly recommend that you review the methods detailed in the Experimental Design literature.

Testing the Normality Assumption

The indices we have just reviewed are only meaningful if, in fact, the quality characteristic that is being measured is normally distributed. A specific test of the normality assumption (Kolmogorov-Smirnov and Chi-square test of goodness-of-fit) is available; these tests are described in most statistics textbooks. A visual check for normality is to examine the probability-probability and quantile- quantile plots for the normal distribution.

Tolerance Limits

Before the introduction of process capability indices in the early 1980's, the common method for estimating the characteristics of a production process was to estimate and examine the tolerance limits of the process (see, for example, Hald, 1952). The logic of this procedure is as follows. Let us assume that the respective quality characteristic is normally distributed in the population of items produced; we can then estimate the lower and upper interval limits that will ensure with a certain level of confidence (probability) that a certain percent of the population is included in those limits. Put another way, given:

1. a specific sample size (n),
2. the process mean,
3. the process standard deviation (sigma),
4. a confidence level, and
5. the percent of the population that we want to be included in the interval,

we can compute the corresponding *tolerance* limits that will satisfy all these parameters. You can also compute parameter-free tolerance limits that are not based on the assumption of normality (Scheffe & Tukey, 1944; Wilks, 1946; Duncan, 1974, Montgomery, 1991).

CONCLUDING REMARK

When monitoring a process via a quality control chart (e.g., the X-bar and R-chart) it is often useful to compute the capability indices for the process. Specifically, when the data set consists of multiple samples, such as data collected for the quality control chart, then one can compute two different indices of variability in the data. One is the regular standard deviation for all observations, ignoring the fact that the data consist of multiple samples; the other is to estimate the process's inherent variation from the within-sample variability. For example, when plotting X-bar and R-charts one may use the common estimator R-bar/D_2 for the process sigma (e.g. Montgomery, 2000). Note however, that this estimator is only valid if the process is statistically stable. For a detailed discussion of the difference between the total process variation and the inherent variation refer to ASQC/AIAG reference manual (ASQC/AIAG, 1991).

When the total process variability is used in the standard capability computations, the resulting indices are usually referred to as process performance indices (as they describe the actual performance of the process), while indices computed from the inherent variation (within- sample sigma) are referred to as capability indices. Capability studies can estimate future process performance only when such performance is consistent over time, i.e. when a stable process is observed.

In summary, it is highly recommended that control charts be used in conjunction with the process capability measures whenever one wants to detect process variations for PACS improvements.

REFERENCES

ASQC/AIAG Task Force (1991). *Fundamental Process Control, Reference Manual.* Automotive Division of the American Society for Quality Control, in collaboration with the Automotive Industry Action Group.

Bohte, K. R. (1988). *World Class Quality: Design of Experiments Made Easier, More Cost Effective Than Spc.* American Management Association Books.

Callahan, C. D., & Barisa, M. T. (2005). Statistical Process Control and Rehabilitation Outcome: The Single-Subject Design Reconsidered. *Rehabilitation Psychology, 50*(1), 24-33.

Bucuvalas, J. C., Ryckman, F. C., Arya, G., Andrew, B., Lesko, A., Cole, C. R., James, B., & Kotagal, U. (2005). A Novel Approach to Managing Variation: Outpatient Therapeutic Monitoring of Calcineurin Inhibitor Blood Levels in Liver Transplant Recipients. *The Journal of Pediatrics, 146*(6), 744-750.

Callahan, C. D., & Barisa, M. T. (2005). *Rehabilitation Psychology, 50*(1), 24-33.

Carey, R. G., & Lloyd, R. C.. (2001). *Measuring Quality Improvement in Healthcare: A Guide to Statistical Process Control Applications.* Milwaukee, WI: American Society for Quality.

Chang, L. K., Cheng, S. W., & Spiring, F. A. (1988). A new measure of process capability: Cpm. *J. Quality Technology, 20,* 162–175.

Doty, L. (1996). *Statistical Process Control.* New York: Industrial Press, Inc.

Gitlow, H., Gitlow, S., Oppenheim, A., & Oppenheim, R. (1989). *Tools and Methods for the Improvement of Quality.* Homewood, IL: Richard D. Irwin

Green, R. S. (1999). The application of statistical process control to manage global client outcomes in behavioral healthcare. *Evaluation and Program Planning, 22*(2), 199-210.

Lewis, N. D. C. (1999). Assessing the evidence from the use of SPC in monitoring, predicting & improving software quality. *Computers & Industrial Engineering, 37*(1-2), 157-160.

Montgomery, D. C. (2000) *Design and Analysis of Experiments.* 5th Edition. New York: Wiley.

Self, C. A. & Enzenauer, R. W. (2004). The application of statistical process control to horizontal strabismus surgery. *Journal of American Association for Pediatric Ophthalmology and Strabismus, 8*(2), 165-170.

Stapenhurst, T. (2005). Comparing surgical complication rates between hospitals. *Mastering Statistical Process Control - A Handbook for Performance Improvement Using SPC Cases (*pp. 91-101). Oxford:Butterworth-Heinemann.

Stockman, T., & Krishnan, S. (2006) Acceptance of PACS utilizing a PACS QI Program. *Radiol Manage., 28*(2), 16-27.

Western Electric: A Brief History. (2008). Available from the Bell System Memorial Home Page, http://www.porticus.org/bell/westernelectric_history.html

Wikipedia. (2008). *Definition of a Control Chart.* Retrieved on 16 January 2008 from http://en.wikipedia.org/wiki/Control_chart

Section IV
Future PACS Directions and Planning of Future Hospitals

Chapter XVI
Quality Management Benefits

BACKGROUND

To illustrate the benefits of implementing QM in PACS, a successful case based on the Six Sigma approach is given below. It involves a project aiming at the 2005 Hong Kong Quality Management Award. A brief description of the Award and its judging criteria is given, followed by an outline of the Grand Award holder's submission and the Project Leader's clarification of project-related issues during the Judging Panel interview.

Hong Kong Quality Management Association and the Hong Kong Productivity Council have jointly organized the "Hong Kong Quality Management Convention" on a bi-annual basis at the Hong Kong Convention and Exhibition Centre since 1991. The Convention is a renowned quality event in Hong Kong with active participation from both Hong Kong and Mainland China (e.g. over hundred of delegates from various cities of China in 2003).

With the rapid development of quality circles in local organizations, the Hong Kong Quality Circle Award was introduced in 1993, being the exclusive award to recognize employees' effort and contribution towards the improvement of productivity in their industry via quality circles. The purpose of the Award is to reward employees' contribution in quality enhancement and to recognize the companies' commitment in quality management. Over the years, award-winners have been recognized for their determination to tackle issues from the grass-root level in pursuit of operational efficiency and effectiveness.

This Award offers the participating companies excellent opportunities to benchmark their quality practice among their counterparts and enhance their competitive advantage in their industry. It also improves their corporate image and enhances the morale of the circle members. Organizations with principal activities based in Hong Kong are eligible to compete for the Award. The final and binding decisions on the award are vested with the Hong Kong Quality Management Association and the Hong Kong Productivity Council. To qualify for the award, the participants have to undergo a stringent adjudication process.

The adjudication criteria are shown in Table 1. The total Awards comprise one Grand QC Award and four QC Awards. Five best teams among the applications would be selected by a panel of judges based on the adjudication criteria to award the QC Award. The panel of judges comprises academic staff from four local universities and public listed company CEOs representing professional bodies such as the Association for the Promotion of Small and Medium Enterprises (SMEs) and the Toy Manufacturers Association. The Government of Hong Kong Special Administration Region has defined a small and medium enterprise (SME) as a manufacturing business that employs fewer than 100 persons or a non-manufacturing business that employs fewer than 50 persons in Hong Kong (HK SAR Government, 2005).

According to the June 2004 figures published by the Census and Statistics Department (HK SAR Government, 2004), more than 98% of the 288,912 business establishments in Hong Kong excluding those in the civil service can be classified as SMEs. It can be seen that the QC Awards cover both the big manufacturers (with production plants located in regions north of Hong Kong) and the SMEs. The Grand QC Award is issued to the most outstanding team within these five teams. Merits are issued to the teams achieved satisfactory level.

Based on the submissions received, there were altogether 23 teams shortlisted for the 2005 QC Awards and based on the Project Leader's clarification of various project-related issues raised during the Judging Panel interview, the following PACS-based project submission forwarded by a local hospital was granted the QC Grand Award. With the agreement of the Project Leader, a modified submission is provided below to illustrate one practical way of applying TQM in the PACS environment. An outline of the questions and answers session during the Judging Panel interview is also given.

Table 1. Judging criteria for the 2005 Quality Circle (QC) Award

QC Activities	Evaluation Criteria	Max. Scores
Team Work	• Meetings are regularly held and with good attendance rate. • Members' suggestions are implemented and adopted for improvement. • Advice or help is sought from internal or external parties.	5
Project Selection	• Project selection based on assessment of background information, organizational constraints and previous statistics. • Project meets sectional or departmental requirements.	5
Problem Identification	• Problems are clearly identified and defined. • Specific targets are formulated.	10
Analytical Techniques	• Analytical techniques and methodology such as graph, Fishbone Diagram, Pareto Diagram, check sheet, chart, etc are effectively used. • Systematic approach in identifying and verifying the most probable causes is adopted, with proper application of the Plan-Do-Check-Action (PDCA) approach.	10
Improvement Initiatives and Implementation	• Alternative solutions are stated. • Solutions are properly evaluated. • Recommended solution is sound and practical. • Solutions are creative and innovative.	15
Results Achieved	• Tangible results have been achieved. • Intangible results have been achieved. • Variation (s) between results and original target (s) is explained.	25
Standardization	• Standardization is realized through changes in procedures or other arrangements. • Follow-up actions are taken to ensure compliance with new procedures.	10
Self-examination and Future Plans	• Teams are aware of their problems. • Difficulties in accomplishing the project are considered. • Teams' next project is stated and sufficient reasons are given. Alternatives to overcome its limitations and problems are considered.	10
Report Presentation	• Professionalism in data collection and analysis are demonstrated.	10
Overall		100

CASE ILLUSTRATION

The title of the 2005 HK QC Grand Award project is, "Improving Medical Imaging Service at Tseung Kwan O Hospital (TKOH) Filmless Radiology".

Team Work

In 1999 a PACS was installed in TKOH. At the beginning, due to immature development of PACS technologies, the radiology service in the TKOH was operating with film printing. A major upgrade was carried out in 2003 for the implementation of server clustering, network resilience, Liquid Crystal Display (LCD), smart card, and Storage Area Network (SAN) technologies. This upgrade has greatly improved the reliability of the system. Since November 2003, TKOH has started filmless radiology service for the whole hospital.

To prepare for the Hong Kong Quality Circle Award, a PACS Team was formed in March 2004 and the composition of the team (names of members were not shown) is shown in Table 2. PACS is a mission-critical component of a hospital. Particularly in the case of large hospitals, the effect of errors in PACS on the institution is tremendous. At a minimum, it may cause patients discomfort, but it may also cause legal problems and economic burdens for the hospital (Smith & Berlin, 2001). Thus, hospitals using PACS should maintain quality control programs to ensure that all the processes and images are defect-free.

The Six Sigma initiative is the latest quality improvement movement. Started at Motorola (Sander, 2001), where it was focused primarily on the reduction of quality defects, it has rapidly propagated into many industries, including hospitals, where it has changed the environment and culture (Ettinger, 2000; Simmons, 2002). In brief, Six Sigma (6σ) is a statistical representation of the variance in a process as compared with the acceptable tolerance window provided by the customer. This level of quality management, referred to as "zero defect," results in only 3.4 ppm outside of the customer specification limits.

In this aspect, Six Sigma is suitable for healthcare because many healthcare processes require a near-zero tolerance for mistakes. However, establishing a Six

Table 2. Members of TKOH PACS Team

Role in the PACS Team	Position	Experience
Head	Chief Of Service	~30 Years
PACS Manager	Medical Physicist	>15 Years
Administrator	Radiographer 1	>10 Years
Administrator	Radiographer 2	>10 Years
Administrator	Radiographer 3	~10 Years
Administrator	Electronic Technician 1	>10 Years
Administrator	Electronic Technician 2	<5 Years

Sigma program requires major human and capital resources for most hospitals. Therefore, the adoption of Six Sigma in the healthcare industry is not as broad as in other industries. Nevertheless, Six Sigma has been adapted for the medical field in several studies. There is also pioneering research in the field of radiology. Benedetto (2003) reported the successful implementation of a project to dramatically improve the performance of its film library. Hence, the PACS team members were given the opportunity to acquire a working knowledge of Six Sigma methods through participation in several local six sigma seminars and workshops.

Filmless Radiology

Filmless radiology is a practice of storing digital radiological images stored in electronic files, which can be viewed and saved on a computer. This technology has many benefits including film-cost saving, increase of efficiencies of clinicians and radiologists, space saving, reduction of film management cost, environmental friendly, and infection control. The common technique in filmless radiology today is using Picture Archiving and Communication System (PACS), which involves the storage of data and database managements. Expanding the practice of filmless radiology into a hospital-wide scale is called "Filmless Hospital". However, the success of a filmless hospital depends on many technical and management issues. These technical issues include user-friendliness, flexibility, reliability, and security of the computer system. The management issues are usually more complex including communication between clinicians and radiologists, sharing of responsibilities, medico-legal aspects, and account and network management.

From 1999 to 2003, numerous technical and operational discussions among clinical departments, radiology department, senior management, and medical physics unit were held in Tseung Kwan O Hospital (TKOH) for the feasibility of filmless hospital project. Key members of the hospital-appointed PACS team were assigned specific activities, as shown in Table 3.

As some preliminary work on PACS implementation has already been carried out since 1999 and the working relationship among all four members is a harmonious one, the Medical Physicist managed to convince other three colleagues to join the competition for the Hong Kong Quality Management Award. He also requested the members to invite other staff to participate in the voluntary project. The DMAIC procedure is shown below.

Problem Identification

Using the six sigma DMAIC approach, the project was selected based on initial findings and was chosen for their alignment with organizational goals and the prob-

Table 3. PACS activities during the period 1999 – 2003

Person responsible	PACS Activity
Chief of Service	Clinical operation
Medical Physicist	Technical issues
Radiographers	Operation
E-Technicians	Maintenance

ability that it will produce results in terms of financial, quality and productivity improvement.

During the Define and Measure phases, it is important that critical elements are clearly identified and that voice of the customer (VOC) information was obtained through stakeholder interviews. Key performance indicators also are gathered, including examination volume, examination duration and room utilization for all modalities; patient, referring physician and staff satisfaction, and staffing to identify current operational performance relative to labor expense, revenue and operational quality metrics. Financial data is pulled from existing systems within the facility and cycle time data needs to be collected manually. Process mapping and sub-process mapping with assigned indicators for selected modalities helps to outline existing procedures within the department.

During the Analyze phase, the project team determines the most critical drivers that may impact the process under examination. Analysis would reveal issues such as slow start-up times in the mornings or scheduling conflicts with physicians. The information also may indicate that a high volume of patients failing to show up for appointments is consuming capacity, or that utilization fluctuates during the day due to bottlenecks in the system or variability in patient arrival patterns. With analysis complete, the team then develops action plans and recommends performance improvement opportunities that are aligned with the organization's strategic objectives. Moving into the Improve phase often is the most challenging, yet most rewarding part of the project. As process changes are actually implemented, long-standing issues are finally addressed and better processes are put in place – changes that will ultimately improve the overall effectiveness of the facility's diagnostic imaging services.

The Control phase begins once process changes have been established and appear to be working. The importance of monitoring results during this phase cannot be underestimated. This is one of the most critical keys to long-term success and a differentiating element for Six Sigma. During this phase, control tools are implemented such as "dashboards" or balanced scorecards to monitor key indicators and ensure that project gains remain on track. It also is important during the Control phase to "institutionalize" the wins, celebrate success and instill ongoing change management capabilities through change management The objective of this project has therefore been found to be "To achieve 90% of hospital-wide filmless radiological service starting from November 1, 2003."

It is understood that most equipment is designed for reliability, but breakdowns can still occur, especially when equipment is used in a demanding environment. A typical situation is what could be called a "single point failure." That is, the entire system fails if only one piece of equipment such as a network switch fails. If some of the processes that the system supports are critical or the cost of a system breakdown is too high, then introducing redundancy into the system is a usual way to overcome the problem. There are many different approaches, each of which uses a different kind of device, for providing a system with redundancy.

The continuous operation of a PACS in a filmless hospital for patient care is a challenging task. The design objectives of a PACS for such a system should be high speed, reliable and user friendly. The main aim of the design is to avoid the occurrence of any single point of failure in the system.

In order to achieve the project objective, the Six Sigma approach was adopted and each member then volunteered specific tasks for the QC Award project and the project duty list is shown in Table 4.

Data Collection

Before the team started a filmless radiology operation, they need to find out the causes of film printing in their hospital. Some team members were assigned to find out all the possible causes of film printing. Due to the difference of job nature and duties, different team members using different techniques collected different source of data.

Table 4. QC project responsibility

Responsibility	Content
Data collection	Medical Physicist Radiographers, E-Technicians
Problem analysis	Medical Physicist
Selection of control	Chief of Service Medical Physicist
Control testing	Radiographers, E-Technicians
Quality Assurance of result	Chief of Service
Reporting	Medical Physicist

In order to measure the benefits of filmless radiology service, some other information were collected by searching the historical record in Radiology Information System, and comparing ours with other existing hospital with similar scale. From Radiology Information System, the yearly film consumptions from 2001 to 2003 were shown in Figure 1.

In a traditional radiology department, the storage space for their films occupies a space of 2,000 to 5,000 sq ft. In TKOH, 3,800 sq ft storage space was assigned for film library. Management and handling of these films also required one clerk and three workmen by comparing with other hospitals.

Data Analysis

The peak X-ray film consumption rate was 100,240 films per year at 2003. It cost about one million Hong Kong dollars. Obviously, this saving can only be achieved by minimizing the causes of the film printing as shown in Table 5.

For a 90% of hospital-wide filmless radiological service, the maximum allowed film-printing rate of the peak X-ray film consumption (100,240 per year) is 10,024 films per year. The daily maximum allowed film-printing rate is equal to 27.5 films per day. Our daily target is to minimize the film consumption to less than 27.5 films per day by minimizing the causes of film printing.

Table 5. Causes for film printing

Duty	Data Source	Measure	Causes of film printing
Medical Physicist	Policy	Document search	*Vendor service contract covers office hours only. Another service contract is required for non-office hours.
	Environment	Site inspection	*Power failure *Water flooding *Hospital network failure
E-Technician	Machines	System, record check	*Computer failure *Network breakdown
	Procedure	Observation and record check	*Wrong image distribution
Radiographers	Human	Meeting	*Clinicians not familiar with the system *Some users have no confidence
	Machines	Observation and record check	*Computer failure *Network breakdown
	Procedure	Observation and record check	*Wrong image distribution

Figure 1. X-ray film consumption: 2001 to 2003

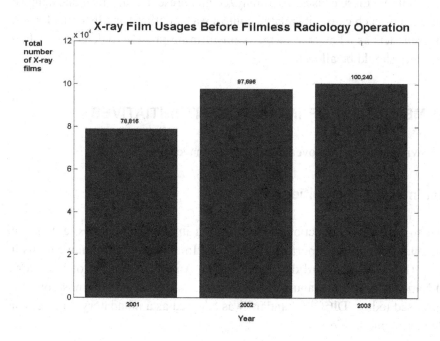

Figure 2. Fishbone diagram of TKOH filmless radiology service

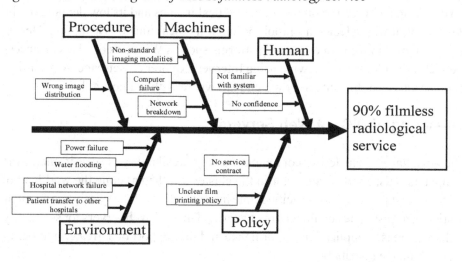

With regard to the data collected as in Table 5, different causes of film printing are presented. All these causes were analyzed and presented in a fishbone diagram as Figure 2. For each cause, its related control was identified and listed in Table 6. The diagram acts as a key map of the brainstorming process to determine where the resources should be allocated.

IMPLEMENTATION OF IMPROVEMENT INITIATIVES

The following process improvement initiatives have been planned:

Digital Imaging Modalities

In order to facilitate connections with different imaging modalities, a common international standard is important. The Digital Imaging and Communications in Medicine (DICOM) standard developed by the American College of Radiology (ACR)-National Electrical Manufacturers' Association (NEMA) is the most common standard used today. DICOM standard was adopted as a mandatory requirement for all imaging modalities.

Web Technology

Since the Web technology can provide a reliable platform for the distribution of various kinds of information including medical images and its low demand on the Web client, it was selected as a tool for major medical image distribution. Hence, any computer running on common platforms such as Windows or Mac can access the Web server for image viewing using Internet Explorer or Netscape. Any clinical user can carry out his duty anytime and anywhere within a hospital.

Clustering of DICOM Web Servers

The advantage of clustering computers for high availability is seen if one of the computers fails; another computer in the cluster can then assume the workload of the failed computer at a pre-specified time interval. Users of the system see no interruption of access. The advantages of clustering DICOM Web servers for scalability include increased application performance and the support of a greater number of users for image distribution.

Clustering can be implemented at different levels of the system, including hardware, operating systems, middleware, systems management and applications. The more layers that incorporate clustering technology, the more complex the whole

Table 6. Film printing causes and associated controls

Causes of film printing	Controls
Vendor service contract covers office hours only. No service coverage is for non-office hours.	Another service contract is required for non-office hours
Power failure	Installation of essential power supply with uninterrupted power supply
Water flooding	Daily inspection
Hospital network failure	Daily inspection and network monitoring. Redundant network for image distribution
Computer failure	• Installation of backup server • Using a cluster of Web servers • RAID Technology • Use of SAN
Network breakdown	• Backup network. • Daily inspection and network monitoring.
Wrong image distribution	• Daily inspection
Clinicians not familiar with the system	• Training • Using Web technology • Smart card system • Barcode system • LCD
Some users have no confidence	• Online help • Barcode system for easy patient search • Smart card system for fast system logon
Non-standard imaging modalities	DICOM standard is set as a mandatory requirement for all imaging modalities
Patient transfer to other hospitals	Network expanding to other hospitals
Unclear film printing policy	• No-film policy • Film printing protocol

system is to manage. To implement a successful clustering solution specialists in all the technologies (i.e. hardware, networking, and software) are required. The way we used for clustering the Web servers is connecting all Web servers using a load-balancing switch. This method has the advantage of low server overhead and requiring no computer processor power.

RAID Technology

In PACS, redundant array of inexpensive disks (RAID) technology can provide protection on the availability of the data in the server. In RAID level 5, no data is lost even during the failure of a single hard disk within a RAID group. This is essential for a patient care information system. Extra protection can be obtained by using additional global spare hard disks for automatic protection of data during the malfunctioning of more than one hard disk. Today, most storage area network (SAN) designed for high capacity storage are built on RAID technology.

Storage Area Network (SAN)

A storage area network (SAN) is a high-speed special-purpose network (or sub-network) that interconnects different kinds of data storage devices with associated data servers on behalf of a larger network of users. Typically, a storage area network is part of the entire enterprise network of computing resources. The advanced features of SAN are its supporting of high speed data transfer, disk mirroring, backup and restore, archival and retrieval of archived data, data migration from one storage

Figure 3. X-ray imaging modalities connected into TKOH PACS using DICOM standard

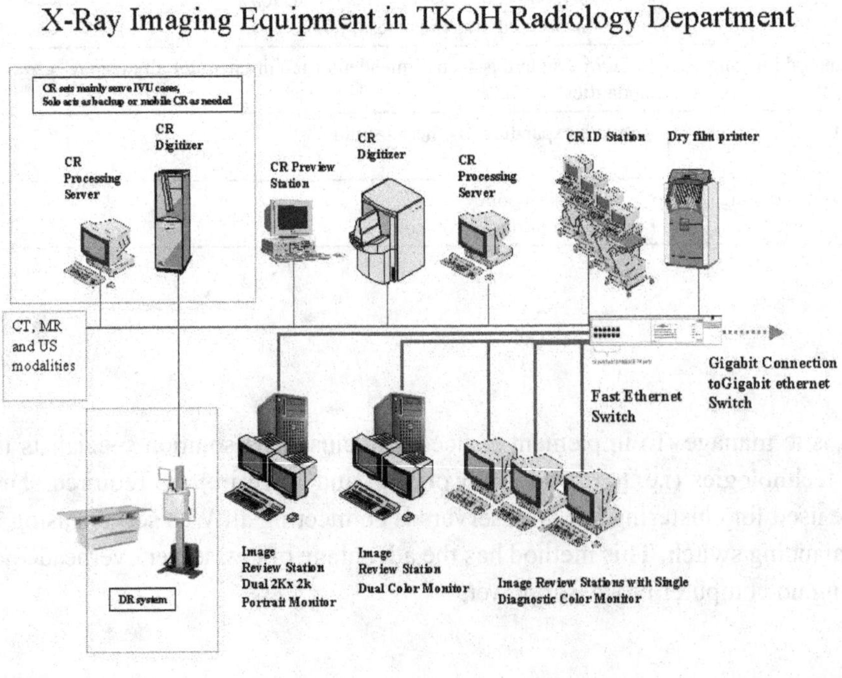

X-Ray Imaging Equipment in TKOH Radiology Department

device to another, and the sharing of data among different servers in a network. SANs can also incorporate sub-networks with network-attached storage (NAS) systems, which are shown in Figure 4.

Redundant Network for Image Distribution

Nevertheless, all of the PACS devices still need to be connected to the network, so to maximize system reliability, a PACS network should be built with redundancy. To build up a redundant network, two parallel gigabit-optical fibers were connected between the PACS and the hospital networks as two network segments using four Ethernet switches (see Figure 5). The Ethernet switches were configured in such as way that one of the network segments was in active mode while the other was in standby mode. If the active network segment fails, the standby network segment will become active within less than 300 ms to allow the system to keep running continuously.

Barcode System

Recognizing that manual data collection and keyed data entry are inefficient and error-prone, bar codes are evolved to replace human intervention. Bar codes are simply a method of retaining data in a format or medium that is conducive to electronic data entry. In other words, it is much easier to teach a computer to recognize simple patterns of lines, spaces and squares than it is to teach it to understand written characters or the English language. Bar codes not only improve the accuracy of entered data, but also increase the rate at which data can be entered.

Barcode system includes printing and reading of the barcode labels. In most Hospital Information System, barcode system is commonly adopted as a part of the information system for accurate and fast patient data retrieval. In PACS, barcode labels are mostly used for patient identification and DICOM accession. They are used to retrieve records on patient examinations and studies.

Smart Card System

A smart card is a card that is embedded with either a microprocessor and a memory chip, or only a memory chip with non-programmable logic. The microprocessor card can add, delete, and otherwise manipulate information on the card, while a memory-chip card, such as pre-paid phone cards, can only undertake a pre-defined operation. Smart cards, unlike magnetic stripe cards, can carry all the necessary functions and information on the card. Smart card can also be classified as contact

Figure 4. Design of TKOH PACS

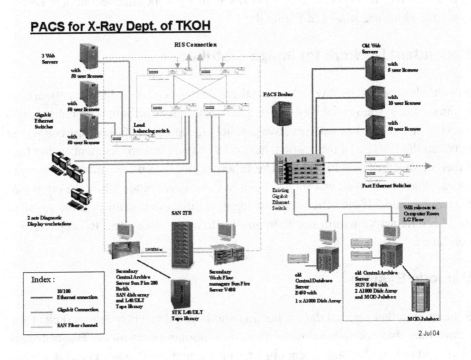

Figure 5. Design of PACS and hospital network interface

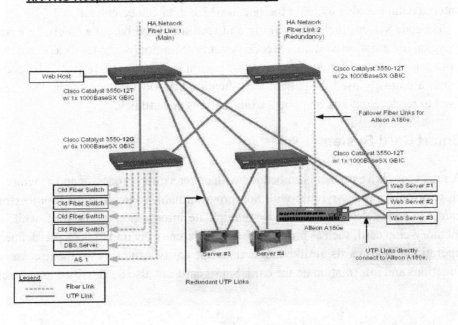

and contactless types. The contactless smart card communicates with the reader using radio frequency (RF) method.

In the TKOH PACS, a contactless smart card system was installed for authentication of the user. The information about the user name, login time and location are stored in a remote server through a computer network.

No-Film Policy

No film is printed when the patients are still under the care of TKOH. Films are printed only when the patient is transferred to another hospital. Under the no-film policy, the chance of spreading infectious disease through films is also reduced.

Embedded Liquid Crystal Display (LCD) Monitor

For the display of medical images in TKOH, LCD monitors are installed on the walls in ward areas in place of the existing light boxes. The LCD monitors are installed in pairs to facilitate comparison of a large number of medical images. They are also configured in portrait mode for the display of chest X-ray CR images (see Figure 6).

In the design of the TKOH PACS (Figure 3), all Computed Tomographic (CT), Magnetic Resonance (MR), Ultrasound (US), Digital Radiology (DR), and Computed Radiographic (CR) images were archived in image servers of the PACS (Figure 4). The capacity of the image servers was about 5 Terabytes using a 2.3 Terabyte Storage Area Network (SAN) technology and a DICOM compression of 2.5 compression rate. The image distribution to the clinicians was sent through a cluster of WEB servers, which would provide a high availability of the service. The connection between the PACS and hospital network was through a cluster of automatic fail-over switches as shown in Figure 5. Our users can use a WEB browser for X-ray image viewing for the diagnosis or follow up of patients. The WEB-based X-ray image viewers were set up in the computers in all wards, intensive care unit and specialist outpatient departments to provide a filmless radiological service. The design of the computers for X-ray image viewing in wards is shown in Figure 6. These computers were built using all the above technologies for performance and reliability.

User trainings were provided for all clinicians regularly. Online help, smart card system, and barcode system were installed for improving the efficiency of the clinician. For management of the system, no-film policy and the objective of the project was declared and explained in departmental meeting. Vendor service contract was rearranged to cover 24 hours of service and seven days a week.

Finally, the international standard ISO27000/BS7799 was implemented. After internal and external audits, our PACS has obtained the BS7799 certificate since 2004.

RESULTS

From the Radiology Information System, the film consumptions for the year 2004 and the first quarter of 2005 were obtained. The total film consumption for 2005 can be projected from this first quarter data. The comparison of total film consumptions is shown as in Figure 7.

Assuming the peak film consumption rate to be 100,240 films per year, the percentage of filmless radiology service for the years of 2004 and 2005 are 92.1 and 91.5 respectively.

The % of filmless radiology service at 2004
= (100,240-7,959)/100,240
= 92.1%

Figure 6. X-ray image viewer in wards

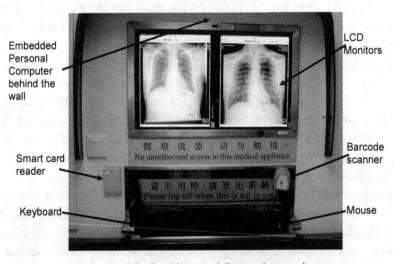

Medical Image Viewer in ward

The % of filmless radiology service at 2005
= (100,240-8,540)/100,240
= 91.5%

Besides achieving the project objective, other tangible and intangible benefits resulting from the project include:

Film-Cost Saving

The film-cost saving for TKOH is about 0.9 million dollars per year. The labour cost for the administration of the films is about 0.5 million per year. Similar film-less radiology technology can be transfer and apply to 44 other public hospitals under the administration of Hospital Authority. The projected film-cost with related labouring cost are about 22-23 million dollars per year. The saving on staff cost is around another 5 million dollars per year.

Infection Control

Since filmless radiology service minimized the amount of film transfer, it reduced the chance for spreading of highly infectious disease through health-care staff. No staff from the radiology department in TKOH was infected during the outbreak of Severe Acute Respiratory Syndrome (SARS) in Hong Kong during 2003.

Space Saving

In TKOH, 3,800 sq ft film storage space has been saved. In other hospitals with a radiology department, similar saving can easily be achieved. The estimated space saving should be not less than 76,000 sq ft for the whole Hospital Authority.

Increase Efficiency

Since the use of filmless radiology technology, no film waiting time and film loss were identified. Remote consultation using digital images was allowed. The efficiencies of radiologists and clinicians were improved.

Environmental Friendliness

Filmless radiology reduces the use of a large amount of films and chemicals. It helped to promote an environmental friendly image to the local community.

Promotion of Hospital Image

Both the Chief of Service and the Medical Physicist are invited to join the Hospital Authority PACS Technology Advisory Group as Committee Members, a major role of this Group is to standardize the image distribution technique for other public hospitals,

PROJECT REVIEW AND FUTURE PLAN

The whole system is reviewed regularly through internal and ISO27000/BS7799 audits. The purposes of these audits are to identify the potential risks of the PACS system in confidentiality, integrity and availability of data. The major difficulties encountered are:

- Some of the users are temporary staff transferred from other hospitals. Even the human resource department may find it difficult to track their movements. It is difficult for the PACS team to review the status of each user account. At this moment, the user account review has to be done manually within the Human Resource Department.

Figure 7. X-ray film consumption: 2001 to 2005

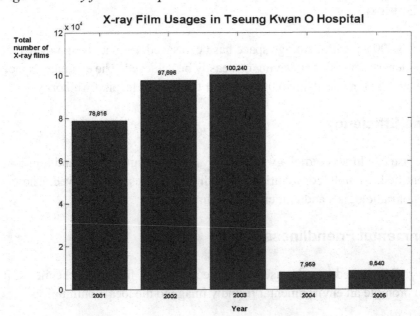

- Although the PACS team has acquired some basic knowledge of quality management and six sigma, they were of the view that they were weak in the following areas:
  - ° Hardware and software reliability evaluations;
  - ° Without any previous knowledge on the operating characteristics of PACS equipment and associated software, it is not an easy task to carry out a realistic Failure Mode and Effect Analysis;
  - ° Method of assessing the existing organizational culture, as they found that the speed of implementing various changes is rather slow.

It was planned that in future, standardization of user information and storage format in clinical departments, human resource department, and radiology department would be pursued. This can facilitate physicians' review of the status of each temporary user.

Conclusion

In conclusion, the TKOH Filmless Radiology Project was successful through the application of Six Sigma methodology and the target of 90% of the proposed filmless radiology service has been achieved.

JUDGING PANEL Q & A

During the Judging Panel interview, the PACS Project Leader was asked to clarify following issues:

- The way of generating the project action plan and how to solve any difficulty encountered.

The reply was:

"Improving quality of services is best done with voluntary, multifunctional and multidisciplinary teams, where each PACS team member has specific responsibility and share the project target of achieving 90% of hospital-wide filmless radiological service towards end of 2003. All team members have been encouraged to communicate more with each other since they have different duties and functions and are at different levels in the organization."

The following procedure was used to generate an action plan:

1. Conduct a Force Field Analysis with the group.
2. Generate alternatives: Bearing in mind the forces, use brainstorming to generate possible strategies to fulfill the project mission.
3. Viability Analysis: After defining several possible strategies, review them to see if they are viable (possible) and align with the Project objective. Determine whether the necessary resources exist to carry out each strategy. Also, analyze to see if the strategies are politically viable.
4. Pugh Matrix: The Pugh matrix was used to prioritize various feasible designs for testing and development.
5. Plan of Action: Develop a plan of action by putting in writing each defined strategy and the time line for each strategy. To test the plan of action, compare it to the following criteria:
   - each action should be no more than four to five lines
   - each line gives clear guidelines of when and how it will be completed
   - each strategy helps fulfill the project objective
   - each strategy takes advantage of the driving forces and helps overcome the forces of resistance.
6. Practice of problem-solving: He has also encouraged members to practise TRIZ and Shewhart's Plan-Do-Check-Act (PDCA) techniques.

The Project Leader then informed the Judging Panel that the QC project team structure (with some new members) was hierarchical rather than egalitarian, since working in a non-hierarchical manner have been challenging for the team members and the Project Leaders. Indeed during the very first meeting on causes of film printing, there was no consensus reached.

Having consulted a management consultant, the Project Leader was advised to use the Affinity Technique to deal with the difficult situation. The operating principle of the technique was then outlined:

1. **First stage—Individual work:**
   - The leader asked the group a specific question.
   - Request each PACS team member to write their ideas on four or five cards (size similar to the cue cards used in presentations).
   - Each card should have only one idea containing five to seven words.
2. **Second Stage—Ordering of cards:**
   - The cards are placed on a long table, and the ideas are reordered in groups, by "affinity" (category). People can move any cards to group them into a category, until all members agree about the grouping of ideas.

3. **Third Stage—Group consensus:**
   - When the cards are not being moved anymore, he and the group try to summarize the central idea of each group of cards into one simple and short phrase. If the summary is longer than one phrase, it is probable that the groupings are too broad. Then the groupings would need to be subdivided into smaller categories.
   - After summarizing each group of ideas, he then put the central ideas in sequence to form a series of phrases, to answer the main question.

- The PACS Project Leader was asked to offer his way of dealing with any conflict that might arise during the project period. He cited the following seven steps to resolve any conflict in the team:
   1. As the Leader, avoid jumping to a solution before fully analyzing the problem.
   2. Describe the facts in detail:
      - What is the unsatisfactory situation?
      - What is the context of the conflict?
      - Who is involved?
      - What is each person's point of view?
   3. Define the conflict: Where is the contradiction between the different points of view? Analyze each team member's viewpoint by speaking to him or her individually about the situation.
   4. Diagnose the conflict:
      - What preceded the conflict?
      - What are the individual interests?
      - What advantages does each party have?
      - What are the power issues?
   5. Consider the alternatives, for there is no "best" solution. Sometimes, when the conflict is due to a misunderstanding, explaining the situation in an explicit way may help to resolve the conflict. In other circumstances, the differing points of view cannot be changed, only accepted.
   6. Implement the solution that has been chosen.
   7. Evaluate the solution. If the unsatisfactory situation still exists, the above process (i.e. Steps 1 to Step 6) would have to repeat.
- Since the PACS comprises a lot of equipment, what is the failure density model that has been used to describe the "single point failures" and why use the model?
   He replied that as there is no reliability expertise within the hospital, he had submitted all equipment data to his research partner in a local university for

failure data modeling purposes. He was informed that the Weibull distribution is the most suitable candidate as it relates to the "weakest link" concept.

- The Project Leader was asked why the cause-effect diagram had been used instead of Failure Mode and Effect Analysis. His answer was that most of the team members did not have PACS operating experience and not all of them have received training on this analytical technique. However, with his research partner's help, a FMEA project has recently been initiated in his hospital.
- In view of the rapid development of teleradiology, what is the reason for not introducing relevant initiatives in the project plan? His explanation was that he noted that the rate of implementing the proposed changes had been slightly slow and he was of the view that the skeptical attitude of some colleagues might be due to the effect of organization culture in different departments of the hospital.

CONCLUDING REMARK

From the above-mentioned case, one can see that depending on the expertise available within the PACS team, various TQM tools could be applied to a PACS project and as shown in the above case, these include:

- Force Field Analysis
- Brainstorming
- Six Sigma Method: Define, Measure, Analysis, Improve and Control (DMA-IC)
- QFD – VOC
- Pugh Matrix
- TRIZ and Shewhart's Plan-Do-Check-Act (PDCA) problem solving techniques
- Affinity Technique
- Conflict Management
- FMEA/ Cause and effect diagram
- Reliability Modeling - Effect of non-normal statistical distributions
- HFE - Organization culture evaluation

One can also see that besides the tangible and intangible benefits obtained, another benefit of adopting TQM approach is the generation of systematic information in a standardized way, which simplifies answering questions such as "Where are you in the project timeline?", "Why is there so much effort on one particular sub-system?",

"What are you trying to achieve by testing the software again?". In addition, those members not directly responsible for a given specific element of PACS development, or those who cannot understand the derivation of system reliability by looking at a combination of components, can then learn and understand the reliability relationships between components and sub-assemblies. This systematic approach also helps in influencing the attitude of other hospital staff who usually believes that PACS development is so advanced that only external experts should be involved. With proper leadership and support, TQM tools can thus help the important area of team building and knowledge sharing.

REFERENCES

Benedetto A. R. (2003). Adapting manufacturing-based Six Sigma methodology to the service environment of a radiology film library. *J Healthc Manag, 48,* 63 -280.

Ettinger, W. H. (2001). Six Sigma: Adapting GE's lessons to healthcare. *Trustee, 54,* 10 -15.

Sander, W. (2000). Six Sigma: The breakthrough management strategy revolutionizing the world's top corporations. *Qual Prog, 33,* 106 -107.

Simmons, J. C. (2002). Using Six Sigma to make a difference in healthcare quality. *Qual Lett Healthc Lead, 14,* 2-10.

Smith, J. J., & Berlin, L. (2003). Picture archiving and communication systems (PACS) and the loss of patient examination records. *AJR 2001, 176,* 1381-1384.

Chapter XVII
Epilogue

Today's filmless radiology through PACS provides greater speed and superior image quality. However, when workflow is encumbered by inefficiencies, the benefit to the organization – and ultimately the patients – may not be fully realized. Even with the latest equipment installed, many organizations face delays in report-turnaround time and a backlog of patients waiting for appointments. Diminished security and quality can lead to a variety of problems for filmless radiology facilities or departments, including:

- Delay in diagnosis and treatment
- Emergency department bottlenecks
- Increased length of stay
- Patient dissatisfaction
- Referring physician dissatisfaction
- Potential loss of outpatient business
- Loss of revenue
- Poor public image

To optimize PACS performance, technology, and the associated security, issues must not only be leading edge, it also must be appropriately aligned with the people and process steps involved in the delivery of safe and cost-effective patient care. One approach that has proven to be effective involves the implementation of technical and management strategies incorporating PACS data security management, QFD, reliability modelling, internet flow control, and human factor techniques to accelerate change and build acceptance.

In the digital revolution in healthcare industry came with the PACS, many new Information and Communication Technologies such as clustering technology, high resolution LCD monitors, high speed networking technology, large volume storage, and new data compression techniques have been applied. Management of a PACS for filmless radiology operation is a practical problem. This involves information security, workflow, quality control, quality assurance, and standardization. In this book, the authors have adopted ISO27000 information security management standard as a framework for security management in PACS.

The concept of total quality management (TQM) has been around for several decades, but its adoption has been hindered by the lack of a clear way to implement it in the healthcare industry. Most hospital administrators have been looking for a simple, direct method of bolting it onto what they have been doing. By now, it is clear that the TQM concept is incompatible with business as usual. With the realization that a new way must be found to implement TQM came the question of how. TQM must be implemented with a management method, which has the opportunity for continuous improvement and customer sensitivity built into it. A synergetic model comprising Six Sigma, reliability and human factor engineering methods is a prime candidate for being this vehicle.

Every component of this comprehensive PACS model is designed to facilitate the development and operation of complex medical systems such as the PACS. To the authors' knowledge, there are no books that specifically focus on applying both Security and Quality Management Systems concomitantly to PACS development and operation. The main purpose is to address the following PACS operation problems:

- Information security on PACS is a new area of research, which involves technology, workflow redesign, management, and social engineering. ISO27000 can be used as a framework in this topic.
- Implementation of a filmless hospital project involves design, planning, and project management.
- PACS Quality Assurance (QA) is an overarching topic that covers all aspects of system design and implementation, embracing everything from information governance to network performance.
- Reliability prediction of PACS hardware and software often deviates by more than ten percent from manufacturers' recommendations.

- A quick method of determining PACS failure characteristics is lacking. This hinders the formulation of cost-effective and proactive maintenance strategy for PACS in general.
- Field performances of PACS are quite different from those identified by hardware manufacturers and software suppliers.

As mentioned earlier, this is mainly because all information security, hardware, and software reliability predictions were catered for individual components in a laboratory environment. Thus, the combined effects of (i) information security, (ii) hardware and software integration, and (iii) system networking, and (iv) human factors have rarely been considered in the PACS operating environment.

It is expected that through this book the readers will acquire the necessary working knowledge on (i) the setting up of a secure information system, (ii) the prediction of PACS overall reliability, (iii) modelling the failure modes and effects of key components individually and jointly on the integrated system, (iv) applying flow control method such as AQM in PACS network, and (v) eclectic use of various human factor and cultural tools in the development and operation of PACS systems, such that they are better prepared to make an educated decision regarding their PACS projects. The quality award winning case has demonstrated how a small PACS project team could achieve both significant tangible and intangible results through their continuous improvement spirit and whole-hearted endeavour.

The HSSH-based TQM approach should be considered a philosophy rather than simply a methodology; it assumes no endpoints in improvement efforts and does not attempt to replace the older concepts of QA and QC but rather to reap their benefits and take them to a higher conceptual level. The PACS-TQM model has 5 foci: (1) to determine and meet the needs of patients and customers (internal and external), (2) to approach quality improvement holistically on the basis of the identification of the underlying cause of poor performance, (3) to apply data-based management and scientific methodology, (4) to consider organization culture and human factors in PACS development and management, and (5) to empower its practitioners to improve quality on a daily basis.

FUTURE TREND

Introduction of ISO 27799

ISO/IEC 27799 is a part of a growing family of ISO/IEC ISMS standards, the 'ISO/IEC 27000 series' is an information security standard being currently developed by the International Organization for Standardization (ISO) and the International

Electrotechnical Commission (IEC). Its current draft title is Information Security Management in Health using ISO/IEC 27002. It has now reached 'committee draft' stage within its development cycle. The purpose of ISO/IEC 27799 is providing guidance to health organizations and other holders of personal health information on how to protect such information via implementation of ISO/IEC 27002. It specifically covers the security management needs in this sector, with respect to the particular nature of the data involved.

The standard takes account of the range of models of service delivery within the healthcare sector, and provides additional explanation with respect to those control objectives within 17799/27002 that require it. A number of additional requirements are also listed.

Contents of ISO 27799

The content sections of ISO 27799 include the followings:

Scope
References
Terminology
Symbols
Health information security overview
1.   Information security within information governance
2.   Information governance within corporate and clinical governance
3.   Health information to be protected:
- personal health information
- pseudonyms data derived from personal health information
- statistical and research data, including anonyms data derived by removal of personally identifying data
- clinical / medical knowledge not related to specific patients (e.g., data on adverse drug reactions)
- data on health professionals and staff
- information related to public health surveillance
- audit trail data that are produced by health information systems containing personal health information or data about the actions of users in regard to personal health information
- system security data, e.g.: access control data and other security related system configuration data for health information systems.
4.   Threats and vulnerabilities in health information security
- 25 threats to health info security are described

Practical Action Plan for Implementing ISO/IEC 27799

1.   Taxonomy of the 17799 and 27001 standards
2.   Management commitment to implementing ISO/IEC 17799
3.   Establishing, operating, maintaining and improving the information security management system (ISMS)
     •   Planning: establishing the ISMS
     •   Doing: implementing and operating the ISMS
     •   Checking: monitoring and reviewing the ISMS
     •   Acting: maintaining and improving the ISMS

Healthcare Implications of ISO/IEC 27799

1.   Information security policy
     •   Information security policy document
     •   Review of the information security policy document
2.   Organizing information security
     •   Internal organization
         ◦   Management commitment to information security, information security co-ordination, and allocation of security responsibilities
         ◦   Authorization process for information processing facilities
         ◦   Confidentiality agreements
         ◦   Contact with Authorities, contact with special interest groups, and independent review of security
     •   Third parties
         ◦   Identification of risks related to external parties
         ◦   Addressing security when dealing with customers
         ◦   Addressing security in third party agreement
3.   Asset management
     •   Responsibility for health information assets
     •   Health information classification
         ◦   Classification Guidelines
         ◦   Information labelling and handling
4.   Human resources security
     •   Prior to employment
         ◦   Roles and responsibilities
         ◦   Screening
         ◦   Terms and conditions of employment
     •   During employment
         ◦   Management responsibilities

- ○ security awareness, education and training
- ○ Disciplinary process
- Termination or change of employment
  - ○ Termination of responsibilities and return of assets
  - ○ Removal of access rights
5. Physical and environmental security
   - Secure areas
     - ○ Physical security perimeter
     - ○ Physical entry controls; securing offices, rooms and facilities; protecting against external and environmental threats; and working in secure areas
     - ○ Public access, delivery and loading areas
   - Equipment security
     - ○ Equipment siting and protection
   - Supporting utilities, cabling security, and equipment maintenance
   - Security of equipment off-premises
   - Secure disposal or reuse of equipment
   - Removal of property
6. Communications and operations management
   - Operational procedures and responsibilities
     - ○ Documented operating procedures
     - ○ Change management
     - ○ Segregation of duties
     - ○ Separation of development, test and operational facilities
   - Third-party service delivery management
   - System planning and acceptance
     - ○ Capacity management
     - ○ System acceptance
   - Protection against malicious and mobile code
     - ○ Controls against malicious code
     - ○ Controls against mobile code
   - Backup
     - ○ Health information backup
   - Network security management
     - ○ Network controls
     - ○ Security of network services
   - Media handling
     - ○ Management of removable computer media
     - ○ Disposal of media

- ° Information handling procedures
- ° Security of system documentation
- Exchanges of information
  - ° Health information exchange policies and procedures, and exchange agreements
  - ° Physical media in transit
  - ° Electronic messaging
  - ° Health information systems
- Electronic health information services
  - ° Electronic commerce, and online transactions
  - ° Publicly available health information
- Monitoring
  - ° Audit logging
  - ° Protection of log information
  - ° Clock synchronization Structure

7. Access control
- Requirements for access control in health
  - ° Access control policy
- User access management
  - ° User registration
  - ° Privilege management
  - ° User password management
  - ° Review of user access rights
- User responsibilities
- Network access control, and operating system access control
- Application and information access control
  - ° Information access restriction
  - ° Sensitive system isolation
- Mobile computing and teleworking
  - ° Mobile computing and communications
  - ° Teleworking

8. Information systems acquisition, development, maintenance
- Security requirements of information systems
  - ° Security requirements analysis and specification
- Correct processing in applications
  - ° Uniquely identifying subjects of care
  - ° Input data validation
  - ° Control of internal processing
  - ° Message Integrity
  - ° Output data validation

- Cryptographic controls
  - ° Policy on use of cryptographic controls, and key management
- Security of system files
  - ° Control of operational software
  - ° Protection of system test data
  - ° Access control to program source code
- Security in development and support processes, and technical vulnerability management

9. Information Security incident management
  - Reporting information security events and weaknesses
  - Management of incidents and improvements
    - ° Responsibilities and procedures
    - ° Learning from incidents
    - ° Collection of evidence

10. Business continuity management
  - Information security aspects of business continuity management

11. Compliance
  - Compliance with legal requirements
    - ° Identifying applicable legislation, intellectual property rights, and protection of organizational records
    - ° Data protection and privacy of personal information
    - ° Prevention of misuse of information processing facilities, and regulation of cryptographic controls
  - Compliance with security policies and technical compliance
  - Information systems audit considerations in a health environment

Annexes of ISO 27799

- A: Threats
- B: Tasks and documentation of the ISMS
- C: Potential benefits and tool attributes
- D: Related standards

Good quality information underpins sound decision making at every level in the medical imaging sector and most importantly contributes to the improvement of diagnostic decisions. All too often data quality is still seen as something that is the responsibility of informatics staff alone and is often seen with disinterest by PACS clinicians and administrators, despite being so critical to the quality of the decisions they make. To ensure high quality PACS information, it is considered most likely that a PACS information strategy (PACSIS) for improving the quality of information in the PACS networks (regional or national) would need to be developed in the not too distant future.

The starting point of this strategy is the recognition that efforts to secure quality must be directed appropriately, and that this should start with patient data collected for clinical and operational purposes. Whilst the PACSIS is equally applicable to all information collected and used throughout a local hospital network, the initial focus is on information used to support diagnostic imaging. PACS information quality needs to be addressed within existing procedures and work plans rather than as a stand-alone initiative, though it does need to be managed in a focused way. In particular, the PACSIS should aim to build on the initiatives of (i) the drive to reduce adverse diagnostic incidents and (ii) the modern approach to PACS error prevention and risk management.

Poor quality information is generally due to error and these two initiatives are changing the way that errors are perceived, prevented and corrected. Considerable attention has been focused upon readily measurable aspects of data quality, namely the validity and completeness of data items, whilst harder to measure but perhaps more important aspects in the context of overall information quality, such as timeliness, accuracy and reliability have often been neglected and these aspects should be considered in the PACSIS. Data quality is an important component of PACS information quality but there are other components that influence just how useful the information is to a particular user.

Similarly, one can find that in many instances centrally led initiatives to monitor and improve the quality of information have employed a top-down audit/accreditation approach and largely on administrative or management information. It is proposed that the new PACSIS should focus on building in security quality from the bottom up—at the point that information is collected and recorded—with the clear goal of improving the security and quality of the information used to support diagnostic decisions. The strategy should also reflect recent changes in information management, electronic records, patient access, and the reporting of adverse health events.

It is generally accepted that PACS information quality does not have to be perfect to satisfy some purposes, e.g. PACS management. However, perfect quality must be the aspiration where PACS information directly supports clinical care. This gives rise to the concept of 'fit for purpose', but whilst this is an important concept, it is essential that it be seen in the context of the relevant information 'pathway'.

Radiological imaging information is usually captured for specific purposes associated with patient care and subsequently flows along pathways that branch out at different stages to support different secondary purposes. Where PACS information quality worsens as the information flows along a pathway, this may be acceptable in some circumstances. Where the PACS information quality is, poor at the point of capture or where quality worsens along a pathway that supports diagnostic effectiveness this degradation is most certainly not acceptable. Information flows along pathways from its point of origin to eventual users. The pathway includes the steps taken by the PACS hospital to build appropriate capacity to support PACS information security and quality through leadership, management, training, policies and procedures. It should aim to encompass all of the PACS information processing that takes place between the initial recording of radiological images and its diagnostic use, and goes on to include the benefit derived by users and the use of user feedback to improve processes. There are therefore a number of distinct stages within pathways, the PACS information security and quality needs are to be addressed at every relevant stage of a pathway, and it is necessary to understand the action that would be taken to assure and monitor quality at each point. Some stages may not be relevant within a particular pathway and some may occur at more than one point if an extended pathway is being considered.

For effective implementation, specific PACS policies on major PACS information pathways are needed and these pathways would include:

- **Capture:** Policies that address acquisition/collection will be needed (e.g. how patient information is to be checked, automated data or image validation rules, etc).
- **Transfer:** Policies that address the approach to disclosure of PACS images will be needed.
- **Transcription:** Policies relating to validation and audit will be needed.
- **Extraction:** Policies relating to the validation of PACS information will be required (e.g. cross checking of imaging sources, etc)
- **Presentation:** Policies that address how PACS information is presented will be needed (e.g. reports or screens for different audiences, etc).
- **Feedback:** Policies that relate to the effective application of feedback from end users and learning are required.

Finally, hospital management support for a PACS information security and quality culture is essential if improvements are to be made and sustained.

Section V
Appendices

Appendix A

EXAMPLE POLICY STATEMENT

The following is an example of an Information Security Policy Statement.

Objective

The objective of information security is to ensure business continuity and minimize business damage by preventing and minimizing the impact of security incidents.

Policy

The purpose of the Policy is to protect the **organization's information assets**[3] from **all** threats, whether internal or external, deliberate or accidental. The Chief Executive has approved the Information Security Policy.

- It is the Policy of the organization to ensure that:
  - ○ Information will be protected against unauthorized access;
  - ○ **Confidentiality** of information will be assured ;
  - ○ **Integrity** of information will be maintained[5];

- ° **Availability** of information is ensured as required by the business processes;
- ° Regulatory and legislative requirements will be met[6];
- ° **Business Continuity plans** will be produced, maintained and tested[7];
- ° **Information security training** will be available to **all** staff;
- ° All breaches of information security, actual or suspected, will be reported to, and investigated by the Information Security Manager [11].

- Procedures exist to support the policy. These include virus control, passwords and business continuity.
- Business requirements for the availability of information and information systems will be met.
- The Information Security Manager has direct responsibility for maintaining the Policy and providing advice and guidance on its implementation.
- All managers are directly responsible for implementing the Policy within their business areas, and for adherence by their staff.
- It is the responsibility of each member of staff to adhere to the Policy.

Signed: ....

Title: .... Date: ....

(The Policy will be reviewed by the Information Security Manager, usually I year on from the date signed.)

BUSINESS CONTINUITY PLAN

1.0 Objective

By the practice of BCP, reduce the impact and downtime of Hospital PACS system operation due to some change or failure in the company operation procedure. BCP is used to make sure the critical part of PACS system operation is not affected by critical failure or disaster.

2.0 Responsibilities

- Information security management organization representative monitor the operation of this BCP
- Top Level commitment secured
- Initiate the management process

- Identify the threats and risks
- Manage the risks as part of the Risk Management
- Business Impact Analysis (BIA)
- Develop Strategies
- Developing and implementing the plan
- Test, exercise and maintain the plan

3.0 Scope

- All normal operation procedures in the PACS system

Assumption

The design of this BCP is based on the assumption that the largest disaster is completely breakdown of the PACS room in the radiology department of the hospital. The wards, SOPD, and imaging modalities are all still in functional stage.

4.0 Content

4.1 Business Proces

Business Flow Chart

Process No	Sub-Process	Process Location
1	Patient demographic data retrieval	PACS Broker
2	Image receiving	PACS Servers
3	Image on-line storage	PACS Server, SAN
4	Image verification	PACS Servers
5	Image reporting	Image viewers
6	Image archiving to MOD jukebox	Jukebox
7	Image archiving to tape library	Tape Library
8	Image prefetching from MOD jukebox	Jukebox
9	Image prefetching from tape library	Tape Library
10	Image distribution to clinicians	Web servers
11	Image distribution through Cisco switches	Cisco switches
12	Web server load balancing	Load balancing switch
13	Remote maintenance	RAS server and Cisco router
14	Login the smart card server	Smart card server in Web servers

4.1.1 Risk Identification

According to the PACS operation procedure to find out potential risk and impact. Perform the necessary risk management, transfer (e.g. insurance)

Process No	Process Location	Risk
1	PACS Broker	Hardware failure
2	PACS Servers	Hardware failure
3	SAN	Hardware failure
4	PACS Servers	Hardware failure
5	Image viewers	Hardware failure
6	Jukebox	Hardware failure
7	Tap Library	Hardware failure
8	Jukebox	Hardware failure
9	Tap Library	Hardware failure
10	Web servers	Hardware failure
11	Cisco switches	Hardware failure
12	Load balancing switch	Hardware failure
13	RAS server and Cisco router	System malfunction
14	Smart card servers	Hardware failure

4.1.2 Level Determination

Consider the possibility of risk occurrence and practice the importance.

Process No	Process Location	Risk	Probability	Level of Importance
1	PACS Broker	Hardware failure	1	1
2	PACS Servers	Hardware failure	1	2
3	SAN	Hardware failure	1	2
4	PACS Servers	Hardware failure	1	2
5	Image viewers	Hardware failure	1	2
6	Jukebox	Hardware failure	2	4
7	Tap Library	Hardware failure	1	2
8	Jukebox	Hardware failure	2	4
9	Tap Library	Hardware failure	1	2
10	Web servers	Hardware failure	2	6
11	Cisco switches	Hardware failure	1	3
12	Load balancing switch	Hardware failure	1	2
13	RAS server and Cisco router	System malfunction	1	1
14	Smart card servers	Hardware failure	1	1

4.1.3 Responsibility Determination

Find out the responsibility to that relevant team or personnel according to the operation procedure of PACS.

Process No	Sub-Process	Related Users	Responsible Person
1	Patient demographic data retrieval	Radiographers	Radiographers, ITD
2	Image receiving	Radiographers	PACS Team
3	Image on-line storage	Radiographers	PACS Team
4	Image verification	Radiologists, Clinicians	PACS Team
5	Image reporting	Radiologists	PACS Team, Radiographers
6	Image archiving to MOD jukebox	Radiologists, Clinicians	PACS Team
7	Image archiving to tape library	Radiologists, Clinicians	PACS Team
8	Image prefetching from MOD jukebox	Radiologists, Clinicians	Radiologists, Radiographers
9	Image prefetching from tape library	Radiologists, Clinicians	Radiologists, Radiographers
10	Image distribution to clinicians	Clinicians	Clinicians, Radiographers
11	Image distribution through Cisco switches	Clinicians	Clinicians, Radiographers
12	Web server load balancing	Clinicians	PACS Team
13	Remote maintenance	Contractor	PACS Team
14	Smart card server	Clinicians	PACS Team

4.1.4 Impact Analysis

Found out critical risk which may affect the operation of PACS, and perform risk evaluation to find out the potential impact. This is done by the relevant department/team/personnel.

Process No	Sub-Process	Impact	Impact Level
1	Patient demographic data retrieval	Manual input patient demographic data	1
2	Image receiving	PACS cannot receive new images	2
3	Image on-line storage	No on-line image available in PACS. User still can view the images in the Web servers.	2
4	Image verification	Image data maybe different from in RIS.	1
5	Image reporting	Radiologists cannot view images in the PACS server for advanced image processing and reporting. However, they can still see the images in the Web servers.	2
6	Image archiving to MOD jukebox	Long-term archiving of the images. There is a risk of loss images in the SAN.	2
7	Image archiving to tape library	Another copy of long-term archiving. There is a risk of loss images in the SAN.	2
8	Image prefetching from MOD jukebox	Users cannot see the previous images. They cannot compare the present study with the previous.	2
9	Image prefetching from tape library	Users cannot see the previous images. They cannot compare the present study with the previous.	2
10	Image distribution to clinicians	The clinician cannot make diagnosis without the images.	3
11	Image distribution through Cisco switches	The clinician cannot make diagnosis without the images.	3
12	Web server load balancing	The clinician cannot make diagnosis without the images.	2
13	Remote maintenance	Vendor cannot do maintenance remotely.	1
14	Smart card server	Hardware failure	1

Business Continuity Plan For TKOH PACS

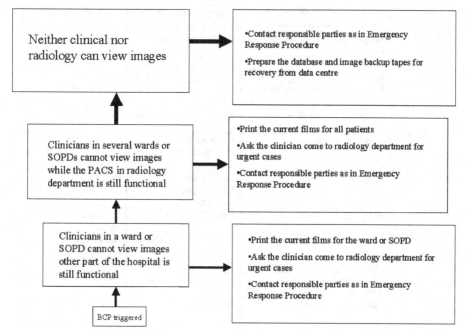

Business Continuity Plan for filmless hospital

4.1.5 Plan Development

1. The criteria for the kick-off of the BCP
    In the condition that if the clinician cannot access the Web servers (Process no 10) more than 30 minutes, the BCP should be start.
2. Emergency Response Procedure:
    a. The procedure during emergency and downtime
    b. The responsible department, team or personnel

    COS of Radiology Department   Dr. Huang
    Or PACS Manager   Dr. Carrison Tong

    c. Perform regular training, test and maintenance
        Yearly, BCP training should be provided.
    d. New BCP procedure should be approved by senior staff

3.   Recovery procedure

Step	Recovering Sub-Process	Responsible Person	Process Location
1	Image distribution to clinicians	PACS Team, contractor	Web servers
2	Image distribution through Cisco switches	PACS Team, contractor	Cisco switches
3	Image on-line storage	PACS Team, contractor	PACS Servers, SAN
4	Image reporting	PACS Team, contractor	Image viewers
5	Image prefetching from MOD jukebox	PACS Team, contractor	MOD Jukebox
6	Image prefetching from tape library	PACS Team, contractor	Tape Library
7	Image receiving	PACS Team, Radiographers, contractor	PACS Servers
8	Image verification	PACS Team, Radiographers, contractor	PACS Servers
9	Web server load balancing	PACS Team, contractor	Load balancing switch
10	Image archiving to MOD jukebox	PACS Team, contractor	Jukebox
11	Image archiving to tape library	PACS Team, contractor	Tape Library
12	Patient demographic data retrieval	Radiographers, ITD	PACS Broker
13	Remote maintenance	PACS Team	RAS server and Cisco router

4.   Recovery time

BCP Level triggered	Scope	Recovery time
1	Clinicians in a ward or SOPD cannot view images other part of the hospital is still functional	Half day for the recovering of Sub-process no 10
2	Clinicians in several wards or SOPDs cannot view images while the PACS in radiology department is still functional	One day for the recovering of Sub-process no 10 and 11
3	Neither clinical nor radiology can view images	One week for the recovering of Sub-process no 1 to 13

4.1.6 Plan Implementation

During emergency and downtime, should perform the BCP accordingly. All personnel fail to perform according to the BCP should be recorded down for future liability.

4.1.7. Annual BCP Plan Revision

1. From previous emergency or event, evaluate whether BCP is workable or not.
2. Provide training to the relevant personnel in the BCP
3. Test or check relevant hardware, software, services or system from the supplier or vendor
4. Whenever PACS or hospital has new hardware, software, services or system upgrade or change, the BCP should be re-evaluated.
5. Whenever PACS has new strategy in the operation, BCP should be re-evaluated
6. Whenever the physical location, equipment or resources changes, the BCP should be re-evaluated
7. Whenever there is a relevant change in the law or regulation, BCP should be re-evaluated

4.2 Responsibility Table

Department/ Team/Staff	Responsible Risk area	Responsible staff	Test period	Risk factor
PACS	Water Flood Fire Power Failure Typhoon Electric Strike H/W, S/W, systems check	Dr. Carrison Tong	6 months 6 months quarterly 1 year 1 year 1 year	
PACS	Hacker Computer Virus Network Failure Computer H/W, S/W failure	Dr. Carrison Tong, contractor	6 months 6 months 6 months 6 months	

HEALTH CHECK REPORT OF PACS
IN TSEUNG KWAN O HOSPITAL
DATE: DD/MM/YYYY

During the period of dd - dd mm yyyy, we carried out routine check of PACS system at Tseung Kwan O Hospital. The health check report is summarized in the following table.

PACS Model: IMPAX System

Machine	Result	Potential Problem Found	Corrective Action
TKOAS01	OK	NONE	NONE
TKODB01	OK	NONE	NONE
TKOAS02	OK	NONE	NONE
TKONWG01	OK	NONE	NONE
TKOWEB01	OK	NONE	NONE
TKOWEB02	OK	NONE	NONE
TKOWEB03	OK	None	None
TKOWC01	OK	None	None
TKOWC02	OK	None	None
TKOWC04	OK	None	None
TKOWC05	OK	None	None
TKOWC06	OK	None	None
TKOWC07	OK	None	None
TKOWC08	OK	None	None
TKOWC09	OK	None	None
TKOWC10	OK	None	None
TKOWC11	OK	None	None
TKODP01	OK	None	None
TKODP02	OK	None	None
TKODP03	OK	None	None
TKODP04	OK	None	None
TKODP05	OK	None	None
TKODP07	OK	None	None
TKODP08	OK	None	None
TALKSERVER	OK	None	None
BROKER	OK	None	None
Router SR2100	OK	None	None

Switch A	OK	None	None
Switch B	OK	None	None
Switch C	OK	None	None
Switch D	OK	None	None
Shiva RAS	OK	None	None
Switch E	OK	None	None
Switch F	OK	None	None
Switch G	OK	None	None
Switch H	OK	None	None
Switch I	OK	None	None

Action List of PACS System

1. The SUN E450 machines of both TKOAS01 and TKODB01 are shutdown and start-up in PM check. No error is found in boot up log file, /var/adm/messages.

   The disk usage is summarized as below.

Disk Usage at TKOAS01

File system	Kbytes	used	avail	capacity	Mounted on
/dev/vx/dsk/rootvol	1492070	139499	1292889	10%	/
/dev/vx/dsk/usr	1986439	1182101	744745	62%	/usr
/proc	0	0	0	0%	/proc
mnttab	0	0	0	0%	/etc/mnttab
fd	0	0	0	0%	/dev/fd
/dev/vx/dsk/var	963869	294419	611618	33%	/var
swap	813944	104	813840	1%	/var/run
swap	814144	304	813840	1%	/tmp
/dev/vx/dsk/export	1986439	700104	1226742	37%	/export
/dev/dsk/c3t5d0s7	104262624	99658173	3561825	97%	/cache1
/dev/dsk/c5t5d0s7	104262624	99658026	3561972	97%	/cache2

Disk Usage at TKODB01

Filesystem	Kbytes	used	avail	capacity	Mounted on
/dev/vx/dsk/rootvol	962571	136558	768259	16%	/
/dev/vx/dsk/usr	4032142	1178942	2812879	30%	/usr

/proc	0	0	0	0%	/proc
mnttab	0	0	0	0%	/etc/mnttab
fd	0	0	0	0%	/dev/fd
/dev/vx/dsk/var	1985043	308643	1616849	17%	/var
swap	2730032	104	2729928	1%	/var/run
swap	2730240	312	2729928	1%	/tmp
/dev/vx/dsk/export	7059201	3529636	3458973	51%	/export
/dev/dsk/c2t5d0s7	17372586	4100089	13098772	24%	/dbase/data1
/dev/dsk/c2t5d1s7	17372586	10252273	6946588	60%	/dbase/index1
/dev/dsk/c2t5d2s7	17372586	2154983	15043878	13%	/dbase/arch
/dev/dsk/c2t5d3s7	17372586	2522450	14676411	15%	/dbase/system

Disk Usage at TKONWG01

Filesystem	Kbytes	used	avail	capacity	Mounted on
/dev/md/dsk/d2	2053605	449532	1542465	23%	/
/dev/md/dsk/d11	4127845	1116200	2970367	28%	/usr
/proc	0	0	0	0%	/proc
mnttab	0	0	0	0%	/etc/mnttab
fd	0	0	0	0%	/dev/fd
/dev/md/dsk/d8	8148810	856551	7210771	11%	/var
swap	10890104	112	10889992	1%	/var/run
/dev/dsk/emcpower0h	103245937	99290946	2922532	98%	/cache25
/dev/dsk/emcpower1h	103245937	97310671	4902807	96%	/cache20
/dev/dsk/emcpower2h	103245937	97411261	4802217	96%	/cache21
/dev/dsk/emcpower3h	103245937	99288762	2924716	98%	/cache26
/dev/dsk/emcpower4h	103245937	96745011	5468467	95%	/cache22
/dev/dsk/emcpower7h	103245937	99300240	2913238	98%	/cache28
/dev/dsk/emcpower6h	103245937	96681812	5531666	95%	/cache23
/dev/dsk/emcpower5h	103245937	99292372	2921106	98%	/cache27
/dev/dsk/emcpower9h	103245937	99299833	2913645	98%	/cache29
/dev/dsk/emcpower11h	103245937	59475977	42737501	59%	/cache31
/dev/dsk/emcpower8h	103245937	99290890	2922588	98%	/cache24
/dev/dsk/emcpower14h	103245937	59478400	42735078	59%	/cache34
/dev/dsk/emcpower10h	103245937	59475914	42737564	59%	/cache30
/dev/dsk/emcpower12h	103245937	59476249	42737229	59%	/cache32
/dev/dsk/emcpower17h	103245937	59475856	42737622	59%	/cache37

/dev/dsk/emcpower15h	103245937	59475837	42737641	59%	/cache35
/dev/dsk/emcpower13h	103245937	59477697	42735781	59%	/cache33
swap	10889992	0	10889992	0%	/tmp
/dev/dsk/emcpower18h	103245937	59475888	42737590	59%	/cache38
/dev/dsk/emcpower16h	103245937	59475891	42737587	59%	/cache36
/dev/dsk/emcpower19h	103245937	59474911	42738567	59%	/cache39
/dev/md/dsk/d14	12386458	775983	11486611	7%	/export

Disk Usage at TKOAS02

Filesystem	Kbytes	used	avail	capacity	Mounted on
/dev/md/dsk/d2	8068013	417596	7569737	6%	/
/dev/md/dsk/d11	16136042	1133575	14841107	8%	/usr
/proc	0	0	0	0%	/proc
mnttab	0	0	0	0%	/etc/mnttab
fd	0	0	0	0%	/dev/fd
/dev/md/dsk/d8	18155018	231800	17741668	2%	/var
swap	3345144	112	3345032	1%	/var/run
/dev/dsk/emcpower0h	103245937	63438824	38774654	63%	/cache14
/dev/dsk/emcpower1h	103245937	101135420	1078058	99%	/cache10
/dev/dsk/emcpower2h	103245937	63437704	38775774	63%	/cache16
/dev/dsk/emcpower3h	103245937	63437974	38775504	63%	/cache17
/dev/dsk/emcpower4h	103245937	101129811	1083667	99%	/cache11
/dev/dsk/emcpower6h	103245937	63440972	38772506	63%	/cache18
/dev/dsk/emcpower8h	103245937	63440495	38772983	63%	/cache19
/dev/dsk/emcpower5h	103245937	101265465	948013	100%	/cache12
/dev/dsk/emcpower7h	103245937	101265809	947669	100%	/cache13
swap	3345032	0	3345032	0%	/tmp
/dev/dsk/emcpower9h	103245937	63440036	38773442	63%	/cache15
/dev/md/dsk/d14	24204072	1996152	21965880	9%	/export

The Dell PowerEdge 4650 machine of TKOWEB01 server was shutdown and start-up successfully in PM check. The MVF database was checked with no problem. Anti-virus definition was updated. The disk usage was as follows.

	Total (GB)	Used (GB)	Free (GB)	Capacity
Dell Server (C:)	9.95	7.12	2.83	28.4%
Database (E:)	49.9	29.8	20.1	40.3%

2. The Dell PowerEdge 4650 machine of TKOWEB02 server was shutdown and start-up successfully in PM check. The MVF database was checked with no problem. Anti-virus definition was updated. The disk usage was shown as follows.

	Total (GB)	Used (GB)	Free (GB)	Capacity
Dell Server (C:)	9.95	7.82	2.13	21.4%
Database (E:)	49.9	33.9	16.0	32.1%

3. The Dell PowerEdge 4650 machine of TKOWEB03 server was shutdown and start-up successfully in PM check. The MVF database was checked with no problem. Anti-virus definition was updated. The disk usage was as follows.

	Total (GB)	Used (GB)	Free (GB)	Capacity
Dell Server (C:)	9.95	7.34	2.61	26.2%
Database (E:)	49.9	36.8	13.1	26.3%

4. The Dell PowerEdge 1300 machines and Dell Precision 340 machines of DS3000 Review workstations are shutdown and start-up in PM check
5. The system time of WEB1000 1, WEB1000 2, WEB1000 3 are synchronized (synchronized time: dd/mm/yyyy mm:ssss)
6. The UPS are checked

Brand and model	Serial Number
Liebert 2K UPS	0223400024AF041
Liebert 3K UPS	0325900002AF491
Liebert 2K UPS	0320900002AF101
APC 2200 UPS	GS9903002683

PACS System Information

Health Check Summary of Oracle Database, MVF

ORACLE TABLESPACES
Report Date: dd/mm/yyyy

Tablespace	Filename	Size (Mb)
MVF	/usr/mvf/data/dbase/data1/mvf01.dbf	2000
	/usr/mvf/data/dbase/data1/mvf02.dbf	2000
MVFINDX	/usr/mvf/data/dbase/index1/mvfindx01.dbf	2000
	/usr/mvf/data/dbase/index1/mvfindx02.dbf	2000
	/usr/mvf/data/dbase/index1/mvfindx04.dbf	2000
	/usr/mvf/data/dbase/index1/mvfindx05.dbf	2000
	/usr/mvf/data/dbase/index1/mvfindx06.dbf	2000
SYSTEM	/usr/mvf/data/dbase/system/system01.dbf	250
TEMP	/usr/mvf/data/dbase/system/temp01.dbf	2000
TOOLS	/usr/mvf/data/dbase/index2/tools01.dbf	5
UNDO	/usr/mvf/data/dbase/rbs/undo01.dbf	60
	/usr/mvf/data/dbase/rbs/undo02.dbf	60
	/usr/mvf/data/dbase/rbs/undo03.dbf	60

Tablespace	Free(Mb)	Current Used (Mb)	Avg. Weekly Used (Mb)	Expected Size in 6 Months	Weeks Left
MVF	872.8	3127.2	15.0	3517.2	58.2
TEMP	2000.0	0.0	0.0	0.0	N/A
UNDO	158.6	21.4	-17.8	-442.1	N/A
TOOLS	5.0	0.0	0.0	0.0	N/A
SYSTEM	68.3	181.7	0.0	181.7	N/A
MVFINDX	1805.8	8194.2	73.0	10091.8	24.7

Health Check Summary of Root Disks under Volume Manager, Archive Server

DEVICE	TYPE	DISK	GROUP	STATUS
C0t0d0s2	sliced	bootdisk0	rootdg	online
C0t1d0s2	sliced	bootdisk1	rootdg	online

System Check of Archive Server, Tkoas01

System Configuration: Sun Microsystems sun4u Sun Enterprise 450 (4 X UltraSPARC-II 296MHz)
System clock frequency: 99 MHz
Memory size: 1024 Megabytes

========================= CPUs =========================

| | | Run | Ecache | CPU | CPU | |
Brd	CPU	Module	MHz	MB	Impl.	Mask
SYS	0	0	296	2.0	US-II	2.0
SYS	1	1	296	2.0	US-II	2.0
SYS	2	2	296	2.0	US-II	2.0
SYS	3	3	296	2.0	US-II	2.0

======================= Memory =======================

Memory Interleave Factor = 2-way

| | Interlv. | Socket | Size | |
Bank	Group	Name	(MB)	Status
0	0	1901	128	OK
0	0	1902	128	OK
0	0	1903	128	OK
0	0	1904	128	OK
1	0	1801	128	OK
1	0	1802	128	OK
1	0	1803	128	OK
1	0	1804	128	OK

========================= IO Cards =========================

| | Bus | Freq | | | |
Brd	Type	MHz	Slot	Name	Model
SYS	PCI	33	1	TSI,gfxp	GFXP
SYS	PCI	33	2	network-pciclass,020000	SUNW,pci-gem
SYS	PCI	33	3	scsi-pciclass,001000	Symbios,53C875
SYS	PCI	33	4	scsi-pciclass,001000	Symbios,53C875
SYS	PCI	33	5	pci108e,1000-pciclass,068000	
SYS	PCI	33	5	SUNW,hme-pci108e,1001	SUNW,cheerio
SYS	PCI	33	5	SUNW,isptwo-pciclass,010000	QLGC,ISP1040B

No failures found in System
============================

========================= Environmental Status =========================

System Temperatures (Celsius):

AMBIENT   19
CPU 0   43
CPU 1   44
CPU 2   42
CPU 3   42
==================================

Front Status Panel:

Keyswitch position is in On mode.

System LED Status: POWER   GENERAL ERROR   ACTIVITY
                     [ON]   [OFF]   [ON]
                     DISK ERROR THERMAL ERROR POWER SUPPLY ERROR
                     [OFF]   [OFF]   [OFF]

Disk LED Status: OK = GREEN   ERROR = YELLOW
                     DISK 2: [EMPTY]   DISK 3: [EMPTY]
                     DISK 0: [OK]   DISK 1: [OK]
==================================

Fans:

Fan Bank Speed Status
-------   ----- ------
CPU   31   OK
PWR   31   OK

```
Power Supplies:
----------------
Supply   Rating   Temp   Status
------   ------   ----   ------
0        550 W    31     OK
1        550 W    33     OK

=========================== HW Revisions ===========================

ASIC Revisions:
----------------
STP2223BGA: Rev 4
STP2223BGA: Rev 4
STP2223BGA: Rev 4
STP2003QFP: Rev 1
STP2205BGA: Rev 1
FEPS: SUNW,hme Rev c1

System PROM revisions:
----------------------
  OBP 3.26.0 2002/05/06 16:05   POST 6.1.0 2002/05/06 16:06
```

```
System Check of Database Server, Tkodb01

System Configuration:  Sun Microsystems  sun4u Sun Enterprise 450 (4 X UltraSPARC-II 296MHz)
System clock frequency: 99 MHz
Memory size: 1536 Megabytes

========================= CPUs =========================

           Run  Ecache  CPU   CPU
Brd  CPU  Module  MHz    MB   Impl.  Mask
---  ---  ------  -----  -----  ------  ----
SYS   0    0     296    2.0  US-II   2.0
SYS   1    1     296    2.0  US-II   2.0
SYS   2    2     296    2.0  US-II   2.0
SYS   3    3     296    2.0  US-II   2.0


========================= Memory =========================

    Interlv.  Socket  Size
Bank  Group   Name   (MB)  Status
----  -----   ------  ----  ------
 0    none    1901    256   OK
 0    none    1902    256   OK
 0    none    1903    256   OK
 0    none    1904    256   OK
 1    none    1801    128   OK
 1    none    1802    128   OK
 1    none    1803    128   OK
 1    none    1804    128   OK


========================= IO Cards =========================

    Bus  Freq
Brd  Type MHz  Slot  Name                 Model
---  ---- ----  ---  -------------------------------  ----------------------
SYS  PCI   33    1   TSI,gfxp                 GFXP
SYS  PCI   33    2   network-pciclass,020000       SUNW,pci-gem
SYS  PCI   33    3   scsi-pciclass,001000          Symbios,53C875

No failures found in System
============================

========================= Environmental Status =========================

System Temperatures (Celsius):
------------------------------
AMBIENT   17
CPU 0    42
CPU 1    43
CPU 2    44
CPU 3    42
==================================

Front Status Panel:
-------------------
Keyswitch position is in On mode.

System LED Status:   POWER    GENERAL ERROR    ACTIVITY
              [ ON]      [OFF]         [OFF]
              DISK ERROR THERMAL ERROR  POWER SUPPLY ERROR
              [OFF]       [OFF]        [OFF]

Disk LED Status:    OK = GREEN    ERROR = YELLOW
          DISK  2: [EMPTY]    DISK  3: [EMPTY]
          DISK  0:  [OK]      DISK  1:  [OK]
==================================
```

```
Fans:
-----
Fan Bank  Speed  Status
--------  -----  ------
CPU        31    OK
PWR        31    OK


Power Supplies:
---------------
Supply  Rating  Temp  Status
------  ------  ----  ------
  0     550 W    32   OK
  1     550 W    32   OK

===================== HW Revisions =====================

ASIC Revisions:
---------------
STP2223BGA: Rev 4
STP2223BGA: Rev 4
STP2223BGA: Rev 4
STP2003QFP: Rev 1
STP2205BGA: Rev 1

System PROM revisions:
----------------------
  OBP 3.26.0 2002/05/06 16:05  POST 6.1.0 2002/05/06 16:06
```

Health Check Summary of Root Disks under Volume Manager, Database Server

DEVICE	TYPE	DISK	GROUP	STATUS
C0t0d0s2	sliced	bootdisk0	rootdg	online
C0t1d0s2	sliced	bootdisk1	rootdg	online

Health Check Summary of A1000 Storage Arrays that are Connected to Archive Server, TKOAS01

Health Check Summary Information

bc007_005:	Optimal
bc007_004:	Optimal

Health check succeeded!

Health Check Summary of A1000 Storage Arrays that are Connected to Database Server, TKODB01

Health Check Summary Information

bc007_002:   Optimal

Health check succeeded!

MONTHLY MOD TAPE TEST

May-06

Study Date	Accession Number	No. of images	DLT no	MOD no	Result
2006 MAY 21	TKO0004725060	3	TK0208/209	V1604/1605	Succeeded

Jun-06

Study Date	Accession Number	No. of images	DLT no	MOD no	Result
2006 JUN 10	TKO000477577W	2	TK0210/211	V1624/1625	Succeeded

Jul-06

ADC COMPACT

Type 5145

Operating procedure for order no.

TKO Hospital

System components to be inspected:

- ☐ ADC - DIGITIZER SN 1435 , 1446   Counter level...
- ☐ ID / PRID - Station SN No 1 to No. 8   SN............................. SN ....
- ☐ (V)DIPS SN ....
- ☐ Preview Station SN No. 1 to No. 8

Maintenance must be carried out in compliance with the maintenance instructions (DD+DIS110.98E).
Maintenance should be carried out *every 6 months or every 30000 cassette cycles!*

	Range	Test Point - Maintenance Point	OK	not OK
1	Complete System	• Talk to the operators about possible problems. • Talk to the physician in charge about the image processing parameters in the various menus.	✓	
2	Digitizer	Check overall condition of the machine.	✓	
3	Digitizer	Vacuum the inside and wipe it.	✓	
4	Digitizer - Output buffer	Clean both transport rollers.	✓	
5	Digitizer - IP transport units	Check both outer toothed belts, replace the belts every year. Check also the corresponding double toothed belt pulley. Replace, if defective.	✓	
6	Digitizer - Robot	Check visually: The movement of the suction shaft must not be impeded by cables or hoses.	✓	
7	Digitizer - Robot	Install the springs (8 x) of the hoses, if they not exist. Visual check at the robot carriage; the vacuum hoses must not be bent or blocked in any position of the robot.	✓	
8	Digitizer - Robot	Clean the suction cups. Replace defective suction cups	✓	
9	Digitizer - Cassette units	Replace the transport rollers.	✓	
10	Digitizer - Erasure unit	Clean the erasure unit.	✓	
11	Digitizer - Erasure unit	Check the KG2 filters for damage, replace defective parts.	✓	
12	Digitizer - Erasure unit	Check the lamp socket for burning marks and replace if necessary.	✓	
13	Digitizer - Erasure unit	Insert new lamps.	✓	
14	Digitizer - Scan unit	Remove the upper rubber roller on both sides and clean them.	✓	
15	Digitizer - Scan unit	The lower rubber rollers must be cleaned inside the machine. (The rollers must be driven manually via the slow scan motor.)	✓	
16	Digitizer - Scan unit	Check the clutch of the slow scan motor visually.	✓	
17	Digitizer - Scan unit	Operate the cleaning brushes several times. Check the operation of the cleaning brushes (stability of the steel wire).	✓	
18	Digitizer - Scan unit	Check the discharge brush for visible damage and dirt. Clean, replace if necessary.	✓	
19	Digitizer - Vacuum pump	Replace the air filter.	✓	
20	Digitizer	Check the function of the safety switch.	✓	
21	Digitizer	Check the function of the VME fan manually.	✓	
22	Digitizer	Check the cassette transport with all formats with the Service Program <Test cycle>.	✓	

DRYSTAR 5000
Type 5361

Work instruction for order number	SN	Film cycle status
TKO Hospital	2829. 3430	

Maintenance must be carried out every 12 months or always after 15,000 prints according to the maintenance instructions DD+DIS237.01E.

Machine ON:

Diagnostics		OK	n.OK
Problem analysis	Discussion with the customer	☑	☐
Infocounter analysis	Check, make an analysis	☑	☐
The problems which are detected during the analysis have priority during maintenance!!!		☑	☐

Preparations		OK	n.OK
	Print a SMPTE and a flatfield test image to compare them afterwards with the test prints exposed after the maintenance	☑	☐

Machine OFF:

General		OK	n.OK
Everything	Check all cables, cable connections, and plugs visually for damage.	☑	☐

Film feed		OK	n.OK
Film feed	Clean the film feed	☑	☐
	Clean the feed rollers		
	Replace the film feed rollers after one year or after 50,000 prints		
Light barriers	Check the light barriers for tight mounting (4 plastic clips each)	☑	☐
Cables	Check the cable for mechanical damage, especially the cable between the film feed and the PMC1	☑	☐

Print engine		OK	n.OK
	Clean the rubber of the transport rollers and the print drum with a cloth soaked in alcohol	☑	☐
	Check the metal frame and the plastic parts for damage and for sharp edges which might damage the film	☑	☐
	Check the rubber of the print drum for damage (by turning the outer gear by hand)	☑	☐
	Clean the print drum	☑	☐
	Check the transport roller springs visually	☑	☐
Thermal head	Clean the thermal print head with an eraser for ink	☑	☐
	Clean the thermal print head with alcohol and a cloth	☑	☐
	Check the thermal head visually / Check the cable connections	☑	☐
Anti-static brushes	Check the anti-static brushes for wear and replace if necessary	☑	☐
Decurl unit	Clean the IR temperature sensor in the decurl unit with a cloth and alcohol (this applies only to machines with temperature sensors which can be removed separately).	☑	☐

Maintenance Instructions   DD+DIS237.01E

VME rack		OK	n.OK
	Remove all dust from the VME rack	☑	☐

Machine ON:

Print quality		OK	n.OK
	Print a flatfield test image and evaluate the print quality	☑	☐
	Measure and note Dmin and Dmax of the SMPTE test print	☑	☐
	Print a test image of every host system and check for artifacts	☑	☐
	Execute the "registration calibration" and the "density meter calibration" ①	☑	☐
	If an external Densitometer on site is used for checking the quality, execute the "reference density calibration" ①	☑	☐
	If the flatfield test print is not uniform enough, execute the TH profile calibration	☑	☐
	If the maximum density is outside the tolerance range of 3.0 ± 0.2 O.D., execute the Dmax calibration	☑	☐
	If the customer activates the film-sensito-calibration with every new film batch, execute a film-sensito-calibration ①	☑	☐

① must only be made if SW Release ≥ 1.7 is installed

Completion of the maintenance		OK	n.OK
Completion of the maintenance	Print a SMPTE and a flatfield test image, to compare them with the test print exposed at the beginning of the maintenance	☑	☐
	Exit from the IMOS Drystar. Click on the box "Preventive Maintenance" as soon as the Service Report window is displayed.	☑	☐
	Execute a reset and print an image from the host system	☑	☐
	Explain the completed maintenance actions to the customer.	☑	☐

Study Date	Accession Number	No. of images	DLT no	MOD no	Result
2006 JUL 01	TKO000483040Y	2	TK0212/213	V1640/1641	Succeeded

Aug-06

Study Date	Accession Number	No. of images	DLT no	MOD no	Result
2006 AUG 15	TKO0004943262	2	TK0218/219	V1677/1678	Succeeded

Sep-06

Study Date	Accession Number	No. of images	DLT no	MOD no	Result
2006 SEPT 10	TKO0005008222	4	TK0220/221	V1700/1701	Succeeded

Oct-06

Study Date	Accession Number	No. of images	DLT no	MOD no	Result
2006 OCT 15	TKO000509868Z	2	TK0222/225	V1728/1729	Succeeded

Nov-06

Study Date	Accession Number	No. of images	DLT no	MOD no	Result
2006 NOV 29	TKO000521421S	2	TK0230/231	V1770/1771	Succeeded

Dec-06

Study Date	Accession Number	No. of images	DLT no	MOD no	Result
2006 DEC 24	TKO000527376W	2	TK0232/233	V1790/1791, V1792/V1793	Succeeded

Jan-07

Study Date	Accession Number	No. of images	DLT no	MOD no	Result
2007 JAN 15	TKO000532709S	3	TKO236/237	V1812/1813	Succeeded

Feb-07

Study Date	Accession Number	No. of images	DLT no	MOD no	Result
2007 FEB 10	TKO0005395781	2	TKO238/239	V1834/1835	Succeeded

Appendix B

PACS QUALITY FUNCTIONAL BLOCK DIAGRAMS

Figure 1. Functional block diagram for PACS hardware

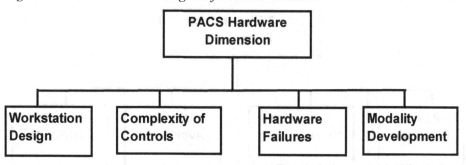

Figure 2. Functional block diagram for PACS software

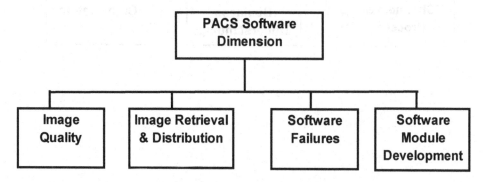

Figure 3. Functional block diagram for PACS system integration

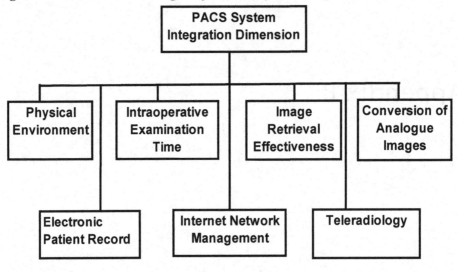

Figure 4. Functional block diagram for PACS human factors

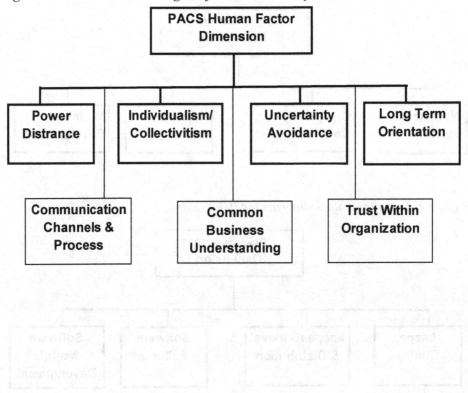

Appendix C

APPENDIX C1 VALUES OF $\{\Gamma[1+(1/B)]\}^2 / \Gamma[1+(2/B)]$

β	0.00	0.01	0.02	0.03	0.04	0.05	0.06	0.07	0.08	0.09
0.10	0.000	0.000	0.000	0.000	0.000	0.000	0.001	0.001	0.002	0.003
0.20	0.004	0.005	0.007	0.009	0.012	0.014	0.017	0.021	0.025	0.029
0.30	0.033	0.038	0.043	0.048	0.054	0.060	0.066	0.071	0.078	0.085
0.40	0.092	0.099	0.106	0.113	0.121	0.128	0.136	0.143	0.151	0.159
0.50	0.167	0.174	0.182	0.190	0.198	0.206	0.214	0.221	0.229	0.237
0.60	0.244	0.252	0.260	0.267	0.275	0.282	0.290	0.297	0.304	0.311
0.70	0.319	0.326	0.333	0.340	0.347	0.353	0.360	0.367	0.373	0.380
0.80	0.386	0.393	0.399	0.405	0.411	0.417	0.423	0.429	0.435	0.441
0.90	0.447	0.452	0.458	0.463	0.469	0.474	0.479	0.485	0.490	0.495
1.00	0.500	0.505	0.510	0.515	0.519	0.524	0.529	0.533	0.538	0.542
1.10	0.547	0.551	0.556	0.560	0.564	0.568	0.572	0.576	0.580	0.584
1.20	0.588	0.592	0.596	0.599	0.603	0.607	0.610	0.614	0.617	0.621
1.30	0.624	0.628	0.631	0.634	0.638	0.641	0.644	0.647	0.650	0.653
1.40	0.656	0.659	0.662	0.665	0.668	0.671	0.674	0.676	0.679	0.682
1.50	0.684	0.687	0.690	0.692	0.695	0.697	0.700	0.702	0.705	0.707
1.60	0.709	0.712	0.714	0.716	0.719	0.721	0.723	0.725	0.727	0.730
1.70	0.732	0.734	0.736	0.738	0.740	0.742	0.744	0.746	0.748	0.750

1.80	0.752	0.753	0.755	0.757	0.759	0.761	0.763	0.764	0.766	0.768
1.90	0.769	0.771	0.773	0.774	0.776	0.778	0.779	0.781	0.782	0.784
2.00	0.785	0.787	0.788	0.790	0.791	0.793	0.794	0.796	0.797	0.798
2.10	0.800	0.801	0.803	0.804	0.805	0.806	0.808	0.809	0.810	0.812
2.20	0.813	0.814	0.815	0.817	0.818	0.819	0.820	0.821	0.822	0.824
2.30	0.825	0.826	0.827	0.828	0.829	0.830	0.831	0.832	0.833	0.834
2.40	0.835	0.836	0.837	0.838	0.839	0.840	0.841	0.842	0.843	0.844
2.50	0.845	0.846	0.847	0.848	0.849	0.850	0.851	0.852	0.852	0.853
2.60	0.854	0.855	0.856	0.857	0.858	0.858	0.859	0.860	0.861	0.862
2.70	0.862	0.863	0.864	0.865	0.866	0.866	0.867	0.868	0.869	0.869
2.80	0.870	0.871	0.871	0.872	0.873	0.874	0.874	0.875	0.876	0.876
2.90	0.877	0.878	0.878	0.879	0.880	0.880	0.881	0.881	0.882	0.883
3.00	0.883	0.884	0.885	0.885	0.886	0.886	0.887	0.888	0.888	0.889
3.10	0.889	0.890	0.890	0.891	0.891	0.892	0.893	0.893	0.894	0.894
3.20	0.895	0.895	0.896	0.896	0.897	0.897	0.898	0.898	0.899	0.899
3.30	0.900	0.900	0.901	0.901	0.902	0.902	0.903	0.903	0.904	0.904
3.40	0.905	0.905	0.905	0.906	0.906	0.907	0.907	0.908	0.908	0.909
3.50	0.909	0.909	0.910	0.910	0.911	0.911	0.911	0.912	0.912	0.913
3.60	0.913	0.913	0.914	0.914	0.915	0.915	0.915	0.916	0.916	0.917
3.70	0.917	0.917	0.918	0.918	0.918	0.919	0.919	0.919	0.920	0.920
3.80	0.921	0.921	0.921	0.922	0.922	0.922	0.923	0.923	0.923	0.924
3.90	0.924	0.924	0.925	0.925	0.925	0.925	0.926	0.926	0.926	0.927
4.00	0.927	0.927	0.928	0.928	0.928	0.929	0.929	0.929	0.929	0.930
4.10	0.930	0.930	0.931	0.931	0.931	0.931	0.932	0.932	0.932	0.933
4.20	0.933	0.933	0.933	0.934	0.934	0.934	0.934	0.935	0.935	0.935
4.30	0.935	0.936	0.936	0.936	0.936	0.937	0.937	0.937	0.937	0.938
4.40	0.93	0.938	0.938	0.939	0.939	0.939	0.939	0.940	0.940	0.940
4.50	0.940	0.940	0.941	0.941	0.941	0.941	0.942	0.942	0.942	0.942
4.60	0.942	0.943	0.943	0.943	0.943	0.943	0.944	0.944	0.944	0.944
4.70	0.945	0.945	0.945	0.945	0.945	0.946	0.946	0.946	0.946	0.946
4.80	0.947	0.947	0.947	0.947	0.947	0.947	0.948	0.948	0.948	0.948
4.90	0.948	0.949	0.949	0.949	0.949	0.949	0.949	0.950	0.950	0.950
5.00	0.950	0.950	0.950	0.951	0.951	0.951	0.951	0.951	0.952	0.952
5.10	0.952	0.952	0.952	0.952	0.952	0.953	0.953	0.953	0.953	0.953
5.20	0.953	0.954	0.954	0.954	0.954	0.954	0.954	0.955	0.955	0.955
5.30	0.955	0.955	0.955	0.955	0.956	0.956	0.956	0.956	0.956	0.956
5.40	0.956	0.957	0.957	0.957	0.957	0.957	0.957	0.957	0.958	0.958
5.50	0.958	0.958	0.958	0.958	0.958	0.958	0.959	0.959	0.959	0.959
5.60	0.959	0.959	0.959	0.959	0.960	0.960	0.960	0.960	0.960	0.960
5.70	0.960	0.960	0.961	0.961	0.961	0.961	0.961	0.961	0.961	0.961
5.80	0.962	0.962	0.962	0.962	0.962	0.962	0.962	0.962	0.962	0.963
5.90	0.963	0.963	0.963	0.963	0.963	0.963	0.963	0.963	0.964	0.964

6.00	0.964	0.964	0.964	0.964	0.964	0.964	0.964	0.965	0.965	0.965
6.10	0.965	0.965	0.965	0.965	0.965	0.965	0.965	0.966	0.966	0.966
6.20	0.966	0.966	0.966	0.966	0.966	0.966	0.966	0.967	0.967	0.967
6.30	0.967	0.967	0.967	0.967	0.967	0.967	0.967	0.967	0.968	0.968
6.40	0.968	0.968	0.968	0.968	0.968	0.968	0.968	0.968	0.968	0.969
6.50	0.969	0.969	0.969	0.969	0.969	0.969	0.969	0.969	0.969	0.969
6.60	0.969	0.970	0.970	0.970	0.970	0.970	0.970	0.970	0.970	0.970
6.70	0.970	0.970	0.970	0.971	0.971	0.971	0.971	0.971	0.971	0.971
6.80	0.971	0.971	0.971	0.971	0.971	0.971	0.972	0.972	0.972	0.972
6.90	0.972	0.972	0.972	0.972	0.972	0.972	0.972	0.972	0.972	0.972
7.00	0.973	0.973	0.973	0.973	0.973	0.973	0.973	0.973	0.973	0.973
7.10	0.973	0.973	0.973	0.973	0.974	0.974	0.974	0.974	0.974	0.974
7.20	0.974	0.974	0.974	0.974	0.974	0.974	0.974	0.974	0.974	0.974
7.30	0.975	0.975	0.975	0.975	0.975	0.975	0.975	0.975	0.975	0.975
7.40	0.975	0.975	0.975	0.975	0.975	0.975	0.976	0.976	0.976	0.976
7.50	0.976	0.976	0.976	0.976	0.976	0.976	0.976	0.976	0.976	0.976
7.60	0.976	0.976	0.976	0.977	0.977	0.977	0.977	0.977	0.977	0.977
7.70	0.977	0.977	0.977	0.977	0.977	0.977	0.977	0.977	0.977	0.977
7.80	0.977	0.977	0.978	0.978	0.978	0.978	0.978	0.978	0.978	0.978
7.90	0.978	0.978	0.978	0.978	0.978	0.978	0.978	0.978	0.978	0.978
8.00	0.978	0.979	0.979	0.979	0.979	0.979	0.979	0.979	0.979	0.979
8.10	0.979	0.979	0.979	0.979	0.979	0.979	0.979	0.979	0.979	0.979
8.20	0.979	0.979	0.980	0.980	0.980	0.980	0.980	0.980	0.980	0.980
8.30	0.980	0.980	0.980	0.980	0.980	0.980	0.980	0.980	0.980	0.980
8.40	0.980	0.980	0.980	0.980	0.980	0.981	0.981	0.981	0.981	0.981
8.50	0.981	0.981	0.981	0.981	0.981	0.981	0.981	0.981	0.981	0.981
8.60	0.981	0.981	0.981	0.981	0.981	0.981	0.981	0.981	0.981	0.981
8.70	0.982	0.982	0.982	0.982	0.982	0.982	0.982	0.982	0.982	0.982
8.80	0.982	0.982	0.982	0.982	0.982	0.982	0.982	0.982	0.982	0.982
8.90	0.982	0.982	0.982	0.982	0.982	0.982	0.983	0.983	0.983	0.983
9.00	0.983	0.983	0.983	0.983	0.983	0.983	0.983	0.983	0.983	0.983
9.10	0.983	0.983	0.983	0.983	0.983	0.983	0.983	0.983	0.983	0.983
9.20	0.983	0.983	0.983	0.983	0.983	0.984	0.984	0.984	0.984	0.984
9.30	0.984	0.984	0.984	0.984	0.984	0.984	0.984	0.984	0.984	0.984
9.40	0.984	0.984	0.984	0.984	0.984	0.984	0.984	0.984	0.984	0.984
9.50	0.984	0.984	0.984	0.984	0.984	0.984	0.984	0.985	0.985	0.985
9.60	0.985	0.985	0.985	0.985	0.985	0.985	0.985	0.985	0.985	0.985
9.70	0.985	0.985	0.985	0.985	0.985	0.985	0.985	0.985	0.985	0.985
9.80	0.985	0.985	0.985	0.985	0.985	0.985	0.985	0.985	0.985	0.985
9.90	0.985	0.985	0.986	0.986	0.986	0.986	0.986	0.986	0.986	0.986
10.00	0.986	0.986	0.986	0.986	0.986	0.986	0.986	0.986	0.986	0.986

APPENDIX C2 VALUES OF Γ[1+(1/Β)]

β	0.00	0.01	0.02	0.03	0.04	0.05	0.06	0.07	0.08	0.09
0.10	3628800	445506	82834	20985	6731	2594	1155	578	318	189
0.20	120.000	80.358	56.331	41.058	30.942	24.000	19.087	15.514	12.853	10.829
0.30	9.261	8.024	7.035	6.234	5.575	5.029	4.571	4.184	3.853	3.569
0.40	3.323	3.109	2.921	2.756	2.609	2.479	2.362	2.257	2.163	2.077
0.50	2.000	1.930	1.865	1.806	1.752	1.702	1.657	1.614	1.575	1.538
0.60	1.505	1.473	1.444	1.416	1.390	1.366	1.344	1.322	1.302	1.284
0.70	1.266	1.249	1.233	1.218	1.204	1.191	1.178	1.166	1.154	1.143
0.80	1.133	1.123	1.114	1.105	1.096	1.088	1.080	1.073	1.066	1.059
0.90	1.052	1.046	1.040	1.034	1.029	1.023	1.018	1.013	1.009	1.004
1.00	1.000	0.996	0.992	0.988	0.984	0.981	0.977	0.974	0.971	0.968
1.10	0.965	0.962	0.959	0.957	0.954	0.952	0.949	0.947	0.945	0.943
1.20	0.941	0.939	0.937	0.935	0.933	0.931	0.930	0.928	0.927	0.925
1.30	0.924	0.922	0.921	0.919	0.918	0.917	0.916	0.915	0.914	0.912
1.40	0.911	0.910	0.909	0.909	0.908	0.907	0.906	0.905	0.904	0.903
1.50	0.903	0.902	0.901	0.901	0.900	0.899	0.899	0.898	0.898	0.897
1.60	0.897	0.896	0.896	0.895	0.895	0.894	0.894	0.893	0.893	0.893
1.70	0.892	0.892	0.892	0.891	0.891	0.891	0.890	0.890	0.890	0.890
1.80	0.889	0.889	0.889	0.889	0.888	0.888	0.888	0.888	0.888	0.888
1.90	0.887	0.887	0.887	0.887	0.887	0.887	0.887	0.886	0.886	0.886
2.00	0.886	0.886	0.886	0.886	0.886	0.886	0.886	0.886	0.886	0.886
2.10	0.886	0.886	0.886	0.886	0.886	0.886	0.886	0.886	0.886	0.886
2.20	0.886	0.886	0.886	0.886	0.886	0.886	0.886	0.886	0.886	0.886
2.30	0.886	0.886	0.886	0.886	0.886	0.886	0.886	0.886	0.886	0.886
2.40	0.886	0.887	0.887	0.887	0.887	0.887	0.887	0.887	0.887	0.887
2.50	0.887	0.887	0.887	0.888	0.888	0.888	0.888	0.888	0.888	0.888
2.60	0.888	0.888	0.888	0.889	0.889	0.889	0.889	0.889	0.889	0.889
2.70	0.889	0.889	0.890	0.890	0.890	0.890	0.890	0.890	0.890	0.890
2.80	0.890	0.891	0.891	0.891	0.891	0.891	0.891	0.891	0.891	0.892
2.90	0.892	0.892	0.892	0.892	0.892	0.892	0.892	0.893	0.893	0.893
3.00	0.893	0.893	0.893	0.893	0.894	0.894	0.894	0.894	0.894	0.894
3.10	0.894	0.894	0.895	0.895	0.895	0.895	0.895	0.895	0.895	0.896
3.20	0.896	0.896	0.896	0.896	0.896	0.896	0.896	0.897	0.897	0.897
3.30	0.897	0.897	0.897	0.897	0.898	0.898	0.898	0.898	0.898	0.898
3.40	0.898	0.899	0.899	0.899	0.899	0.899	0.899	0.899	0.899	0.900
3.50	0.900	0.900	0.900	0.900	0.900	0.900	0.901	0.901	0.901	0.901
3.60	0.901	0.901	0.901	0.902	0.902	0.902	0.902	0.902	0.902	0.902
3.70	0.902	0.903	0.903	0.903	0.903	0.903	0.903	0.903	0.904	0.904
3.80	0.904	0.904	0.904	0.904	0.904	0.904	0.905	0.905	0.905	0.905
3.90	0.905	0.905	0.905	0.905	0.906	0.906	0.906	0.906	0.906	0.906

4.00	0.906	0.907	0.907	0.907	0.907	0.907	0.907	0.907	0.907	0.908
4.10	0.908	0.908	0.908	0.908	0.908	0.908	0.908	0.909	0.909	0.909
4.20	0.909	0.909	0.909	0.909	0.909	0.910	0.910	0.910	0.910	0.910
4.30	0.910	0.910	0.910	0.911	0.911	0.911	0.911	0.911	0.911	0.911
4.40	0.911	0.912	0.912	0.912	0.912	0.912	0.912	0.912	0.912	0.912
4.50	0.913	0.913	0.913	0.913	0.913	0.913	0.913	0.913	0.914	0.914
4.60	0.914	0.914	0.914	0.914	0.914	0.914	0.914	0.915	0.915	0.915
4.70	0.915	0.915	0.915	0.915	0.915	0.915	0.916	0.916	0.916	0.916
4.80	0.916	0.916	0.916	0.916	0.916	0.917	0.917	0.917	0.917	0.917
4.90	0.917	0.917	0.917	0.917	0.918	0.918	0.918	0.918	0.918	0.918
5.00	0.918	0.918	0.918	0.918	0.919	0.919	0.919	0.919	0.919	0.919
5.10	0.919	0.919	0.919	0.920	0.920	0.920	0.920	0.920	0.920	0.920
5.20	0.920	0.920	0.920	0.921	0.921	0.921	0.921	0.921	0.921	0.921
5.30	0.921	0.921	0.921	0.922	0.922	0.922	0.922	0.922	0.922	0.922
5.40	0.922	0.922	0.922	0.923	0.923	0.923	0.923	0.923	0.923	0.923
5.50	0.923	0.923	0.923	0.923	0.924	0.924	0.924	0.924	0.924	0.924
5.60	0.924	0.924	0.924	0.924	0.925	0.925	0.925	0.925	0.925	0.925
5.70	0.925	0.925	0.925	0.925	0.925	0.926	0.926	0.926	0.926	0.926
5.80	0.926	0.926	0.926	0.926	0.926	0.926	0.927	0.927	0.927	0.927
5.90	0.927	0.927	0.927	0.927	0.927	0.927	0.927	0.927	0.928	0.928
6.00	0.928	0.928	0.928	0.928	0.928	0.928	0.928	0.928	0.928	0.928
6.10	0.929	0.929	0.929	0.929	0.929	0.929	0.929	0.929	0.929	0.929
6.20	0.929	0.929	0.930	0.930	0.930	0.930	0.930	0.930	0.930	0.930
6.30	0.930	0.930	0.930	0.930	0.931	0.931	0.931	0.931	0.931	0.931
6.40	0.931	0.931	0.931	0.931	0.931	0.931	0.931	0.932	0.932	0.932
6.50	0.932	0.932	0.932	0.932	0.932	0.932	0.932	0.932	0.932	0.932
6.60	0.933	0.933	0.933	0.933	0.933	0.933	0.933	0.933	0.933	0.933
6.70	0.933	0.933	0.933	0.934	0.934	0.934	0.934	0.934	0.934	0.934
6.80	0.934	0.934	0.934	0.934	0.934	0.934	0.934	0.935	0.935	0.935
6.90	0.935	0.935	0.935	0.935	0.935	0.935	0.935	0.935	0.935	0.935
7.00	0.935	0.936	0.936	0.936	0.936	0.936	0.936	0.936	0.936	0.936
7.10	0.936	0.936	0.936	0.936	0.936	0.936	0.937	0.937	0.937	0.937
7.20	0.937	0.937	0.937	0.937	0.937	0.937	0.937	0.937	0.937	0.937
7.30	0.937	0.938	0.938	0.938	0.938	0.938	0.938	0.938	0.938	0.938
7.40	0.938	0.938	0.938	0.938	0.938	0.938	0.938	0.939	0.939	0.939
7.50	0.939	0.939	0.939	0.939	0.939	0.939	0.939	0.939	0.939	0.939
7.60	0.939	0.939	0.939	0.940	0.940	0.940	0.940	0.940	0.940	0.940
7.70	0.940	0.940	0.940	0.940	0.940	0.940	0.940	0.940	0.940	0.941
7.80	0.941	0.941	0.941	0.941	0.941	0.941	0.941	0.941	0.941	0.941
7.90	0.941	0.941	0.941	0.941	0.941	0.941	0.942	0.942	0.942	0.942
8.00	0.942	0.942	0.942	0.942	0.942	0.942	0.942	0.942	0.942	0.942
8.10	0.942	0.942	0.942	0.942	0.943	0.943	0.943	0.943	0.943	0.943

8.20	0.943	0.943	0.943	0.943	0.943	0.943	0.943	0.943	0.943	0.943
8.30	0.943	0.943	0.944	0.944	0.944	0.944	0.944	0.944	0.944	0.944
8.40	0.944	0.944	0.944	0.944	0.944	0.944	0.944	0.944	0.944	0.944
8.50	0.944	0.945	0.945	0.945	0.945	0.945	0.945	0.945	0.945	0.945
8.60	0.945	0.945	0.945	0.945	0.945	0.945	0.945	0.945	0.945	0.945
8.70	0.945	0.946	0.946	0.946	0.946	0.946	0.946	0.946	0.946	0.946
8.80	0.946	0.946	0.946	0.946	0.946	0.946	0.946	0.946	0.946	0.946
8.90	0.946	0.947	0.947	0.947	0.947	0.947	0.947	0.947	0.947	0.947
9.00	0.947	0.947	0.947	0.947	0.947	0.947	0.947	0.947	0.947	0.947
9.10	0.947	0.947	0.948	0.948	0.948	0.948	0.948	0.948	0.948	0.948
9.20	0.948	0.948	0.948	0.948	0.948	0.948	0.948	0.948	0.948	0.948
9.30	0.948	0.948	0.948	0.948	0.949	0.949	0.949	0.949	0.949	0.949
9.40	0.949	0.949	0.949	0.949	0.949	0.949	0.949	0.949	0.949	0.949
9.50	0.949	0.949	0.949	0.949	0.949	0.949	0.950	0.950	0.950	0.950
9.60	0.950	0.950	0.950	0.950	0.950	0.950	0.950	0.950	0.950	0.950
9.70	0.950	0.950	0.950	0.950	0.950	0.950	0.950	0.950	0.950	0.950
9.80	0.951	0.951	0.951	0.951	0.951	0.951	0.951	0.951	0.951	0.951
9.90	0.951	0.951	0.951	0.951	0.951	0.951	0.951	0.951	0.951	0.951
10.00	0.951	0.951	0.951	0.951	0.952	0.952	0.952	0.952	0.952	0.952

Glossary

ACRONYMS

ADT	Admission, delivery, and transfer
ACR	American College of Radiology
AHP	Analytic Hierarchy Process
AQM	Active Queue Management
AS/NZS	Australian and New Zealand
ATM	Asynchronous Transfer Mode
BCP	Business Continuity Plan
BSI	British Standards Institution
CAS	Computer Assisted Surgery
CD	Compact Disk ROM
CIA	Confidentiality, Integrity, Availability
CT	Computed Tomography
DDL	Digital Driving Level
DF	Digital fluorography
DICOM	Digital Imaging and Communications in Medicine
DIN/PACS	Digital Imaging Network and Picture Archiving and Communication System

DLT	Digital Linear Tape
DMAIC	Define, Measure, Analysis, Improve and Control
DT	Drop Tail
ePR	electronic Patient Record
FBD	Functional Block Diagram
FMEA	Failure Mode and Effects Analysis
GSDF	Grayscale Standard Display Function
HFE	Human factors engineering
HIS	Hospital Information System
HL7	Health Level 7
HOQ	House of Quality
HTML	hypertext markup language
HTTP	hypertext transfer protocol
IDV	Individualism
ISMS	Information Security Management System
ISO	International Organization for Standardization
IT	Information Technology
ITU	International Telecommunication Union
JCAHO	Joint Commission on Accreditation of Healthcare Organizations
JND	Just Noticeable Differences
LAN	Local Area Network
LCD	Liquid Crystals Displays
LTO tape	Linear Tape-Open
LTO	Long-Term Orientation
MCL	Multiple Congested Links
MCSP	Multiple Computer Single Processor
MRI	Magnetic resonance imaging
NAS	Network Attached Storage
NEMA	National Electrical Manufacturers Association
NM	Nuclear Medicine
OD	Optical Disk
ODJ	Optical Disk Jukebox
OSI	Open Systems Interconnection
OTTFP	One Time Two Factor Password
PACS	Picture Archiving and Communications System
PDCA	Plan, Do, Check, Act
PDI	Power Distance Index
PET	Positron Emission Tomography
QA	Quality Assurance

QC	Quality Control
RAID	Redundant Array of Inexpensive Disks
RED	Random Early Detection
RFP	Request For Proposal
RIS	Radiology Information System
RPN	Risk Priority Numbers
RTT	Round Trip Times
SAN	storage area network
SCMP	Single Computer Multiple Processors
SoA	Statement of Applicability
SPC	Statistical Process Control
SQL	Structured Query Language
SRD	Short-range Dependent
TCP/IP	Transmission Control Protocol/Internet Protocol
TD	Tail-Drop
TQM	Total Quality Management
TRIZ	The Theory of Inventive Problem Solving (Russian acronym)
UAI	Uncertainty Avoidance Index
UR	User Requirements
US	Ultrasound
VOC	The Voice of the Customer
WAN	Wide Area Network

GLOSSARY

Active Queue Management (AQM): In Internet routers, Active Queue Management is a technique that consists in dropping or marking packets before a router's queue is full. Typically they operate by maintaining one or more drop/mark probabilities, and probabilistically dropping or marking packets even when the queue is short. This technique is intended to achieve high link utilization with a low queuing delay.

Concurrent Engineering: Concurrent engineering is a business strategy which replaces the traditional product development process with one in which tasks are done in parallel and there is an early consideration for every aspect of a product's development process. This strategy focuses on the optimization and distribution of a firm's resources in the design and development process to ensure effective and efficient product development process.

Congestion: A state occurring in part of a network when the message traffic is so heavy that it slows down network response time.

Cracker: A cracker is a hacker who uses their proficiency for personal gains outside of the law. Example: stealing data, changing bank accounts, distributing viruses etc.

Critical to Quality (CTQ): The key measurable characteristics of a product or process whose performance standards or specification limits must be met in order to satisfy the customer. They align improvement or design efforts with customer requirements. CTQs represent the product or service characteristics that are defined by the customer (internal or external). They may include the upper and lower specification limits or any other factors related to the product or service. A CTQ usually must be interpreted from a qualitative customer statement to an actionable, quantitative business specification.

Cultural Dimensions: Cultural dimensions are the mostly psychological dimensions, or value constructs, which can be used to describe a specific culture.

Data Compression: The process of encoding information using fewer bits (or other information-bearing units) than an unencoded representation would use through use of specific encoding schemes.

Digital Image: A digital image for the purpose of this monograph is defined as a raster, 2-dimentional, rectangular array of static data elements called pixels, intended for display on a computer monitor or projected with a digital data projector. Images may be acquired on traditional film and scanned to an electronic file, or acquired electronically with a digital camera.

Drop Tail (DT) or Tail Drop: A queue management algorithm used by Internet routers to decide when to drop packets. In drop tail all the traffic is not differentiated. Each packet is treated identically. With drop tail, when the queue is filled to its maximum capacity, the newly arriving packets are dropped until the queue has enough room to accept incoming traffic.

Flow Control: In communications, the process of adjusting the flow of data from one device to another to ensure that the receiving device can handle all of the incoming data. This is particularly important where the sending device is capable of sending data much faster than the receiving device can receive it.

Failure Mode and Effects Analysis (FMEA): A systematic method for documenting potential failure modes, determining effects, identifying causes of failures, developing plan, team concurrence, and take action.

Hacker: A hacker is a person who is proficient with computers and/or programming to an elite level where they know all of the in's and out's of a system. There is NO illegality involved with being a hacker.

House of Quality (HOQ): House of Quality is a graphic tool for defining the relationship between customer desires and the firm/product capabilities. It is a part of the Quality Function Deployment (QFD) and it utilizes a planning matrix to relate what the customer wants to how an institution (that provides the healthcare service) is going to meet those wants. It looks like a House with correlation matrix as its roof, customer wants versus service features as the main part, competitor evaluation as the porch etc. It is based on the belief that healthcare service should be designed to reflect customers' desires and preferences.

Human Factors: Human factors are considered in this monograph as the environmental, organizational and job factors, and cultural dimensions that influence behavior at work.

Individualism (IDV): A cultural dimension focuses on the degree to which an organization reinforces individual or collective achievement and interpersonal relationships. If a healthcare institution has a high Individualism score, this indicates that individuality and individual rights are dominant. Individuals in these organizations tend to form relationships with larger numbers of people, but with the relationships being weak. A low Individualism score points to an organization that is more collectivist in nature. In such organizations the ties between individual members are very strong and the staff lean towards collective responsibility.

Local Area Network (LAN): A computer network that spans a relatively small area. Most LANs are confined to a single building or group of buildings. However, one LAN can be connected to other LANs over any distance via telephone lines and radio waves. A system of LANs connected in this way is called a wide-area network (WAN).

Long Term Orientation (LTO): A cultural dimension refers to how much an organization values long-standing - as opposed to short term - traditions and values. In healthcare institutions with a high LTO Index, service delivering on social obligations and avoiding "loss of face" are considered very important.

Kano Customer Satisfaction Model: The Kano model was originally developed in the 80's by Noriaki Kano to classify and recognize the importance of different types of customer needs. It provides insights into the dynamics of customer preferences and the thoroughness of their needs in order to ensure successful products and services. In the present context the main application should be to proactively uncover and classify 3 main categories of needs and take action to effectively integrate all 3 types of these needs into the PACS Services. PACS attributes may be classified as: threshold, performance, and excitement. A competitive service meets basic attributes, maximizes performances attributes, and includes as many excitement attributes as possible at a cost the public can bear.

Metadata: Data about data. Metadata describes how and when and by whom a particular set of data was collected, and how the data is formatted.

Packets: A piece of a message transmitted over a packet-switching network. One of the key features of a packet is that it contains the destination address in addition to the data. In IP networks, packets are often called datagrams.

Packet Switching: Refers to protocols in which messages are divided into packets before they are sent. Each packet is then transmitted individually and can even follow different routes to its destination. Once all the packets forming a message arrive at the destination, they are recompiled into the original message.

Picture Archiving and Communication System (PACS): A system that acquires, transmits, stores, retrieves, and displays digital images and related patient information from a variety of imaging sources and communicates the information over a network.

Pixel Dimensions: The number of pixels along the height and width of a digital image.

Power Distance: A cultural dimension relates to the degree of equality/inequality between people in a particular organization. A healthcare institution with a high Power Distance Index (PDI) both accepts and perpetuates inequalities between staff. A low PDI indicates that the institution does not emphasize differences in staff position, power or salary. Equality is seen as the collective aim of the organization and upward mobility is common.

Protocols: An agreed-upon format for transmitting data between two devices. The protocol determines: (a) the type of error checking to be used, (b) data compression method, if any, (c) how the sending device will indicate that it has finished sending a message, and (d) how the receiving device will indicate that it has received a message

Quality Function Deployment (QFD): A method originally developed by Yoji Akao in 1966 when the author combined his work in quality assurance and quality control points with function deployment used in Value Engineering. In the present context QFD may be regarded as a method to transform user demands into design quality, to deploy the functions forming quality, and to deploy methods for achieving the design quality into subsystems and component parts, and ultimately to specific elements of the PACS process. QFD is designed to help planners focus on characteristics of a new or existing product or service from the viewpoints of market segments, company, or technology-development needs. The technique yields graphs and matrices

Reliability Modeling: Reliability modeling is the process of predicting the reliability of a component or system. Two different ways of investigation are common: The physics of failure approach uses an understanding of the failure mechanisms involved, such as crack propagation or material fatigue. The parts stress modeling approach is an empirical method for prediction based on counting the number and type of components of the system, and the stress they undergo during operation. For systems(hardware or software) with a clearly defined failure time, the empirical distribution function of these failure times can be determined.

Redundancy: Redundancy in PACS engineering is the duplication of critical components of a system with the intention of increasing reliability of the system, usually in the case of a backup or fail-safe. Redundancy in PACS software engineering is the number of bits used to transmit a message minus the number of bits of actual information in the message. In other words, it is the amount of wasted space used to transmit certain data. Data compression is a way to reduce or eliminate unwanted redundancy, while checksums are a way of adding desired redundancy for purposes of error detection when communicating over a noisy channel of limited capacity.

Resolution: The resolution of an image is determined by the number of pixels per inch printed on a page.

Radiology Information System (RIS): An information system used by radiology departments to store, manipulate and distribute patient radiological data and imagery. The system generally comprises of patient tracking and scheduling, result reporting and image tracking capabilities.

Routers: Routers are network layer devices used to interconnect different networks. An Internet router typically maintains a set of queues, one per interface, that hold packets scheduled to go out on that interface. Their primary role is to switch packets from input links to output links. In order to do so a router must be able to determine the path that every incoming packet needs to follow, and decide which outgoing link should it be switched to.

Six Sigma: A business management strategy that seeks to identify and remove the causes of defects and errors in manufacturing and business processes. It uses a set of quality management methods, including statistical methods, and creates a special infrastructure of people within the organization ("Black Belts", etc.) who are experts in these methods.

Transmission Control Protocol/Internet Protocol (TCP/IP): The basic communication language or protocol of the Internet. It can also be used as a communications protocol in a private network (either an intranet or an extranet). TCP/IP is a two-layer program. The higher layer, TCP, manages the assembling of a message or file into smaller packets that are transmitted over the Internet and received by a TCP layer that reassembles the packets into the original message. The lower layer, IP, handles the address part of each packet so that it gets to the right destination. Each gateway computer on the network checks this address to see where to forward the message. Even though some packets from the same message are routed differently than others, they will be reassembled at the destination.

TRIZ: The Russian acronym for the "Theory of Inventive Problem Solving". It is a problem solving method based on logic and data, not intuition, which accelerates the project team's ability to solve these problems creatively. TRIZ also provides repeatability, predictability, and reliability due to its structure and algorithmic approach. More than three million patents have been analyzed to discover the patterns that predict breakthrough solutions to problems.

Uncertainty Avoidance: A cultural dimension concerns the level of acceptance for uncertainty and ambiguity within an organization. A healthcare institution with a high Uncertainty Avoidance Index (UAI) will have a low tolerance towards uncertainty and ambiguity. As a result it is usually a very rule-orientated organization and follows well defined and established institution policy, regulations and controls.

Wide Area Network (WAN): A computer network that spans a relatively large geographical area. Typically, a WAN consists of two or more local-area networks (LANs).

About the Authors

Dr. Tong graduated from Southampton Institute of Higher Education, Southampton University in engineering and obtained his MSc in Engineering Computation from Queen's University of Belfast. He finished his PhD in Medical Imaging at the Royal Postgraduate Medical School, Imperial College, UK. Dr. Tong is a fellow member of British Computer Society, professional member of Institution of Mechanical Engineers, Chartered Engineer and Scientist. He has published more than forty papers in the area of medical imaging and modelling.

Dr. Tong was been working as a Medical Physicist and Picture Archiving and Communication System (PACS) Manager for Tseung Kwan O Hospital and Pamela Youde Nethersole Eastern Hospital, Hospital Authority since 1996. He has built various medical imaging networks for different specialties including Nuclear Medicine Departments, Radiology Departments, Neurosurgery Departments, Ear Noise Throat Department, and Oncology Department for surgical and treatment purposes. From 1999 to 2003, Dr. Tong was appointed medical physicist in-charge for the building of the Tseung Kwan O Hospital as the first filmless hospital project in Hong Kong and PR China which project has awarded the ISO27000 certificate and a gold award in Hong Kong Information & Communication Technology (HKICT) Awards 2006. In 2007, Dr. Tong was appointed for the development of a Surgical Virtual Reality Laboratory for surgical department. This project has awarded three prizes including gold, silver, and bronze awards in the HK ICT Awards 2007. Being one of the big winners in ICT field, Dr. Tong has been invited to represent Hong Kong for the competition of Asia Pacific Information & Communication Technology Awards 2006 and 2007. Internationally, Dr. Tong has won a finalist certificate in the Science and Engineering Visualization Challenge 2006 organized by National Science Foundation and Science. As a scientist, Dr. Tong has been appointed as a subject expert by Hong Kong Council for Accreditation of Academic & Vocational Qualifications and Education Bureau.

Dr. Eric Wong received his MSc degree in Plant Engineering from the Loughborough University(UK) and PhD degree from the Leicester University(UK). Prior to joining the Mechanical Engineering Department of the Hong Kong Polytechnic University, he worked for the Hong Kong Civil Aviation Department in the area of flight crew licensing and examinations, as well as aviation safety. His research interests include: aviation management, risk modeling, Picture Archiving and Communications System, virtual organization trust, and quality management. He has been a Member of the China Council for the Promotion of Six Sigma since 2004. He is a Fellow of the Royal Aeronautical Society (UK), a Fellow of the HK Quality Management Association, and a Council Member of the China Association for Quality. He was Vice-Chairman of the HK Institute of Marine Technology (2002), the Organizing Committee Chairman of the 11th Hong Kong Quality Management & the 1st Six Sigma Convention(2005). He is also the Program Chair of the ISSAT Internatioal Conference on Modeling of Complex Systems and Environments (2007) at Ho Chi Minh City, Vietnam. He is an editorial board member of the International Journal of Industrial Engineering – Theory, Application and Practice and has published over 100 book chapters, refereed journal articles and conference papers. He is also one of the editors of the book "Quality Management: A New Era".

Index

J

K

L

thallium drifted sodium iodide NaI(Tl) 17
Theory of Inventive Problem Solving 165
Theory of Inventive Problem Solving
      (TRIZ) 164
thin-film transistor (TFT) 105
threat 66
threats 63
TKOH filmless radiology service 274
TKOH PACS 280
TKOH PACS, design of 279
TKOH PACS team 269
tolerance limits 261
total quality management 139
total quality management (TQM) 290
TQM approach 246
TQM method 231
transmission control protocol (TCP)
      144, 147
transmission control protocol (TCP) net-
      work 212
transmission control protocol/Internet pro-
      tocol (TCP/IP), definition 338
TRIZ, definition 339
Tseung Kwan O Hospital 6
Tseung Kwan O Hospital (TKOH) 270

U

ultrasound (US) 18, 280
uncertainty avoidance, definition 339
uncertainty avoidance index (UAI)
      232, 236
United Lincolnshire NHS Trust 5
upper control limit (UCL) 253
user requirements (UR) 159

V

variable costs 77
variables data 251, 252
video scanning 13
virtual HDD 48
voice of customers (VOC) 157
voice of PACS customers (VOPC) 149
voice of the customer (VOC) information
      271

vulnerabilities 63
vulnerability 66

W

Web-based file server 22
Web server 22
Web servers loading (WSL) 74
Web technology 43, 275
Weibull analysis 182
Weibull assumption 177
Weibull distribution 172
Weibull distribution function 174
Weibull estimation 178
Weibull parameters 176
whole body imaging technique 18
wide area network (WAN) 2, 94
wide area network (WAN), definition 339
wide area networks (WAN) 25
workflow analysis 118
workflow plan 72, 87
worklist management supervision 125
workstations 81, 125
write once read many (WORM) 103
wrong patient operations 193
wrong procedure 193
wrong site surgery 193

X

X-Bar 251
x-ray film 1
X-ray film consumption 273
x-ray image 1
X-ray image viewer 281
X-ray imaging modalities 277
x-ray procedure 13
x-ray tube assembly 13
X and Moving Range (XmR) control
      charts 256